the pregnancy quiz

Try the quiz at the start of your pregnancy and then again at the end, and see how far you've come.

1 Colostrum is:
a) a very attractive ruin in Rome
b) stuff that comes out of your bosoms before you breastfeed
c) that strange blue goo that newborn babies are covered in
d) a thrash-trance band from near Brighton

2 Can you retain fluid and be dehydrated at the same time?
a) don't be ridiculous
b) oh, lordy, yes
c) it depends on what star sign you are

3 Should you try to get time off before the baby arrives, rather than work until the due date?
a) yes
b) uh-huh
c) ooh, yeah
d) damn straight

4 Which is the most relaxing birth support team?
a) a midwife, an obstetrician and your partner, sister or friend
b) a film crew, a live-on-the-internet technical support team, a stills photographer, your children, parents and second cousins, all the girls from work and somebody called Arthur who took a wrong turn on the way to the canteen
c) nobody at all

5 Inducement is:
a) a very large diamond ring and a holiday in the Bahamas
b) an artificial medical process to stimulate labour
c) holding a Kit Kat at the end of the vagina to coax the baby out
d) a technical term for the placement of the placenta

6 Braxton Hicks is:

a) that lantern-jawed bloke who slept with his aunty on *The Bold and the Beautiful*

b) a term coined by NASA astronauts for a false alarm, named after an over-excited engineer on the *Apollo 12* mission

c) practice labour contractions

d) a combination of the two most popular baby names in Kentucky in 1897

7 Palpation is:

a) what happens to your cervix when you have an orgasm

b) a pretentious word for 'having a feel'

c) the medical term for the faster heart rate you attain towards the end of a pregnancy

d) the opposite of temptation or craving: something that makes you nauseated

8 Placenta is:

a) the most popular girl's name after Sarah, Rebecca and Emily

b) the geographical location where you have your baby

c) a big gloopy item that looks like a liver and keeps the baby alive with nutrients and oxygen

d) a terrific marketing opportunity if you put it through a blender, whack it in a moisturiser and give it a French name

9 The easiest way of giving birth is by:

a) taking all the drugs you can get your hands on and shouting a lot at random

b) imagining you're in a perfectly charming wheat field having sex with Brad Pitt

c) having a general anaesthetic and paying someone to look after the baby for the first ten years

d) whatever means are necessary at the time

e) just like they do it in the movies

10 Women who say childbirth doesn't really hurt are:

a) lucky

b) deluded

c) insane

d) men

11 A primigravida is:

a) one of those ballerinas who doesn't eat enough

b) a woman giving birth for the first time

c) the first time you feel the baby move inside you

12 Living with a newborn baby is:

a) just like a lovely holiday

b) exhausting

c) what was the question again?

13 **If you don't have a husband, you can:**

a) get help from relatives and friends

b) just go straight to hell, you flaunty Miss Jezebel person

c) claim benefits and be involved in special re-employment and study programmes provided by the government

14 **Post-partum means after the birth. Antenatal means:**

a) prenatal, or before the birth

b) you're against the whole idea of pregnancy, or being in any way slightly natal

c) another word for childbirth

15 **Sex is:**

a) really a tremendously heightened sensual experience all through pregnancy

b) just asking for trouble

c) apparently something that single, childless people do in their spare time.

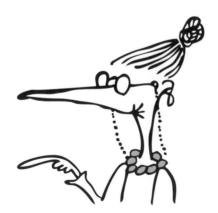

MRS FANNY BRAXTON HICKS

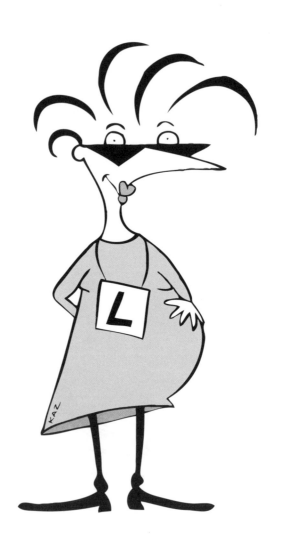

The ROUGH GUIDE to

Pregnancy
and birth

by
KAZ COOKE

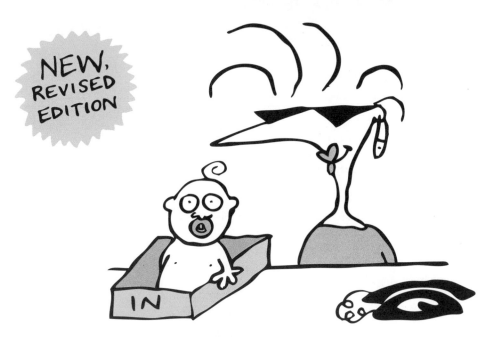

ROUGH
GUIDES

www.roughguides.com

CREDITS

The Rough Guide to Pregnancy and Birth
Editor: Ruth Tidball
Typesetting: Dan May
Proofreading: Susanne Hillen
Index: Jonathan Burd
Production: Rebecca Short

Rough Guides Reference
Editors: Kate Berens, Peter Buckley, Tracy Hopkins, Matthew Milton, Joe Staines, Ruth Tidball
Director: Andrew Lockett

PUBLISHING INFORMATION

First published as *Up The Duff* by Penguin Group Australia, 1999 and 2009
This revised third edition published April 2010 by Rough Guides:
80 Strand, London WC2R 0RL, UK
Email: mail@roughguides.com

Distributed by the Penguin Group:
Penguin Books Ltd, 80 Strand, London WC2R 0RL, UK

Typeset in Shannon and Minion 11.5 pt to an original design by Sandy Cull and Elissa Christian © Penguin Group (Australia)

Printed and bound in Singapore by Toppan Security Printing Pte. Ltd.

Text and illustrations © Kaz Cooke 1999, 2010

496 pages; includes index

A catalogue record for this book is available from the British Library

ISBN 13: 978-1-84836-559-9

1 3 5 7 9 8 6 4 2

for Oofty Goofty

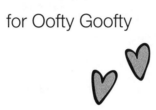

CONTENTS

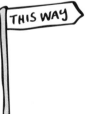
THIS WAY

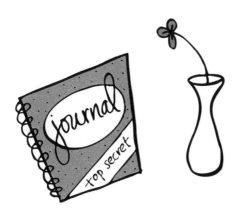
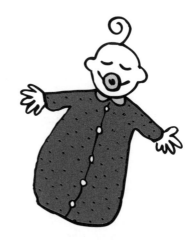

INTRO

Well, here it is: the new edition of *The Rough Guide to Pregnancy and Birth*.

'Wait a minute', I hear you say, rather suspiciously, with narrowed eyes, pausing in your reach for another HobNob. 'What's wrong with the last edition? Did it tell women a baby was going to come out of their ear?'

Nope, although I think I may have thought it would before I started my original research and writing for the first edition. Since then, I've kept updating the book with the latest medical info. Eventually, though, it was time for a big overhaul (and a new cover colour – sunshiny yellow instead of limy, well, lime).

I've added new stuff for partners (signalled by a heart in the book's margins), and made sure all the latest on medical tests is included, covering what they are, when to have them, why they're done, and how to interpret the results. I've badgered a whole new lot of experts working at the coalface of caring for pregnant women, helping them through birth, and looking after new babies. They've checked the facts, provided all the latest info and made suggestions.

The book now kicks off with a new chapter on getting ready for pregnancy and closes with a bigger, better Help part at the back, featuring added chapters on fertility troubles and assisted conception (including IVF) as well as an updated contacts and resources chapter for pregnancy and after the baby is born. Throughout the book there's also loads more info on everything from which fish you can eat safely to when you can have sex after the baby's birth (any time Johnny Depp knocks on the door).

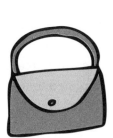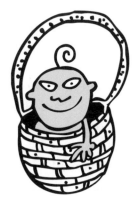

But back to basics: why did I write this book in the first place? Aren't there enough pregnancy gurus already? For a start, the last thing you need when you're pregnant is a bossy-boots insisting you 'should' feel this and 'must' do that. Who wants to have, or be, a guru? Not me.

Okay, so first, I got up the duff. Then realised I had no idea what I was in for.

I bought a squillion pregnancy books and discovered they often contradict each other on key points; they're only relevant in Idaho; or they're written by rich women who think you should get a sink installed in your child's 'nursery' (I ask you), or by people pushing their own personal theory, which may or may not involve giving birth in a wading pool full of lavender water and the dog.

The other thing pregnancy books tend to do is describe the size of the developing fetus through comparisons with food. One week it's a brazil nut, then a plum, then an aubergine. At one point I became convinced I was going to give birth to a giant fruit and nut bar.

And most of the books finish at exactly week 40, when the baby is due. In real life, while you're pregnant, you can't think any further than the birth. But the very minute you have a baby you can hardly remember a thing about the pregnancy. It's suddenly entirely irrelevant and you have to deal IMMEDIATELY with a tiny person who depends on you completely (and also do stuff with your bosoms they don't even ask from exotic dancers).

For some reason I had always imagined that being pregnant would just be like being me with a big bump out the front. It hadn't occurred to me that the reality of being pregnant would eventually be felt constantly in every physical part of my body, and in every recess of what I fondly used to call my mind. Even though I had heard about nausea and fluid retention and vagueness and a ferzillion other things, for some dumb reason I thought they were part of an old-fashioned pregnancy, relegated to history along with the concept of 'confinement' and Mrs Spinoza's mechanical home-perm-and-gherkin-bottling machine.

I'm a career woman, I thought. I'm over 30. I've always pretended to be in control of my life, and that doesn't have to stop just because I'm pregnant. I'll just live my life the way it has always been (without getting wasted and having a few fags at the weekend). Work will go on as normal, life at home will be just the same, only I'll need bigger shirts at some point. My life will only completely change once the baby comes out.

WELL.

Apparently not.

I had not bargained on the body taking control of itself. The power of the mind? Pah, and furthermore, snorty snonking sound. As far as my body was concerned, its major priority was growing a healthy baby. Several times I felt my legs going off along the corridor for a lie down when I thought my torso should have been elsewhere. I woke up in the middle of the night compelled to eat banana sandwiches and drink glasses of soy milk. I had become a host organism.

My first thoughts every morning and my last thoughts at night were about being pregnant, and there was a fair whack of it in between. (This is as well as the other stuff you usually have to be on top of in your normal life.) Would I be a good mother? What if something went wrong? Was it too late to have second thoughts? Should I feel guilty about having second thoughts? Where do we stand on third and subsequent thoughts? Where the hell are my keys? Why is the Marmite in the freezer? Did I do that? What the hell has happened to my HAIR? What's that weird bump forming on my gums? Do stretch marks stay that fetching shade of royal purple forever? Will I ever want to have sex again? What do people mean when they say 'pregnancy hormones'? Is it true some aromatherapy can

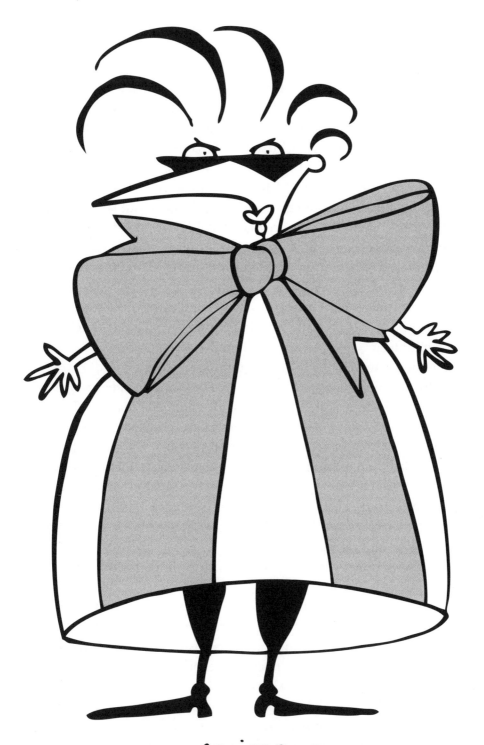

'VERTICAL STRIPES FLATTER THE MATERNAL FIGURE' - SALES ASSISTANT make you have a miscarriage? Is it any wonder they keep making horror movies about motherhood and creatures inside us? Isn't this miraculous? Isn't this uncomfortable? Isn't this terrifying, and wonderful, and fascinating, and boring as batshit, all at the same time? Am I supposed to feel serene, or just seasick? If you don't do your pelvic-floor exercises will your fanny fall out? Why can't I feel the baby move yet? Could the baby stop moving for a while and give me a rest? What about those cigarettes I had before I realised I was pregnant? Will I ever be able to be alone again? How can I tell people I don't want my career back? How can I get my career back? When does a fetus become a baby? Does that mean if it's born then it will survive? Could I get any fatter? What's pre-eclampsia and how do you get it? What can you see on an ultrasound screen? What if labour goes on forever and nothing comes out? Could somebody get me a cup of tea?

And then when I had a baby the questions really started.

So to find out what's what I wrote *The Rough Guide to Pregnancy and Birth* (and the sequel, *The Rough Guide to Babies and Toddlers*). The researchers and I went to work, and then experts checked everything written about their special area and suggested new bits, and then the editor asked a gadzillion questions and in the normal course of events I would have had a huge tantrum but I was too tired because by that time I'd had a baby, so instead we checked it all over again and took bits out and put bits in and waved it all about. And now, ten years later, here it is still – updated to the eyeballs and raring to go.

It is always rather disconcerting when somebody introduces me as a 'pregnancy and parenting expert'. For one thing, I used to think you could squirt breast milk out of one hole in your breast like a firefighter's hose (but more on that later). In fact, the real reason I wrote the book was total cluelessness. If there's one thing that journalism training teaches you, it's that you can bowl up to some tippety-top experts and say 'please help me, I don't understand anything'. That's why I'm so grateful to all the various medical experts who've helped with this and previous editions of *The Rough Guide to Pregnancy and Birth*.

If you read everything in the book you might think pregnancy is a terrible minefield of bizarre health complaints. Don't freak out: lots of the pregnancy problems are rare – they're included 'just in case'. If you do have a special interest or problem, though, this book will give you the basics. And if there's something you need to know more about, you can find a phone number, website or book pointing you in the right direction recommended in the 'More Info' lists at the end of each chapter or chapter section, or in Contacts and Resources at the end of the book.

_Kaz

PS One last thing: the Diary entries you'll find in each chapter include many aspects of my own experience, with a few stories from other people thrown in and the odd embellishment, but it is not quite my story. A woman has to try to cling to some sense of mystery (especially when she's got baby vomit up her nose). (Oh, don't ask.)

PPS Now if you'll excuse me I have to go and write *The Rough Guide to Babies and Toddlers*. Because I have to consult an expert to find out if toddlers come with removable batteries.

You'll Need to Know

definitions

There's no medical rule about when an embryo starts to be a fetus and a fetus graduates to a baby. This book goes with:

⊚ **embryo** – from conception to week 10

⊚ **fetus** – week 10 to week 28

⊚ **baby** – from week 28.

From week 28 most premature babies are likely to survive with major-hospital care. (Many survive an earlier birth, particularly from week 24 on.)

Trimesters   Doctors, websites and books differ on when one trimester ends and the next begins ('trimester' means three months). Check with your doctor and midwife: they may say the first trimester is to the end of week 12. In this book:

⊚ **the first trimester** is to the end of week 13

⊚ **the second trimester** is from week 14 to the end of week 26

⊚ **the third trimester** is from week 27 until birth.

Other words you'll hear

⊚ **antenatal**, or **prenatal** – before the birth

⊚ **postnatal** – after the birth

⊚ **GP** – general practitioner (your local or family doctor)

⊚ **obstetrician** – a doctor who's a specialist in gynaecology, pregnancy and childbirth and qualified to perform surgery

⊚ **midwife** – a qualified practitioner who cares for women during pregnancy, birth and the early postnatal period.

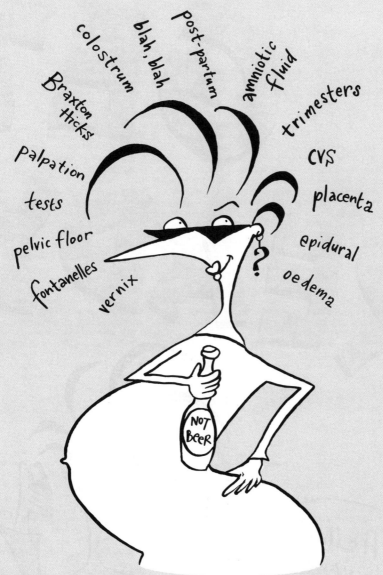

colostrum
blah, blah
post-partum
amniotic fluid
Braxton hicks
trimesters
Palpation
CVS
tests
placenta
pelvic floor
epidural
fontanelles
vernix
oedema

NOT BEER

dates

This book, like doctors, will **count pregnancy from the first day of your last normal period**. Technically, this means you'll be having a period in the first week of your pregnancy, so at the end of week 1 you're 'one week pregnant', at the end of week 15 you'll be '15 weeks pregnant', and so on.

GET READY

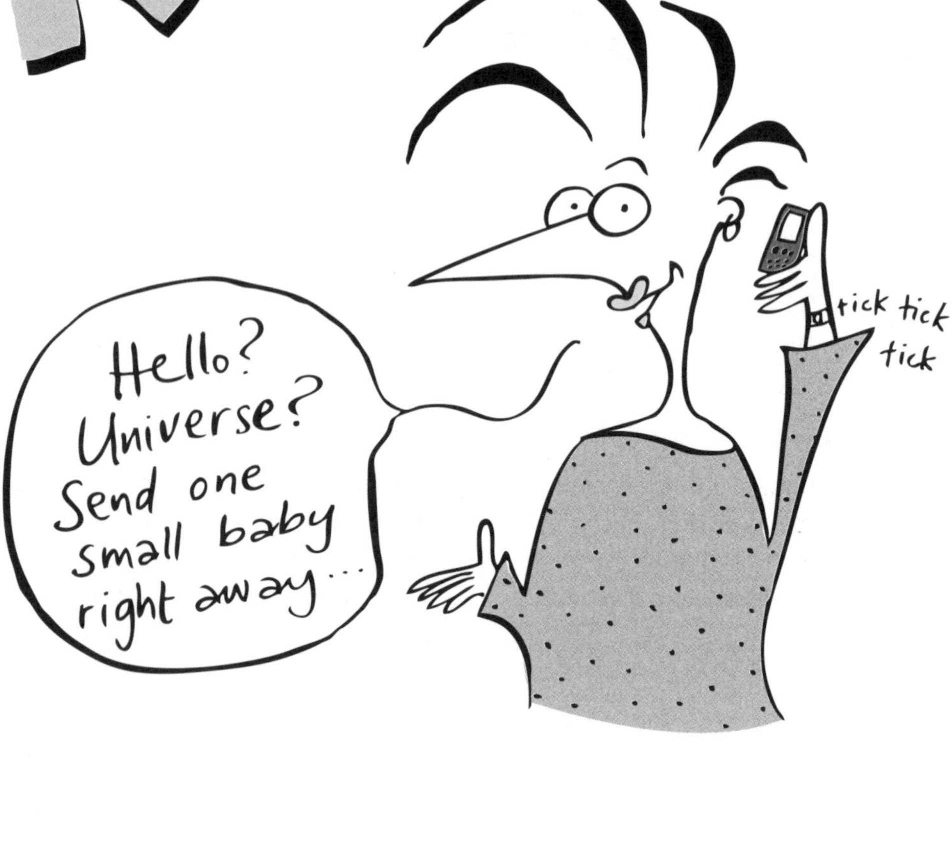
Hello? Universe? Send one small baby right away...
tick tick tick

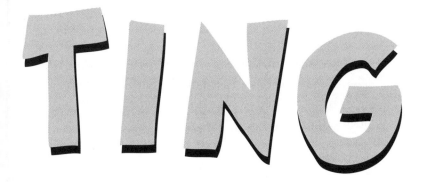

TING

what's going on You're thinking about maybe, possibly, one day, ooh, not yet, doing a feasibility study on, let's not rush into it, conceivably (ha!), perchance, who knows, er, **getting pregnant**. Or you've decided it's definitely time to saddle up, grasp the nettle, go full steam ahead, put on your 'trying' hat, get your ducks in a row, mix the metaphors, get into gear, and give it a **red-hot go.**

This chapter will give you some ideas about how to prepare for being pregnant and help protect you, your relationships and your future baby with some healthy changes, financial strategies and realistic plans. If you're **already pregnant,** never mind: these are still good hints that will help you get up to speed with the practical stuff.

Okay, hold onto that hat. Here we go . . .

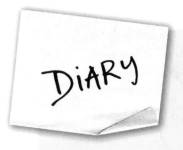
DIARY

I took an inventory of my life recently, and wrote it down with an eyebrow pencil on the back of a brown paper bag that used to have a muffin in it. It pretty much came out this way.

✳ Name: Kaz Cooke.

✳ Age: 32.

✳ Unglamorous designer for small south London fashion company, Real Gorgeous Ltd (we make the Real Women Wear label, sizes 8–18).

✳ Sagittarius (tactless and jovial).

✳ Hobbies: eating, sleeping, buying shoes.

✳ Accoutrements: perfectly decent boyfriend called Geoff, a landscaper who works in a garden shop and has some clients on the side. Small house in Clapham with crippling mortgage. Nice sofa. Some ageing white goods. £1600 in the bank.

✳ Shape: not unlike that of the fruit known colloquially as a pear. With legs. Unusually fat knees. Never mind. Rest of self reasonably overweight, but nothing that a lot of exercise and a little less reliance on chocolate and cheese wouldn't cure.

✳ Medical history: long tussle with endometriosis, a menstrual condition that often causes infertility, which I have controlled by taking the Pill full-time without a break. Haven't had a period for four years.

✳ Doctor's advice last time I went: if you want to get pregnant, take some vitamins for three months, come off the Pill and start bonking like a rabbit (or words to that effect).

Geoff and I had a talk about six months ago. I said I wanted to have kids and he said it was too soon (he's only 31, my toyboy). Recently, though, he'd thought about it and said he was as ready as he'd ever be, particularly since I'd told him that, given my medical history, nothing at all might happen, or it might take two years to get everything working again. I told Geoff there were a few things to sort out: like what would we do if a test during pregnancy showed that there was something wrong with the baby? And how would he feel if the kid grew up to be a gay man?

Geoff put his head on the side and thought for a moment. 'As long as he plays midfield for Palace I can't see the problem.'

We each made a list of stuff we'd have to do before I got pregnant. Mine said:

✳ See GP about tests to do before come off Pill.

✳ Lose weight.

✳ Get fit.

✳ See Beck (that's my herbalist and medical adviser and fellow champagne admirer) about what naturopathy things I should do.

✳ Buy Lotto ticket.

✳ Stop smoking.

✳ Stop drinking.

✳ Get driver's licence.

✳ Don't roll about in pesticide-soaked paddocks, stop eating junk food, cook magnificently cunning little low-fat dishes from primary food sources, stop saying fuck so much, get legs waxed, organise the sanding of the floor of our new house without actually breathing in any of that polyurethane topcoat.

I gaffer-taped the list of things to do onto the fridge. Then I took it off and replaced it with a note on a small piece of the muffin bag saying 'Change entire life immediately', and threw my packet of fags in the bin in a rather melodramatic fashion.

There was absolutely nothing on Geoff's list except:

✳ Buy milk and bread.

✳ Have sex.

info

before you start

You might think that preparing for pregnancy is as simple as stopping contraception or as complicated as needing a massive checklist of stuff you have to do first (increase folic acid intake, learn yoga, inherit mansion, find Mr Right). Either way, you'd be sort of correct. Not all the things listed in this chapter HAVE to be done before you get pregnant, but if you have time to plan they'll probably make your life easier – and a few of the hints will help protect the baby you're thinking of starting.

Because this is a book for a fairly general readership, let's presume for the moment that you're a woman with a male partner and you have no reason to believe either of you has a fertility problem. There is info specially for blokes scattered throughout this chapter and the book: wherever you see a heart symbol in the margin it's a special pit stop for men – or other partners. (If you're a lesbian or a single woman exploring the options, or you're considering a surrogate to go through a pregnancy for you, the Assisted Conception chapter in the Help part at the end of the book has info relevant for you.)

When you're planning to have a baby there's emotional and mental stuff to think about, as well as lifestyle changes that could help you become more fertile and will make you healthier and more resilient for the full-on physical demands of pregnancy, childbirth and being a parent. And there are things you can do, aside from bank robbery, to improve your financial readiness.

mental and emotional homework

Time for a long, hard look at yourself. And a Big Talk with your partner. You don't necessarily have to have all the answers to the following questions, but it's probably a good idea to have thought about them together.

⑥ Are you both ready to try?

⑥ Why do you want to have a baby? Do you share the same reasons for having kids?

⑥ Do you want a toddler and a teenager (that's what babies become)?

⑥ What if you don't get pregnant? Would you try in-vitro fertilisation (IVF)?

⑥ If you postpone the decision, does that mean you might later be trying to get pregnant when your fertility is declining rapidly?

⊚ What are your views on antenatal (also referred to as prenatal) testing?

⊚ What would you do if you found out your unborn child had a severe abnormality or a disabling condition? How would you cope with the idea of terminating the pregnancy, or living with a baby who will grow up always having special needs?

⊚ Would you consider circumcising your child? Why?

⊚ Do you have similar religious or ethical values?

⊚ Do you share the same feelings about the possibility of your child growing up to be gay, or a stockbroker?

⊚ Do your views differ on discipline and the issue of hitting children?

⊚ Do you have a good support network of family and friends? Have any of them had recent experience with babies?

⊚ Are you both go-with-the-flow sorts of people or do you like to plan for the future?

⊚ Are you really ready to make the transition from up-for-anything-at-a-moment's-notice to 'slave-to-baby'-parent-who-hasn't-had-time-to-shower-in-two-days-and-whose-every-outing-must-be-planned-with-a-military-precision-that-needs-to-be-totally-flexible-for-if-the-baby-wakes-up/won't-wake-up/cries/vomits/needs-feeding/poos-on-the-mobile-phone?

Many of these issues are explored in this book, and you can look up topics such as antenatal testing and circumcision in the index.

SPECIAL HINTS FROM A MOTHER

Before you decide to have a baby:

• spend time with friends who already have a baby, or older children, and observe and ask about how their life has changed
• spend at least a full day from dawn until late with a mother and a small baby; it's impossible to imagine just how much work is involved until you are in the thick of it.

If either of you needs to talk to someone about any concerns you may have about prospective parenthood, try Parentline Plus's helpline, 0808 800 2222.

A DIFFICULT RELATIONSHIP

Some people think that having a baby will bring them closer together. In some ways that can be true, but in reality having a baby is probably the most stressful thing you'll ever do. It's not something to do as a last resort to keep a couple together. As writer Nora Ephron once said, 'A baby is a hand grenade thrown into a marriage'. If your partnership is already stressful, pregnancy and a baby will add to that.

Many abusive or controlling partners become more so during pregnancy. You could also be putting your future child at risk of abuse or an unhappy childhood. If you're in a relationship that makes you feel bad or sad and you think 'This is as good as it gets' or 'I deserve to be punished or treated badly', you need help, not a baby. Your GP can recommend a counsellor to talk things through with you, and the 'Family and Partner Abuse and Violence' section in the Contacts and Resources chapter at the end of the book has names and contact details of supportive organisations that offer practical help.

physical health homework

A trip to the GP   Three months before you start the festival of bonking you both need to go to your GP, say you're planning to get pregnant and ask for a check-up. You need some general health checks before you stop contraception, and you might have a simple infertility problem that could be easily identified and taken care of. Make separate GP appointments as there may be different issues for the two of you and the sessions may be longer than usual.

Gentlemen, get:

◎ a full 'physical'

◎ a rubella (German measles) vaccination and any other ones you might need; a blood test will show whether you have immunity to German measles from the usual childhood measles-mumps-rubella jab – rubella can cause birth defects, including blindness and deafness, if contracted by a pregnant woman

◎ a sperm test if you're getting older or you're in a hurry to have a baby, although this is something you're more likely to have if you're having problems conceiving (there's more on this in the Fertility Troubles chapter in the Help part of the book)

◎ a test for any sexually transmitted infections (STIs) – some infections, such as chlamydia and gonorrhoea, can be contracted years before you meet your partner and show no recognisable symptoms but still cause really major problems in the baby-making department for both men and women and also affect the baby ('Protecting Your Pregnancy' in Week 4 has info on this).

Ladies, get the works, including:

◎ a breast check

◎ a smear test

◎ a rubella vaccination if you know you haven't had one, or a blood test if you don't know whether you're covered – you need to have the vaccination or a booster three months before you stop contraception so that your system has time to destroy the live virus (Week 4 has more info)

◎ an ovulation check – you can't get pregnant if you're not ovulating (releasing an egg, ready to be fertilised by any lurking sperm). Almost all women who have periods on a regular 26- to 35-day cycle will be ovulating. Most ovulation tests are performed 21 days after the last period began, but that will only confirm the ovulation of a woman who has a 28-day cycle. Tell your doctor how long your cycle usually is to help them pinpoint when you're likely to ovulate. Most women don't bother with an ovulation test unless they have trouble conceiving

◎ a test for STIs. Don't freak at the idea of either of you having one. It has nothing to do with the loyalty of your partner or where you are on the slutty scale (okay, there is no slutty scale – if there was, gee, I wish I'd been an 11)

◎ a pregnancy vitamin and mineral complex that includes folic acid (also called folate) and iodine. Folic acid, which doctors say you should start taking three months before you stop contraception, helps guard against some kinds of birth defects (see 'Eating and Supplements' in Week 2). Do not buy cheap stuff at an obscure discount shop. Buy a specific pre-conception or pregnancy vitamin and mineral pill from your chemist, supermarket or health food shop. A standard women's or general multivitamin could have too much of some ingredients to be safe for pregnancy, and not enough of some special vitamins and minerals needed for optimum mum and fetal health. Choose a well-known brand.

Vitamins, Minerals & chocolate

THe perfect supplement

Also discuss any ongoing health problems such as asthma with your GP, and talk about how they could be managed during pregnancy and beyond.

Healthy lifestyle

BLOKES

Time to man up in the healthy lifestyle department. Both to support your partner and to have the best chance of making useful sperm:

⑥ limit grog to a couple of standard drinks a day, and not every day

⑥ stop smoking and taking illegal drugs

⑥ eat healthy food – have less fast food from the takeaway shop and ready-made stuff in cans or packets, and go instead for more fresh food, a wider range and extra veggies

⑥ have no more than one coffee or caffeine-based cola or 'energy' drink a day (caffeine is sometimes listed under another name such as guarana).

Or, I think you'll find, ladies will be refusing to have any sex with you because you're a hard-drinking, caffeine-addicted, drug-fiend smoker who hasn't eaten anything green in weeks.

WOMEN

Here's how you can try to increase your general sparkiness and chances of conceiving, and get into some healthy habits you'll need during pregnancy:

⑥ quit cigarettes and illegal drugs ('Protecting Your Pregnancy' in Week 4 explains why), and if that's hard ask for help (doctors are very used to being asked about this) – many people think that knowing they're pregnant or likely to be pregnant will get them to quit an addiction, but that's rarely true so it's best to get help

⑥ limit your alcohol to not drinking every day and not having more than two standard drinks on the same day – many women just stop altogether (because, as explained in Week 4, doctors say that once you're pregnant no amount of alcohol can be assumed to be safe for the developing fetus)

⑥ have a look at your daily caffeine intake – high levels, especially in the first trimester, have been linked to miscarriage. Although most doctors say one coffee or other caffeine drink a day should do no harm (see 'Eating and

HEADS UP: FERTILITY AND PRE-CONCEPTION WEBSITES AND BOOKS

There are many websites and books on pre-conception and fertility based on eating organic foods, often with 'natural' or 'fertility diet' in the title. Some promise 'better babies' or that you can make 'super sperm' or 'eat yourself pregnant'. If you lean towards the 'natural' side of things, these books may be for you.

But be aware that they sometimes make ludicrous and misleading claims along the lines that a healthier life can cure infertility and prevent all birth defects, sick babies, miscarriages and stillbirths, and offer suggestions, such as 'detoxifying' or fasting, that could be dangerous for you and, if you've conceived without knowing it, for your unborn baby. And, like many pregnancy-related books, some are imported from overseas and have 'facts' not relevant to the UK.

Life is often random and unexplained, and eating and living 'naturally' is not a guaranteed way to have a healthy baby nor a cure for fertility problems. Every day, healthy babies are born to women who eat fast food and have never eaten an organic veggie in their life. And some people who 'do all the right things' have babies with problems. That's because these problems are hardly ever anybody's fault or because they did something wrong without knowing it. Bad things can happen to good people.

While supporting the general idea of a healthy lifestyle being ideal for babies and mothers, these books can also worry women with endless charts and promote 'natural remedies' with no evidence that they work. One suggests natural contraception can be achieved by avoiding sex during the phase of the moon in which you were born, and lists scary and deadly possible effects on fertility and health of taking the Pill and pregnancy termination as if these were likely or inevitable. In fact most of these effects are extremely rare.

You can still do all the natural things and have a healthier lifestyle while getting medical help. Doctors say that many women who follow instructions about 'natural fertility' for years without success think they're doing all they can, and come to them too late to get the maximum benefit from assisted conception. So by all means do the natural thing – you'll feel better and be healthier, and that's no small matter – but get medical help after six months or so if you're still not pregnant (see 'Have a Deadline' in Week 1).

Supplements' in Week 2), many women cut down gradually to none before they try to get pregnant to be super-sure

⑥ gain or lose weight to get into the healthy weight range for you if you need to (this is not the weight your Aunty May or *Cosmopolitan* magazine thinks you should be – ask your doctor about it); some women's hospitals have special programmes for overweight or underweight women to increase their chances of getting pregnant

⑥ give yourself a moderate exercise plan – say, a half-hour or one-hour walk each day

⑥ eat healthy food, but don't get hung up on it

⑥ reduce your stress levels – hormones are affected by stress and this can change your chances of fertility.

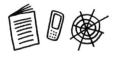

more info on **pre-pregnancy health**

Also see the websites in 'Eating and Supplements' in Week 2.

nhs.uk
> On the main page, type 'pregnancy care planner' into the search option. This will take you to a page where you can choose the 'Before You Are Pregnant' option for lots of info on trying to get pregnant, your health, vitamins and minerals. You can also click on 'Behind the headlines' to find any stories about pregnancy or pre-pregnancy that may be relevant.

Plan to Get Pregnant: 10 Steps to Maximum Fertility by Zita West, Dorling Kindersley, UK, 2008
> A comprehensive round-up of all sorts of things that could affect your ability to get pregnant, including sleep, nutrition, stress, sex drive and health problems, with suggested complementary therapies and strategies (many of which are not recognised as effective in scientific medicine) from acupuncture to 'visualisation'. Should always be used in conjunction with a doctor's advice and a check to try to identify any medical problems that could be dealt with.

financial homework

Health insurance and going private   If you plan to take out private health insurance you need to do it now, before you get pregnant. If you already have insurance, find out exactly what your policy covers in respect of pregnancy. Many policies cover very little in the way of 'routine' care, while other policies will cover a caesarean birth if you need one and/or after care in a private hospital. If you are thinking about using a private midwife (£1000 to £4000), or having a private hospital birth, start looking at the costs right now.

Work entitlements   Check out your entitlement to paid and unpaid parental leave with your employer. In a large company you may be able to do this anonymously by phone if you don't want to flag your intentions. And double-check your entitlement with your union or the Citizens Advice Bureau (see 'More Info' at the end of this section).

Most employees qualify for a year's maternity leave, and Statutory Maternity Pay for 39 weeks. You are also entitled to time off for antenatal appointments. Dads and other partners in employment can take up to two weeks' paid leave following the birth of the baby. Your employer is legally required to offer you the same job or an equivalent-level job on your return from leave. If you're on a contract or are a casual worker you will most likely be entitled to maternity pay but not leave. These are the minimum entitlements. Some employers offer more benefits including extra maternity pay, flexible working arrangements when you return to work, and work-based childcare. If there are two working parents involved, find out whose job offers a better package and childcare arrangements.

Financial plan   Even just taking a pregnancy vitamin once a day will immediately add to your grocery bill, and there will be other, less obvious costs too, so it's good to have some idea of what you're in for financially.

⑥ Do you need to start a savings account especially for emergencies?

⑥ Which partner will give up full-time work, or will both partners keep working and use childcare?

⑥ If only one of you continues paid work, is the other partner's money totally 'ours'? (How do you spell 'budget'?) How would you feel

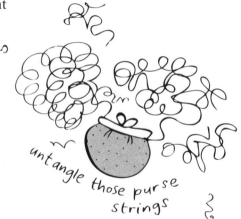

untangle those purse strings

about a joint account? Or about an automatic transferral of money from the income of the paid partner to the account of the one at home with the bub?

⊚ Will both parents contribute to childcare rather than just taking it out of the 'woman's wage'? How much will that cost?

⊚ If you share paid work and both go to part-time, which benefits will you lose? What if those arrangements have to change for some reason?

MAJOR BUYS

Your car If you're thinking about buying a new car (or planning to keep your existing one), check that it has:

- a back seat – babies and children up to the size of an average 12-year-old must travel in the back because airbags, now standard in modern cars, can kill a child in the front (alternatively, you can use a rear-facing baby seat or child seat in the front if there's no airbag or it's been deactivated)
- an anchor point for baby and child restraints (or can have one installed)
- four doors, rather than two, making it heaps more convenient when getting kids in and out.

Don't buy an SUV or a four-wheel drive (this doesn't apply to all-wheel-drive saloons). Apart from their expensive, petrol-guzzling, environment-hurting aspects, four-wheel drives are over-represented in accidents, including those in which small children are hit in their own driveway: a kid hit by a four-wheel drive is statistically very much more likely to die than one hit by a smaller car. (For the same reason – to protect your and other children – *please* remove any bullbar.) Proximity alarms, lenses and video-checking systems are not a guarantee of safety and can promote false confidence, according to car accident authorities. *All* vehicles have blind spots, especially low to the ground.

Wish list Buy a lottery ticket. If you win, check the energy credentials and then buy a new washing machine (and a dryer if you live somewhere very rainy and cold) and a fridge with a freezer at the bottom. A cordless phone you can carry from room to room that has a hands-free speaker function is also really useful when you have a baby. If your home doesn't have a good central heating system, install something energy-efficient. If there's any money left over, get yourself a holiday and an emerald tiara.

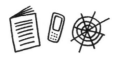

more info on finances

moneymadeclear.fsa.gov.uk
From the main page of the government's Financial Services Authority website, look under 'step-by-step guides' for info on 'moving in together', or 'having a baby'. (You can access the FSA's 'Parent's Guide to Money' online under 'Having a Baby', or get a printed copy from your midwife.) On the main page there are lots of other links to great stuff on making budgets, clearing debts, buying a car, and avoiding rip-offs and scams generally. If you can, it's a good idea to have a look at this stuff before you're a parent, to get a head start.
Advice line: 0300 500 5000.

The Resourceful Mum's Handbook: Baby on a Budget by Elen Lewis, Square Peg Publishing, UK, 2009
If you're the DIY type, you'll like the squillions of hints on how to do things on the cheap, from cheap buying ideas to making your own homewares, toys, games and baby clothes, and recipes for first foods. Links to websites and other handy organisations such as council nappy incentive programmes (where you get 'gifts' to encourage you to use cloth nappies).

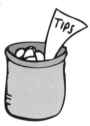

adviceguide.org.uk
The Citizens Advice Bureau is a charity offering free information and advice about legal, money and other matters to the general public. Click on 'Employment', then 'Parental Rights at Work' for information about your rights to maternity leave, maternity pay and other benefits. To find out where your local office is, so that you can call for an appointment or get some info over the phone, visit sister website citizensadvice.org.uk, and type your postcode into the search box.

direct.gov.uk
From the main page of this government website, search 'pregnancy maternity rights' to find out all your entitlements for maternity and paternity leave, pay and other useful stuff.

worksmart.org.uk/rights/maternity_leave
The maternity pages of the Trades Union Congress's Work Smart advice site offer a workers' perspective on your employment rights when you or your partner has a baby. Call the TUC Know Your Rights line (0870 600 4 882) to order printed advice booklets.

MONEY FOR MUMS (AND DADS)

Make sure you know about any financial grants and entitlements from the government for pregnant women or new parents. Some are available to all, regardless of income, while there is extra money for those on low incomes. Visit direct.gov.uk and type 'Expecting or bringing up children benefits' into the search engine, or ask your midwife for your free copy of the Financial Services Authority's *Parent's Guide to Money*.

when to try

There is never a perfect time to have a baby. Some people get pregnant young, without having established qualifications or any money saved up (but have the advantage of a resilient body and heaps of energy). Some people have the 'head start' of an established career and a house on the way to being paid off, then start trying in their mid-to-late thirties and realise they're having trouble conceiving and time is running out. Some people don't have the luxury of deciding, and their pregnancy is the result of a happy or unhappy accident.

It's damned annoying, but even if you are incredibly lucky, full of common sense, prepared to make sacrifices and heir to a brewing fortune – and can find a loyal, supportive, financially secure, good-parent-material partner on cue – you can't simultaneously have a career, achieve all your financial and work goals right on schedule, do further study, get pregnant according to an ideal timetable, produce a child and work full-time.

So I can't tell you how to 'have it all'. But I can tell you that if you do want a family, and you're vaguely thinking 'eventually', you don't have all the time in the world. I'm not saying settle for anybody with a good sperm count the very minute you think you might want kids, just that you might need to think about who and what and when earlier than you might have presumed.

Those 46-year-old movie stars who have twins? They got lucky with in-vitro fertilisation (IVF) – you might not. IVF isn't magic or guaranteed. Its success rate falls away, just as statistical fertility does, as you get older. After 40, your chances of getting pregnant naturally start to plummet – the graphs of available healthy eggs literally look like a drawing of a cliff – and the chance of conceiving with IVF can be very slim indeed after the age of 40, statistically decreasing every year after that. Most IVF clinics won't agree to treat women over about 45. And most mothers will tell you that the very idea of having a baby (or two!) in their forties just makes them feel too shatteringly exhausted to lift an eyebrow. The majority of doctors say that to give yourself the best chance you need to start before you're 36.

Trying   On your mark – ready for Week 1 (where there's info on how long to try without success before you need to get help).

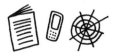

more info on **when to try**

rcog.org.uk
From the home page of the Royal College of Obstetricians and Gynaecologists, search 'maternal age' to see the College report on why it recommends that a woman should try to get pregnant between the ages of 20 and 35 to give herself the best chance. There are links to more information on the subject and a podcast recorded by specialists about related issues including the health of older mothers.

what's going on Not much. By the end of the week you've just finished the last period you'll have for a while. You're into the 'follicular' phase of the menstrual cycle, which means the egg-making and dispatch phase ('follicle' is the name for the tiny sac in which the egg matures). One of your two ovaries is deciding which of the eggs developing in this menstrual cycle will be the one to go forth. (An egg is also known as an ovum, if you want to get all Latin about it.) Your ovaries release 400–500 mature eggs during your 'fertile years'. It only takes one to get pregnant.

Your body is going about its usual hormonal carry-on. Lots of oestrogen (actually several oestrogens, just called 'oestrogen' as an umbrella term) is being produced by your ovaries. This stimulates the uterus (known as the womb) to grow more lining, called the endometrium, to replace the lining that has just left as your last period. This new endometrium is the welcoming surface for the egg if it's fertilised. The egg is extremely weeny: about a tenth of a millimetre in diameter.

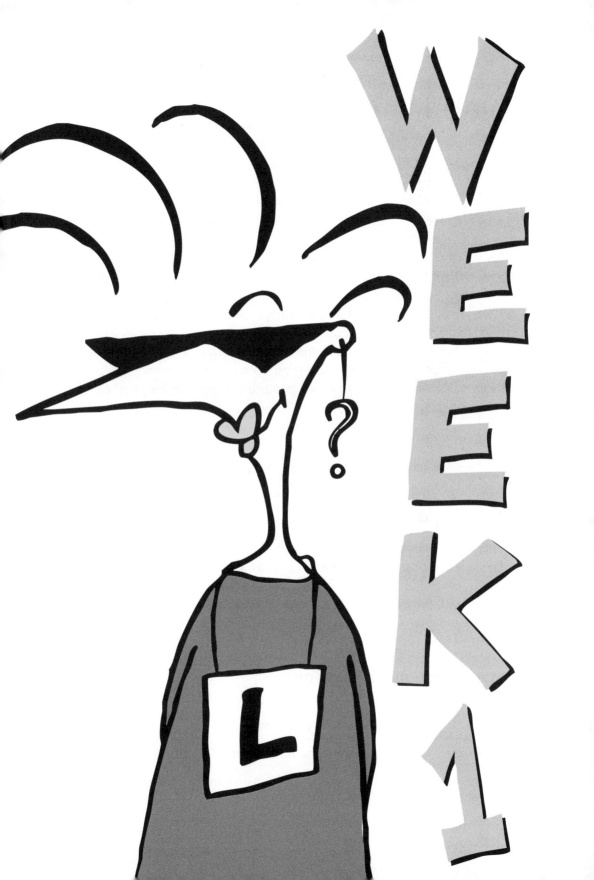

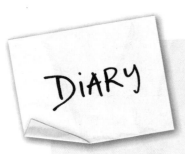

DiARY

I've decided to blow our savings and take Geoff away to a Greek island next week and ravish him constantly. For three months my herbalist, Beck, who's also had years of experience as a hospital midwife, has had me on a tonic and some vitamins that include something called folic acid and heaven knows what other baby-friendly stuff. I've just chucked the Pill in the bin and I'm ready for Operation Up The Duff. Geoff and I both need a holiday to fortify us anyway, having been working like demons to pay for the new house.

I believe there are many ways you can pinpoint the moment of ovulation, involving thermometers, ropes and pulleys, and other implements. I should have got out the calculator and a protractor and a slide rule and a sextant and a sexton and half a sundial to work out when I might ovulate. (Don't know what a sexton is, but it sounds rather raunchy.) Sadly I might not have enough endometrium to have a period because I've been on the Pill for four years, so a menstrual chart's about as much use to me as a stuffed aardvark.

Instead I'll just guess.

info

making a start

Sorry, but it's not just non-stop bonking. You'll need to get the all-clear, dears (yes, blokes too). So if you haven't already, see the previous chapter, Getting Ready, for the physical health checks you'll need. While you're there, have a squiz at all the other things that you may want to think about before you get pregnant or while you're trying, and do the physical health homework outlined in that chapter. Then you can dive in.

start as you mean to go on

From now on, act as if you were already pregnant. That means:

◎ no alcohol, no cigarettes, no illegal drugs

◎ keeping on taking your pregnancy vitamin and mineral supplement

◎ telling your GP about any medications, vitamins or herbal preparations you're taking – a lot of things are okay, but always check with your doctor

⑥ telling pharmacists, natural therapists and herbalists, whenever you buy vitamins, herbal preparations or any legal drugs, that you may be pregnant – normal doses of paracetamol for headaches are considered safe (see the 'Painkillers During Pregnancy' box in Week 4)

⑥ no exposure to suspect chemicals that you know of – make sure your workplace, household appliances and any painting or renovation processes are fetus-friendly, without fumes or leaks.

have a deadline

If you're:

⑥ under 35, try for a year, max, to get pregnant

⑥ over 35, you haven't got as much time to lose, so if you're not pregnant within six months see your doctor.

avoid false assumptions

⑥ It's a myth that being on the Pill means it will take longer for you to get pregnant once you come off it.

⑥ If you're not using contraception, then be prepared to be pregnant. Don't assume you'll have trouble (or won't have any trouble).

⑥ Don't assume that IVF or 'science' will work for you no matter how late you leave it to try.

If you're not pregnant by your loose deadline have a look at the Fertility Troubles chapter in Help at the end of the book.

have sex

Ready, set, go. Whenever you want to (avoid public transport). Two or more times a week would help. (You don't need to worry about complicated charts of vagina temperatures or exact times for having sex – stress or anxiety about getting pregnant is known to make it harder to conceive.)

It'll also help if you have sex around about the time of ovulation. Ask your doctor about how to work out when this is. For most people it's probably a couple of weeks before their next period is due. So, if you have a 28-day cycle (that is, your period usually appears on day 28, when 'day 1' is the first day of your last period), your fertile time is probably around days 10 to 16 (sperm can live for a few days inside you, waiting for an egg to be

GIRL OR BOY?

Every now and then there's another book or 'study' that recommends what to eat or what position to have sex in to statistically increase your chances of choosing your baby's gender. Over the years the recommendations keep changing. By all means eat a banana and stick your legs in the air after bonking, but it doesn't guarantee anything except an amusing sight. Spells, prayers and incantations have about the same success rate.

The only way to know for sure if your unborn baby is male or female is to have a DNA test after the tenth week of pregnancy, which involves taking genetic material from your placenta or amniotic fluid (by amniocentesis or chorionic villus sampling – CVS – which are explained in 'Screening and Diagnostic Tests' in Week 11). These tests carry too much of a risk to be had just to find out if you're having a girl or a boy.

Skilled ultrasound operators can guess the sex but can't guarantee that they're right. Genetic tests on the mother's blood are not yet considered accurate enough to be reliable. Even couples who have paid an IVF clinic to implant only embryos of one sex have found themselves having a baby of the other. Nature's tricky like that. If you have a genetic reason for wanting a particular gender (such as a family history of an illness that affects only boys) talk to your doctor before you try to get pregnant.

The bottom line is that really all you can do is wish. And if it matters so much to you that it means you would welcome a boy less than a girl, or vice versa, maybe you should reconsider having a child. By the time they've carried a baby to full term, most people just want a healthy one, whether or not it has a willy.

released). But everyone is different and some people may ovulate twice, or not at all.

You can usually tell when you're ovulating because your vagina produces more of a slippery fluid (come on in, penis!) that looks clearer than at other times of the month (hey sperm, this is easier to swim through!). You can buy ovulation tests from the chemist, which test the hormone levels in your wee, but they're not very romantic. They are, however, much more accurate than taking your vaginal temperature and keeping charts. The hormone assessment tests measure a hormone that peaks briefly about twenty-four hours before you ovulate, so if you get a result that shows that peak, that's three days of bonking for you, if you feel like it, for the optimum chance of fertilisation.

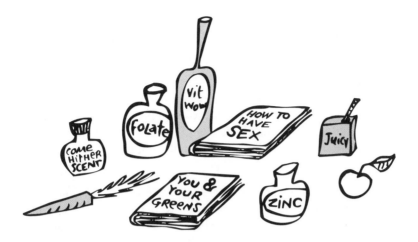

Men, let your partner know if you're starting to feel like an on-call sperm donor. And you can tell her nicely that you don't find 'Quick, my mucus is peaking' a particularly alluring come-on. In exchange, you may have to employ some sexy, go-slow moves and ramp up the romance. (Flowers, I tell you! Massage oils! Doing the dishes!)

PREGNANCY WEBSITES, MAGAZINES AND BOOKS

Also see the websites, mags and books given in Week 43 for more on parenting and childcare.

pregnancy websites and magazines

Make sure you choose a website that's up to date, and watch out for information that has morphed into paid or sponsored advertising – brand names can be a dead giveaway. Some sites – and mags – are very badly written, are based on opinion only, are out of date or exist only to give more credibility to what is mainly advertising. All good reasons why you'll need to check any health info picked up from websites, internet forums, blogs, and mags (especially free ones) with your doctor.

nctpregnancyandbabycare.com

The National Childbirth Trust is a charity set up specifically to help pregnant women and parents. From the main page, choose 'Info centre' for a range of fact sheets, articles and helpful hints for all stages of pregnancy and early parenting. Choose 'Ask our experts' from the main page if you have a specific question, or

'In Your Area' to find local help and services, forums or coffee mornings where you can meet other mums. The shop helps fund their programmes and supplies breastfeeding aids, maternity and kids' clothes, useful books and fact sheets.

babycentre.co.uk

There's a page for each week of pregnancy plus articles on everything from conceiving to naming your new baby. Also supports you after birth, with advice about caring for babies and toddlers and looking after yourself post-baby too. Attractively designed, with lively and friendly chat rooms.

practicalparenting.co.uk

The website of the popular UK magazine *Practical Parenting and Pregnancy* has comprehensive coverage from conception to parenthood, though in-your-face ads can get in the way of finding the best content. Includes pregnancy exercises, recipes, reviews of baby products and a busy forum.

babyworld.co.uk

The website of *Babyworld* magazine features chat rooms, birth stories (always compelling reading when you're pregnant), pregnancy diaries, shopping and an ask-their-expert section. You'll need to register (for free) to access the best bits of the site. As with all commercial sites, make sure you can tell what's an 'article' and what's an 'advertisement' and remember that reviews are unlikely to be critical of products sold by major sponsors or advertisers.

sheilakitzinger.com

UK natural birth activist Sheila Kitzinger may have a habit of comparing the size of a developing fetus to various fruits and vegetables, but she's actually pretty fab. Big on helping mothers and babies whether in a town house or in prison, this site is packed with info on home births, water births, breastfeeding and more. The picture of 'Sheila demonstrating how not to push a baby out' is hilarious.

askamum.co.uk

From the publishers of *Mother and Baby* and *Pregnancy and Birth* magazines. This well-organised site has the usual selection of articles and an active forum, but also offers advice videos you can watch online and audio podcasts.

tommys.org

Helpline: 0870 777 30 60

Tommy's is a charity that funds research into pregnancy complications. Its helpline is staffed by midwives, and its website has info on all sorts of pregnancy stuff, especially potential problems such as pre-eclampsia.

relate.org.uk

Even the strongest of relationships can go through a bit of a wobble at the news a baby is on the way, or it can be a good idea to make sure you're 'on the same 'page' before the new arrival. Relate is the UK's biggest provider of relationship counselling – you can go individually or together.

If you don't mind the 'foreign' aspect, there are some more personal blogs by new mums or fellow travellers on the pregnancy journey. Maybe Brits are just a lot less likely to 'tell all', but many of the popular ones are from the US, including dooce.com, by a woman who's very upfront, funny and rude about the whole caper, and alittlepregnant.com ('madcap misadventures in infertility, pregnancy and parenthood').

pregnancy books

A lot of books are handed to you when you're pregnant. Don't take them. When a friend recommends a book, buy the latest edition of it yourself. Some pregnancy books with out-of-date, even dangerous medical and safety info are passed around. The recommendations below refer to the edition available at the time of going to print; if a newer edition is now available, buy that instead.

New Natural Pregnancy: Practical Wellbeing from Conception to Birth by Janet Balaskas and Gayle Petersen, Gaia Books, UK, 2004

Concentrating on the mother, a holistic look at pregnancy with sections on emotions, nutrition, yoga and exercise, massage, natural therapies and holistic healing. Lots of illustrations of exercises, massage techniques and natural remedies for common pregnancy complaints.

Conception, Pregnancy and Birth by Dr Miriam Stoppard, Dorling Kindersley, UK, 2008

Miriam Stoppard has become the bestselling pregnancy and childcare author in the UK, aided and abetted by the clear Dorling Kindersley illustration-heavy approach. This is a well-researched and up-to-date book covering common worries and queries, from the time before you even know you're pregnant to the first few weeks of parenthood. While nothing is explained exhaustively, Dr Stoppard brings her brisk and basic style to explanations of everything you're likely (or not!) to encounter – from medical diagrams to make-up tips and what sort of sex it's okay to have.

What to Expect When You're Expecting by Heidi E. Murkoff and Sharon Mazel, Simon and Schuster, UK, 2009

This hefty paperback is a look-it-up-when-you-need-to pregnancy guide that includes seemingly everything that can go wrong. Rather too American for most of us.

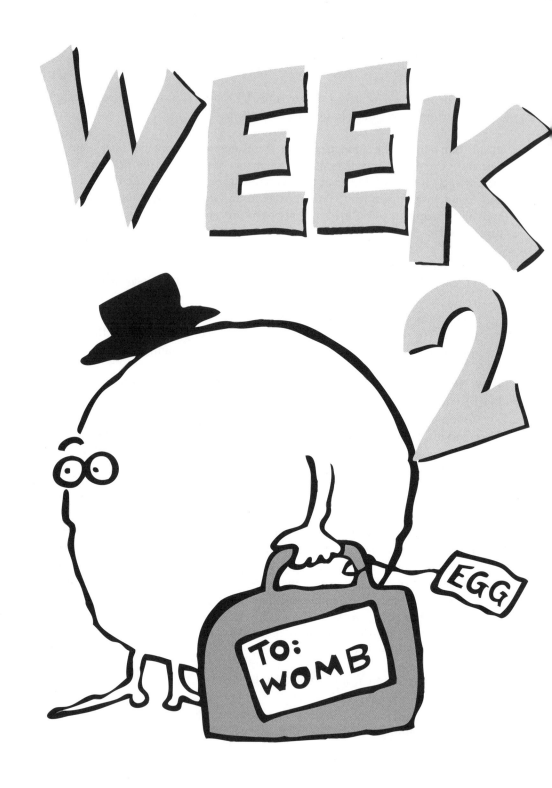

what's going on

By about day 14 (day 1 is the first day of your last period), you've reached the dispatch stage and your body is ready to ovulate. This means this month's 'dominant' egg is released from one of your ovaries, and 'waved' into the nearby opening of a fallopian tube by tentacly-looking bits on the end of the tube. You have two fallopian tubes, one on each side of the uterus, providing the link between each ovary and the uterus. At the time of ovulation, your vaginal mucus (look, you're going to hear a lot worse words and concepts than vaginal mucus in the next nine months so pull yourself together) will usually look like raw egg white, and is known as 'fertile mucus'. And at some point you'll have to get some sperm up there. Most women do this by having sex with a bloke.

Ten days after I've come off the Pill, I am poised for Operation Ravishment. Geoff keeps looking up from his beach towel and science fiction novel and saying, 'Hello, is it that time again?', when he sees the look in my eye, and manfully trailing me back to the hotel. But in between ravishings and drinking champagne (only a glass, even though I can't imagine my body's ready to get pregnant yet), I start to have second thoughts about being pregnant.

This could be a big year for me at work, with even the chance of designing my own small range of clothes. I'm in line for promotion to head designer of Real Women Wear (stuff sold to people you or I might know, in things called 'shops', as opposed to what's known rather unkindly in the industry as 'Sluts on Stilts': the flashier end of the collections called 'couture', the mad, show-offy bits that end up only on catwalk models).

I go over and over the decision, obsessing about all the things I couldn't have if I had a baby: independence, a disposable income, velvet shoes, the chance of being able to walk out the door and catch a plane or go to the shops by myself, vomit-free shoulders, bosoms I can call my own. And I know women whose partners say they'll 'help' instead of 'I'll do half', and house husbands (primary caregivers, thank you very much) who play with the kids but don't cook the dinner or do any washing.

I keep double-checking with Geoff that he really wants to stay home the first year of the baby's life while I go out to work, and that he'll also do the washing. Then I start panicking – as I'm sure most blokes do – that I might have to bring home the bacon and stay employed for the next twenty years. We have long conversations about changing my mind, what it will do to my career, how being childless would be so much easier.

After a particularly well-executed ravishing on the Tuesday morning I lie there looking at the languid ceiling fan with the definite feeling that *that* was exactly the sort of behaviour that would get one pregnant, if one were able to get pregnant. Which of course triggers the decision to go back on the Pill as soon as I get home and postpone the whole thing.

'It's all right, Kaz,' according to Geoff the Ravishee. 'Plenty of time. It's up to you.'

Then he says something terribly sensible, which is that there is never an ideal time to have a baby unless you're the sort of person who has nothing to do all day, vats of money and a spare teddy bear. Neither of us falls into this category, but really it could be worse. We're both in work, we've got somewhere to live and a car and neither of us has a conviction for aggravated assault. And even if things were not so good, we'd work it out somehow. Still, it might be better to just wait and see if I get the promotion before I spend any more energy swinging from the chandelier in the nuddy making diverting remarks about likely ovulation days. Metaphorically speaking.

info

eating and supplements

Be prepared for an onslaught of advice about what you should eat and shouldn't eat when you're pregnant, and why you should shriek at the sight of a shellfish. The truth is it's pretty simple, and not scary. You just need more than the usual amounts of protein and energy foods, and certain vitamins

SHRieKing at SHeLLfisH

and minerals, because you're making another human being (or two). You could well be getting nearly everything you need from the food you already eat (but no, a whisky and pavlova each day does not keep the doctor away).

One of the most important times to eat as well as you can is during the first trimester, when the fetus is making all its parts: bones and kidneys, ears and legs and arms. After that it's pretty much just steady development and lots of growing.

weight gain: relax

It's important for almost everyone to put on weight during pregnancy. This is no time to go on a weight-loss diet or a fast. Either could be very dangerous for your baby and you. Not to mention that you need to get through pregnancy without fainting around the joint and being all gaunt and frazzled.

How many extra calories you need will depend on your age, height, build, weight at the time of conception, current diet, and whether you're a couch potato, but there's no need to count them. You need to add more if you were underweight to start with, you're a teenager, or you're carrying more than one baby.

Who to talk to   You can talk about food with your GP, obstetrician or midwife, a dietician or your natural therapist. It's especially important to get some expert help if you're expecting to remain a vegetarian or a vegan throughout pregnancy (more on that soon).

Do not rely on any of the following for your info: your mother, your sister, your friends, a magazine, a diet website, or the demented ravings of the latest fib-heavy post-pregnancy celebrity.

There's no 'ideal weight gain' to aim for Healthy babies are born to slim women and large ladies. Some pregnant women put on lots of weight, some don't: it's up to the individual body. Don't bother weighing yourself – there's rarely a medical or other useful reason for doing so. If your doctor or midwife does need to weigh you, it can be less stressful if you're not told your weight. This can be especially true for people with a history of eating behaviour worries or disorders.

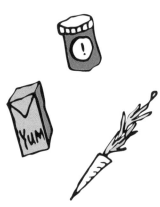

getting the goodies

To give your baby all the goodies it needs, and so you don't get madly hungry, you need to eat quality calories. Fresh, seasonal food provides far more nutrients than highly processed canned and other 'convenience' foods, takeaways or junk food.

Try to make healthy choices, but don't get obsessive and start counting how many milligrams or micrograms a day you're having of various food groups or nutrients. Really it's just a matter of common sense, eating more fresh fruit and veggies from a wide range of colours (the orange and yellows, the whites, the greens, the purples and reds and, ahem, not just the things that are chip-coloured), and not getting the guilts if you have too much cake here and there. Most people can get all the nutrients necessary for a healthy pregnancy from a reasonably varied diet.

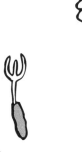

There are a lot of 'you are what you eat' warnings about making sure you eat perfectly balanced meals 'for the baby'. (Listen, if we were what we eat when we're pregnant, I'd be a giant Magnum.) Who's able to always eat a perfectly balanced diet? No one, unless they've got a private chef or all the time in the world. You could be frantically busy and not quite eating what you should. Or throwing up could be leaving you depleted of vital nutrients. Or you might be trying to get through pregnancy on a vegan diet (no animal products), which is just not adequate for fetal development. (You might want to reconsider your vegan status during your pregnancy. Special recommendations for vegans and vegetarians are scattered throughout this section.)

As long as you're listening to your body's needs, you're hydrated enough (doing frequent wees) and you're taking a pregnancy-specific supplement advised by doctors (discussed later), you can eat what you feel like, generally speaking (also see 'Cravings' in Week 8).

Organic   Going organic won't hurt if you can afford it. It will help you know you're not adding to the use of chemicals in farming, but there is no scientific evidence that it's better nutrition for you or your baby. And it's unrealistic for so many books and websites to insist that pregnant women eat only organic food. For some it's too expensive or not available where they live. To remove at least some pesticides, and dirt that may harbour bacteria, you need to thoroughly scrub, rinse or peel *all* fruit and veggies, including organic ones, before eating them. It's important to know that EU regulations forbid the use of hormones in animals raised for meat. Check with your butcher about where your meat comes from and what the animals were fed: 'organic' or 'grass fed' should mean fewer chemicals and additives.

protein
You'll usually need an extra 6 grams a day on top of your non-pregnant requirement. That means you need a total of 5–6 servings of protein a day: 1 serving could be 1 glass of low-fat milk (unless you need the fat); 30 grams of hard cheese; 150 grams of yoghurt; 100 grams of lean meat or fish; or 1 cup of cooked beans, lentils or nuts.

Fish   Pregnant women can be driven bonkers by conflicting info: don't eat fish (mercury and other contaminants) and eat lots of fish (low-fat source of protein and iodine and a good contributor to brain development). Here's the

STAYING VEGGIE

Many medical professionals assert that a vegetarian diet is inadequate for pregnant women, women who are breastfeeding, and babies and children. If you're determined to stick to your guns you'll need to know your stuff, so that you and your child get the right amounts of protein (see above) and other nutrients. Feeling full and healthy may still mean you are deficient in some areas, as pregnant women have a need for more vitamins and minerals than usual. (And many, if not most, women are deficient in some vitamins and nutrients before they're pregnant.)

While not advocating a vegetarian or vegan diet for babies and children, it's important for those who choose that way to be as well-informed as possible. Some vitamins are only found in meat, or only found in useful quantities in meat, so must be supplemented in a veggie diet. Children can appear healthy but not be growing as much as they would with some meat in their diet, and may not be getting all the nutrients needed for brain development. (Of course, all of this also applies to non-vegetarians who may be giving their child a meat-including diet devoid of enough of the vitamins and minerals found in a varied selection of fruit and veg.)

Beware of books and websites offering advice about vegetarian pregnancy: many don't give adequate attention to crucial matters such as recommended daily intake or how to get enough B12 and other nutrients while you're pregnant. To be sure your pregnancy diet is covering everything you need, consult a dietician (see 'More Info' at the end of this chapter).

deal: only some fish, especially big ones that eat lots of smaller fish, are at risk of building up dangerous levels of mercury or other baddies. Tinned fish is considered safe because salmon and sardines are not mercury risks and only smaller tuna are used for canning. For a full list of the fish to limit in your 2–3 servings a week – which includes swordfish, marlin and shark (also called flake) – see 'More Info' coming up.

Protein for vegetarians and vegans Many people have a strongly held moral reason for not eating animal products, but it is a fact that this may not provide enough protein for optimum fetal brain and body development. If you crave meat while you're pregnant, listen to your body and eat meat or fish, provided it doesn't upset you; or answer the call for extra protein with other foods. If you're a vegan you will need to pay very special attention to your protein intake, which may still fall short of ensuring maximum health for your baby.

Protein-rich foods include miso, tofu, seaweeds, nuts, seeds, and (for vegetarians) eggs and dairy foods. You need to be really strict about combining grains with legumes to maximise the quality of your protein intake.

fats

You gotta have 'em for proper fetal development, but steer clear of too much in the way of saturated fats. Use mono-unsaturated vegetable oils, such as extra virgin olive oil, for cooking and salad dressings.

You also need fatty acids, found in linseeds or linseed oil, pumpkin seeds, walnuts, pecan nuts and oily fish (such as canned salmon and tuna); and linoleic acid, found in seeds, seed and vegetable oils and nuts (and also dark green vegetables).

Grill, steam or stir-fry when possible.

sugar and salt

Going for nine months without any sugar is, of course, deeply weird. But do try to avoid stacks of refined sugars where possible, for all the usual reasons. (You probably already know that eating a block of chocolate the size of your head is not considered healthy.)

There's enough natural salt in food without shaking on extra.

fluids

Get onto them! You have more blood pumping around when you're pregnant, and the amniotic fluid surrounding the developing baby is constantly being replaced. (Not to mention the fluid lost with all the sweating and crying that can go on.) Drinking at least two litres of water a day will help you avoid constipation and urinary tract infection.

Steer clear of diuretics (substances that make you wee a lot), such as caffeine and alcohol, which deplete fluids in your body (see the following box). Diuretic drugs are unsafe during pregnancy, even if you have fluid retention (extra fluid in your body that creates puffiness). Instead, you could try plain dandelion-leaf tea (not dandelion-root coffee, which does not have the same diuretic effect). Dandelion-leaf tea looks a lot like lawn clippings.

WHAT NOT TO EAT OR DRINK

Gravel, shampoo and banana-flavoured liqueur. These aside, bear in mind that most of the things you're not supposed to eat are probably okay – if you've already eaten some before knowing you were pregnant don't worry, but if you do feel anxious mention it to your doctor. People get far too worried and start washing their vegetables in detergent and making the sign of the cross if they see some brie. You'd have to eat a lot of something or be extreeeemely unlucky to have a problem: the risks are very small. But there are some things to avoid or have less of. These include large doses of any vitamin or mineral over and above those prescribed in a pregnancy supplement as a recommended daily dose, as discussed later.

High levels of vitamin A   Excessive levels of vitamin A are associated with birth defects ('Protecting Your Pregnancy' in Week 4 has the info). Avoid eating pâté, kidneys, liver or fish liver oils, which have high levels.

Don't take any vitamin A supplement while pregnant, and make sure any multivitamin you are taking doesn't contain the vitamin. Sometimes high levels of vitamin A turn up in unexpected places such as a specific B-group-vitamin supplement.

High levels of vitamin E   High doses can cause several problems in pregnancy. A vitamin E body moisturiser won't cause a problem (and probably won't prevent stretch marks either), but don't take extra vitamin E in a tablet or supplement over and above what's in your everyday pregnancy vitamin and mineral supplement.

Caffeine (most commonly found in coffee but also in energy drinks, tea and colas)   We now know that a high intake of caffeine – above two or three cups or glasses per day – is associated with miscarriage in the first trimester and with low birth weight.

The recommended daily amount has changed over the years – always downwards. Most doctors say one coffee or other caffeine drink a day should be okay, but remember that some shop- or café-bought coffees have enough caffeine for two or more usual ones. You'll have to make up your own mind: maybe you could cut down to none in the first trimester, and one a day after that. Then you'll never have to wonder.

Alcohol   It can damage the embryo and fetus, and cause fetal alcohol syndrome in babies (as discussed in Week 4). Because doctors don't know what level of alcohol is safe for each individual, choosing to have none means you never have to worry about risking your baby's development or think 'What if?'

Other things to avoid eating, especially in the first three months

● Anything you don't want to eat.

● Foods prone to bacteria that (rarely) can cause a listeriosis infection, which is very dangerous to the unborn baby (see Week 4). These include raw, not quite cooked or 'rare' meat; raw or packaged seafood (but tinned fish should be fine); pre-mixed salads, for example in packets or at salad bars; uncooked eggs; unpasteurised milk; pâté; soft-serve ice-cream or soft-serve yoghurt 'ice-cream'; mouldy food and mould-ripened cheeses such as Brie, Camembert and blue vein; and ready-cooked chickens or other meat that has been sitting on a spit or in a bag in a cabinet. Be especially careful about kitchen hygiene, and make sure food is stored and prepared safely.

● Your partner's head, after sex (leave that to the insects, thank you, madam).

vitamins and minerals

The vitamins and minerals described below are essential for the developing unborn baby and a healthy pregnancy. Most vegetarians and vegans will need extra levels of many, although not all, of these.

The nutrients you get in fresh food are always better value than the ones in tablets or capsules, but taking prescribed vitamin and mineral supplements during pregnancy can be a good way of improving your intake if your diet isn't perfect. If your doctor or midwife recommends it, you can have a test for deficiencies in vitamin B12, folic acid and vitamin D. Your iron levels should be routinely checked as part of your blood tests during early pregnancy.

Don't assume that a vitamin or mineral supplement is safe. Remember to talk to your doctor before taking anything prescribed for you by somebody else or that you've bought independently.

ALLERGIES

Obviously during pregnancy you'll want to stay off anything that you're allergic to. But there's no evidence whatsoever that avoiding things such as peanuts will make any difference to whether your baby has an allergy to that type of food. In fact doctors think avoidance to known allergens could deprive a baby of the opportunity to develop immunity to it, so munch away (unless you're allergic yourself).

While the growing rate of childhood allergies still baffles doctors, the agreed general advice now is:

- don't expose a pregnant woman or children to cigarette smoke
- breastfeed if possible
- start solid foods for babies at six months rather than four
- let kids get dirty and hang around with animals to build up their immune system (unless, of course, they have a specific allergy to animals).

Usually the easiest and best way to take supplements is as a daily vitamin and mineral complex especially designed for pregnancy, started if possible three months before trying to conceive to build up useful levels of certain goodies, as the Getting Ready chapter discusses. A pregnancy supplement should be enough on its own unless a health professional advises otherwise. You shouldn't take, say, an additional 'stress multivitamin'. And follow the dose recommendations – more doesn't always mean better and could create a problem. Choose from one of the well-known brands because these companies have researched important factors such as extra components to make the crucial pregnancy vitamins and minerals better absorbed by the body.

calcium

Your tiny offspring is growing bones and teeth and will pinch the very calcium out of your bones if you don't step up your intake. This might mean you're more likely to get osteoporosis later in life. Many natural therapists say that calcium deficiency is one known cause of cramp, while many medical doctors say this is a fallacy and there's no scientific proof.

You'll probably need to have at least 1100 milligrams of calcium a day during pregnancy (3 or 4 glasses of low-fat milk or the equivalent yoghurt or cheese). This is about a third more again than your non-pregnant requirement. Calcium needs are very high during breastfeeding too. Teenagers, who are still growing, will need an especially high calcium allowance during pregnancy. Check with your dietician or doctor.

Some examples of calcium-rich foods are dairy foods (milk, yoghurt and parmesan cheese in particular), spinach or other leafy green vegetables, broccoli, tofu and tinned fish. Some people want to get all their calcium from dairy products, not least because 600 grams of cooked spinach or 1 kilo of cooked broccoli yield the same amount as a glass of milk. (This doesn't mean you can just drink litres of milk and never eat your greens!) But if you want or need to avoid dairy products, your other calcium-packed options include sardines, tinned salmon with the little bones in it, and tahini made from unhulled sesame seeds.

Calcium is better absorbed and retained when accompanied by magnesium and zinc, so a pregnancy supplement is ideal.

magnesium

You need magnesium or you don't get the full effect of the protein, as well as the calcium, you take in. It's also used in prescribed doses to combat pre-eclampsia, a serious pregnancy-related condition (we'll get to that in Week 28). Some good sources of magnesium are whole-wheat flour, muesli, wheatgerm, beetroot leaves, silverbeet, spinach and raw parsley.

iodine

Iodine is a mineral that's only recently been introduced into the pregnancy equation, due to research showing it's important for fetal development generally but especially for putting together a new brain.

There's some iodine in fish and eggs but you won't be eating those every day. And it's been added to some salt (and some breakfast cereals and breads), but we're all told to cut down on salt. So you'll probably need to take iodine in a pregnancy supplement, especially if you're vegetarian or vegan.

vitamin D

Everyone needs vitamin D, and you need extra if you're pregnant or breastfeeding (and extra again if you have dark skin). Vitamin D helps you and the unborn baby absorb calcium, and prevents pregnancy complications and a baby born with its own vitamin D deficiency, which can cause serious health problems for the baby even later in its life.

The best natural way to make enough vitamin D is to absorb some full sunlight five or six days a week (you don't have to take all your kit off, but some exposed skin – face, arms and hands – is necessary). A person with dark skin needs to spend three to six times as long in the sun to make and absorb the same amount of vitamin D as a pale-skinned person.

For pale folk, experts recommend more than half an hour per day of sun – to avoid sunburn, you can get some sun in the morning or afternoon by doing normal things like walking to the Tube or walking to the shops, rather than actually 'sunbathing'. It's easiest to get good sunlight levels between 11 a.m. and 3 p.m., but be aware of the dangers of sunburn especially if it's hot and cloudless, or even hot and cloudy. Remember if you are travelling that other countries can have much stronger sun which burns you more quickly. Exposed face, arms or some of your legs is good enough; you don't have to wear your bikini to the park at lunchtime. People with very dark skin should forget the idea of hats and sunblock and try to expose their arms and legs as much as possible. And anybody who keeps most of their body covered even in summer for religious or other reasons should think about finding a private place and time to expose more of their skin to sunlight – how long will depend on skin colour.

Most pregnancy supplements will have some vitamin D in them (10 micrograms a day is recommended; check with your pharmacist or doctor), but the body absorbs it better from sunshine than from tablets. Never take a single vitamin D supplement without advice from your doctor about the individual dose for you.

zinc

Zinc is one of those minerals that women in general usually don't have enough of and pregnant women can be severely lacking in, so it needs to be increased during pregnancy and breastfeeding. Vegetarians and vegans especially may need extra.

As well as helping calcium to be better absorbed, zinc is needed for enzyme production, brain and nerve formation and building an immune system in the baby. Proper zinc levels have been linked to safer birth weights and less-premature babies. It's found in wheat bran, wheatgerm, ginger, brazil nuts, hazelnuts and peanuts (with lesser levels in other nuts), fresh and dried peas and other legumes, red meat, chicken, fish, wholegrains, and cheeses, especially parmesan.

An iron supplement may interfere with the body's ability to absorb zinc, so if iron's in your supplement make sure zinc is too.

folic acid (folate)

Folic acid is one of the B-group vitamins. (The B-group vitamins in general can help keep up energy levels and are usually included in a pregnancy supplement.) Folic acid is now universally acknowledged as a supplement every woman should take for three months before pregnancy and for three months after conception. It has proved dramatically effective in reducing neural tube defects, such as spina bifida, in babies.

Although folic acid is available in green leafy and yellow vegetables and wholegrain cereals, up to half of it can be lost in cooking or storage. To cover yourself, it's best to take it in a supplement rather than try to make up the folic acid requirement in food every day.

The recommended daily dose is at least 400 micrograms (µg) – *not* 400 milligrams (mg), the more common measurement for many supplements. A 'women's multivitamin' probably won't have enough of this; a pregnancy supplement should. Higher doses may be recommended if you've already had a pregnancy with a neural tube problem or have a relevant family medical history. Some anti-epilepsy drugs interfere with folic acid levels in the body, so if this is relevant to you ask your doctor about boosting your folic acid intake to a useful dose.

B12

B12, another B-group vitamin, only occurs naturally in animal products and is crucial to the development of the baby's nervous system, brain and red blood cells. Vegetarians and vegans will need to take vitamin B12 supplements or drink a lot of soy milk fortified with B12.

iron

Your iron requirement increases during pregnancy: up to one in five pregnant women becomes iron deficient. Extra blood volume – yours and the baby's – means more iron is needed to make more haemoglobin, which your body uses to deliver important stuff such as oxygen via the bloodstream. The placenta gives first priority to the baby's iron requirements, taking it from your blood, and you risk anaemia (a haemoglobin deficiency) if you don't make up the extra iron.

You need 22–36 milligrams of iron per day during the last six months of pregnancy, compared with a non-pregnant requirement of 12–16 milligrams. You're considered to be at a higher risk of developing an iron deficiency if you're carrying twins, you've had children quickly one after another, you've been vomiting a lot during pregnancy or you're a vegetarian or vegan.

Some examples of iron content in 100-gram servings of food are wheat bran (12.9 mg), raw parsley (8 mg), dried peaches (6.8 mg), dried figs (4.2 mg), dried apricots (4.1 mg), lean beef (3.4 mg), spinach (3.4 mg), lentils (2.4 mg), sardines (2.4 mg) and eggs (2 mg). Other good sources include almonds, beans and some breakfast cereals, but check their labels. (If you want a quick boost of iron, have a drink such as Ovaltine or Horlicks, and cop the extra sugar.) Iron absorption is helped by vitamin C and hindered by tea, coffee and antacid medicines.

An extra iron supplement is sometimes recommended from about the thirteenth week of pregnancy to meet that daily requirement of 22–36 milligrams (ask your doctor). Iron supplements may cause constipation or (rarely) diarrhoea. Extra fibre, in for example porridge, and lots of water will help fix the constipation. If they don't, whinge to your doctor.

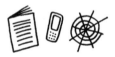

more info on **eating and supplements**

For info on finding qualified herbalists and natural therapists see the 'Natural Health Care' section in the Contacts and Resources chapter in Help at the end of this book.

bda.uk.com
The British Dietetics Association is the official body representing dieticians, which are the only recognised medically trained food experts (no formal qualifications are necessary to call yourself a 'nutritionist', although there are various private courses which offer variations of study in this area). The site has fact sheets, info on weaning and toddler food, and other special interests. You can find a dietician through your GP or hospital or by contacting the Association.

nhs.uk/planners/pregnancycareplanner
The hub of the NHS's online pregnancy information pages. Click on 'Your Pregnancy and Labour', then 'Your health during pregnancy' for advice on foods to eat, foods to avoid, supplements and special diets, as well as guidance on exercise, drugs and other health considerations during pregnancy.

food.gov.uk/multimedia/faq/mercuryfish
> A Q&A page from the Food Standards Agency which explains the government's advice about eating fish during pregnancy.

eatwell.gov.uk/agesandstages/pregnancy
> The Food Standards Agency's pregnancy pages include information about good sources of vitamins and minerals and what foods to steer clear of, as well as foods the Agency says you don't need to worry about. There's a small Q&A section with answers to questions about the safety of specific foods.

Food Facts for Pregnancy and Breastfeeding by Hannah Hulme Hunter and Rosemary Dodds, NCT Publishers, UK, 2003
> A no-nonsense, easy-to-read, info-packed book from the National Childbirth Trust. Far and away the best book on eating (and drinking) during pregnancy and breastfeeding with useful stuff on things like allergies, great quick snack ideas for those ravenous pregnancy munchie-moments and surprising info on fresh versus frozen fruit and veggies.

Babycare Before Birth by Zita West, Dorling Kindersley, UK, 2006
> Lots on looking after yourself and your fetus, and eventually your baby, with Zita West's usual focus on brief, well-illustrated explanations of medical stages and lifestyle issues such as stress, nutrition and physical activity, before, during and after pregnancy.

Beware of books and websites on eating in pregnancy that are from overseas, with all the recipes in pounds and ounces and sometimes unrecognisable ingredients such as cilantro (coriander), zucchini (courgettes) and collard greens (who knows). Some have obsessive average week-by-week weight targets best ignored by actual human beings, or bang on about 'every mouthful counts'. Bollocks.

what's going on

Fertilisation! Inside you, your single-cell egg is tootling slowly down the fallopian tube when it is rather suddenly accosted by an insistent sperm, which wriggles inside it.

The cell splits in two, then those two new cells split in two, and so on, within a surrounding jelly-like coat. This fertilised egg or embryo takes about four days to languidly drift down the tube and into the uterus. A couple of days after arriving, it finally sheds its jelly coating and decides where to park itself, usually in the top, front part of the uterus. By now it's made up of about 200 cells. There's an innie bit that is the embryo; and an outie bit that will become the amniotic sac (which contains the nice, warm amniotic fluid 'bath' the growing baby will float around in) and the placenta (which will sustain the developing baby). The embryo sends out roots – called chorionic villi – to anchor it in the endometrium surface and draw in goodies from your bloodstream. It's this system that develops into the placenta.

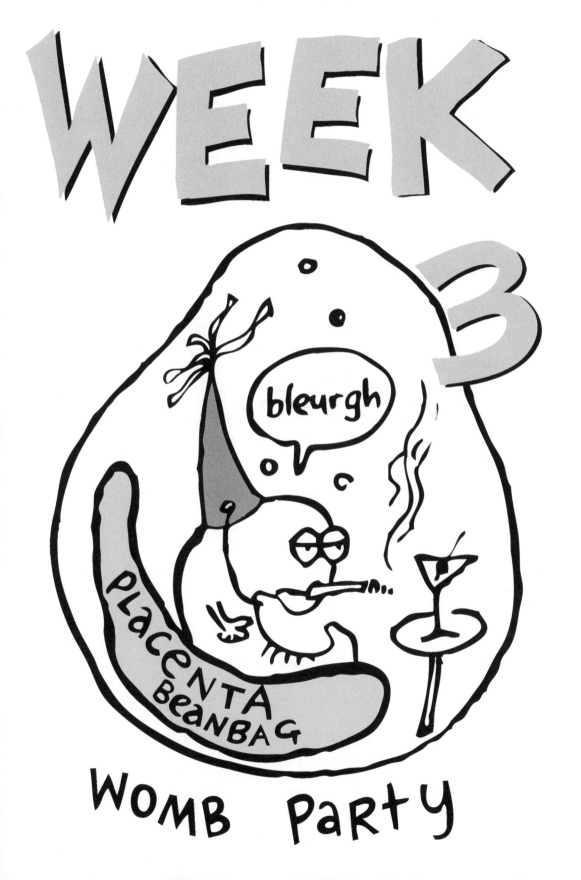

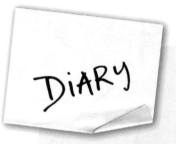
DiARy

We're getting ready to move house. I want everything in its place. Tidy, tidy, tidy. I've been collecting boxes and putting things in them and pretending this means I'm an organised person with a streamlined life. Actually it just means that I'm a disorganised person in possession of a number of boxes.

Geoff bought a small mini-van to transport his azaleas, bay trees and, on really tasteful landscaping jobs, small statues of weeing cherubs. This vehicular purchase, along with moving to a larger house, has led to much unseemly speculation. Combine house purchase, larger car and a hint of an enigmatic smile, which one cultivates to cover a whirling sense of nothing-to-speak-of going on in the brainish region, and there is an immediate up-the-duffian calculation on the part of bystanders.

Some people, almost always the ones who have their own kids and often plenty of them, bang on about it constantly. 'Are you pregnant yet?', 'When are you going to start a family?', as if a baby's just something you send off for with a stamped addressed envelope.

Luckily we don't have the sort of parents who pressure us, given that Mum died before I could remember her, nobody knows who my Dad was, and Geoff's parents are usually off studying lichen on Welsh mountain ranges, rather than demanding that we have some grandchildren to keep them amused. I am constantly amazed by the parents of friends who think it's their perfect right to insist that their offspring hurry up and 'give them grandchildren'.

I'm sure Aunt Julie, who raised me with the help of Uncle Mike before he moved out to live with his secretary, would be chuffed to bits, but at least she isn't leaning on me. Uncle Mike, who has become a born-again eco-nut, would no doubt go all New Age on me. And he ought to know by now that I'm not the Earth Mother type.

Just for fun, Geoff and I have been playing mummies and daddies with a Tamagotchi baby we found at a car-boot sale – it's one of those tiny Japanese digital games that look like a key ring. We turned the game on, called our electronic-screen baby Fred and pressed Start. There was a button to be pressed when Fred produced what the instructions called 'dung'. And buttons to press to see Fred's weight and age; to play paper, scissors, stone with him; to give him rice or a bottle; and to 'discipline' him. (Unfortunately there seemed to be no Childline button.)

Every night Geoff bounds in from a day of demanding clients saying things like 'What about a water feature by the shed?' and 'I've never liked agapanthus' and 'Can't we just patio that bit?' and 'No, I've changed my mind', and asks breathlessly and tenderly, 'How's Fred?'.

And each time, flushed with the bloom of mothering a newborn, baby-purple, extruded-plastic capsule with digital liquid-crystal output screen thingie, I report, 'Haven't seen him all day. Busy', 'Try the cutlery drawer' or 'I left him in a café.' Or more often, the simply poignant diagnosis, 'Well ... Fred's dead.' Bloody depressing game, if you ask me.

No, it has to be said: motherhood is the hardest and most honourable job in the world. Oh well. With my medical history it might take years to get pregnant. If at all. Probably just as well. Let's face it, I'm not likely to get a reference from Fred.

I suppose if I'm going to stay off the Pill, I had better find a friend with a baby and spend a day or so with them. I was off wearing miniskirts in foreign parts when my cousin Amanda's babies were small, and not that interested, really. Now that I am, I realise most of my friends are lesbians or career women who are only just starting to wonder how they might manage it. The only one who's already launched her kayak into the creek is my friend Susanne, and she's only four months pregnant. I guess I can practise on her baby when it arrives. I had better find an instructional video called something like 'A New Baby: Which End Up?'.

We just don't live any more in a tribal society surrounded by a million kids of varying ages and great scads of extended families. My second cousin Chris has six of the blighters, but they live in Spain so there's not much practising to be had there. There should be some kind of library service.

info

sense of smell

Your sense of smell may be far more acute than usual during pregnancy, especially in the first three months. You may even notice this before you know you're pregnant. Perfumes or food smells that previously seemed downright scrumptious may now send you heaving to the bathroom. What's really annoying is that none of the experts seem to be able to say why. Maybe the nausea is a defence mechanism so you're more likely to identify 'off' foods that could harm you or your baby. Maybe it's to compensate for the last two-thirds of a pregnancy often being accompanied by a blocked nose (due to a general increase in bodily secretions you don't want to have to think about yet). Or maybe it's just a meaningless side effect of one of the 'pregnancy hormones'.

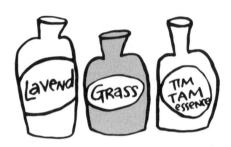

aromatherapy

Aromatherapy, the therapeutic use of essential oils, can make you feel nurtured and relaxed during pregnancy, but some essential oils can harm your unborn baby or bring on labour or even a miscarriage, especially if applied directly to the skin during a bath or massage.

Qualified aromatherapists advise against any aromatherapy applied directly to the skin in this way during pregnancy, especially during the first trimester, without advice from an aromatherapist specialising in pregnancy. Some oils are not even recommended for burning to scent a room when you're pregnant.

Unfortunately some masseurs who use essential oils without being qualified aromatherapists are simply unaware of any risks and will tell you that anything they use is quite safe at whatever concentration they feel like squirting on you. And even the oils considered 'safe' for massage or in the bath should be used at half-strength during pregnancy.

It can be confusing for a layperson to decide what is safe. For example, despite spearmint used directly on the skin being on the 'banned during pregnancy' list given below, some pregnancy magazines recommend it to relieve nausea when used as an infusion to breathe in or to scent a room.

Oils generally considered safe for use during pregnancy include lavender, grapefruit, orange, lemon, tangerine, mandarin, neroli, sandalwood, ylang-ylang, geranium (after the fifth month), bergamot, ginger and tea tree.

Oils that can induce miscarriage (abortifacients) or bring on a period (emmenagogues) must be avoided during pregnancy. They include, but may not be exclusively confined to, yarrow, aniseed, tarragon, caraway, atlas cedarwood, camphor, hyssop, pennyroyal, spearmint, parsley and parsley seed, rosemary, nutmeg, Roman chamomile, German chamomile, myrrh, juniper, lovage, peppermint, basil, Spanish marjoram, clary sage, sage, bay, vetiver, pine, thyme, jasmine, wintergreen and angelica.

Remember that you may be supersensitive to smell, but your nose can also be blocked up during pregnancy and therefore *less* sensitive to smell. So always follow the recipes given by a qualified aromatherapist rather than your schnoz.

And obviously, for your own comfort, don't use anything that makes you feel queasy.

Here are some safe aromatherapy ideas:

⊚ aches and pains – throw a couple of drops of lavender oil in the bath

⊚ fatigue – in a burner to send the smell wafting through the room, two drops of lavender oil, one drop of mandarin oil and one drop of ylang-ylang oil; or one drop of lavender oil, one drop of mandarin oil and two drops of ylang-ylang oil

⊚ nausea – in a burner, one to two drops of lemon oil or lemongrass oil; or make some ginger tea (see 'Nausea' in Week 4) and drink the tea and breathe in the aroma as you go

⊚ insomnia – put three drops of lavender, mandarin or ylang-ylang oil, or a mixture of the three, in the bath; scent your bedroom with two to three drops of lavender or ylang-ylang oil, or a mixture of the two

⊚ stuffy nose – make an inhalation by adding two drops of eucalyptus or tea-tree oil to a bowl of hot water, then stick a towel over your head and breathe in the vapour for a couple of minutes (you can't use many 'cold remedy' drugs during pregnancy so this is a good one to remember)

⊚ bad circulation – in a burner, two drops of grapefruit oil, eucalyptus oil or frankincense.

Many women burn lavender oil when giving birth – but wherever there are oxygen tanks a naked flame is banned. Many hospitals provide electric burners for essential oils during labour. Aromatherapy won't actually help with pain relief.

herbal teas

Many herbs can bring on a period, or cause miscarriage or birth defects. Always check with a trained herbalist. (No more than three cups of any kind of herbal tea should be consumed every day as a habit.)

Herbal teas that are generally considered safe during pregnancy include: peppermint; fresh ginger; lemon balm; chamomile; and dandelion leaf, which is a safe diuretic – dandelion root doesn't have the same effect but isn't considered dangerous. Herbal teas should not be confused with essential oils: an oil extracted from a plant contains very large quantities of components that could be dangerous, whereas a tea made from the plant might not.

medicine and natural therapies

Remember, don't take any medicines, herbs or vitamins without consulting a properly trained doctor or herbalist (see 'Eating and Supplements' in Week 2). Just because your friend took something during her pregnancy that she swears by doesn't mean it's safe for you or your baby. Some preparations can be safe at one time in a pregnancy, but dangerous at another stage. Some preparations are not ever safe during pregnancy. Don't assume that because something is 'natural' it is safe. And always tell your doctor and natural therapist what the other one has prescribed.

Beware of dippy 'natural therapy' or 'diet' advice. Most diets that involve restriction of certain food types are not suitable for pregnancy, and fasting is compleeeeetely out of the question as it could damage the developing baby or even cause miscarriage. (See 'Eating and Supplements' in Week 2 for the lowdown on eating properly during pregnancy.)

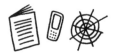

more info on **natural therapies**

Your herbalist should be a member of the National Institute of Medical Herbalists, and should specialise in either fertility or pregnancy. Your natural therapist should be registered with the Complementary and Natural

Healthcare Council. The 'Natural Health Care' section in the Contacts and Resources chapter at the end of the book has contact details for both these organisations.

aromatherapycouncil.co.uk

If in doubt about an aromatherapy oil, or an aromatherapist's credentials, have a rummage on the site of the Aromatherapy Council of the UK, a non-medically regulated body with members across the country.

Natural Pregnancy: Complementary Therapies for Preconception, Pregnancy and Postnatal Care by Zita West, Dorling Kindersley, UK, 2005

This book's first chapter is on the natural things you can do to prepare your body (and his) for trying to get pregnant; most of the book is for when you are pregnant and beyond. The final section is a good wrap-up of complementary medicine, from acupuncture to shiatsu massage. Sensibly, it talks about alternative therapies being used in conjunction with scientific medicine, not always instead of.

Meditation: Exercises and Inspirations for Wellbeing by Bill Anderton, Duncan Baird Publishers, UK, 2002

One of those wee, square books with a yoga-looking lady on the front, this simple and easy introduction to meditation lays out the basic principles and provides some how-to hints and clear instructions for getting started. Alternatives range from concentrating on a flower or a positive affirmation to chanting a mantra, using music or developing 'mindfulness'.

WEEK 4

what's going on

Your period is due. Maybe you've started going wee, wee, wee all the way home. Perhaps you've gone off the smell of alcohol and cigarettes, and foods that you usually like. Now or in the next few weeks, you might start feeling slightly queasy, which in bad cases results in vomiting. (According to one pregnancy book photo, this is when you will wear a hideous smock and an Alice band, and stare out the window holding a cup and saucer like a demented fool.)

The tiny embryo burrows into the wall of the uterus until it's completely embedded, and keeps getting bigger every day. The ovaries are pumping out the hormone progesterone to make the endometrium tough. The sex of your baby, the colour of its hair and eyes, how tall it can grow and whether it has natural footy talent – all these factors have been genetically programmed from the start, and can't be altered. By the end of this week the embryo's way too little to see without using magnifying instruments.

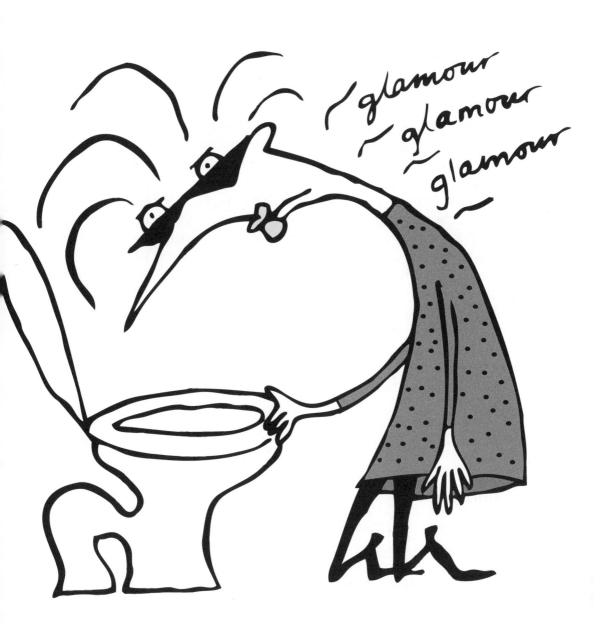

DiARY

Went for a coffee with my old pal Jon, whose wife has been at home with the kids for four years and is now dashing her head against a plywood wall trying to get into the workforce again – the restaurant industry wants her to work split shifts for approximately £6.50 a day. He says that apart from this whole work problem, and vomit and poo, motherhood is INCREDIBLY GLAMOROUS.

I meet with the boss about becoming head designer of Real Women Wear and agree to a schedule of sacred weekly meetings with the new buyers. I sign on the dotted line for my first range. Off to Michelle's party with the girls and had a sneaky fag – it was disgusting – and a glass of a killer punch that tasted like pineapple herbicide. For some reason I don't want to get drunk. Have a bit of a half-hearted dance. I'm feeling kind of tired and out of sorts. Not quite nauseous but squirgly in the tummy.

I've started being absolutely vile to Geoff. I don't know why. I'm quite aware I'm doing it but I can't stop myself: I am the Bitch Queen of the Universe. He comes in the front door and I narrow my eyes looking for a fault. I swear if he came in the door with a bunch of mauve roses and tickets to the Bahamas I'd probably say, 'Wipe those filthy boots!', for all the world as if I had suddenly developed a passion for clean floors. I'm really starting to worry. I think I'm turning into a gorgon.

Oh, how could I be so STUPID? It must be PMT. I've just forgotten what it's like after four years on the Pill.

info

nausea

Some people still call it morning sickness, but it isn't, so they shouldn't. It can get you at any time of the day, even all day. Not everybody gets it, but most pregnant women experience some form of nausea, usually in the first trimester, and half will throw up at least once. It can range from a slightly queasy feeling to full-on, head-in-a-bucket, serious vomiting. For some very unlucky women it persists after the fourteenth week, and even all through the pregnancy.

The cause has not been absolutely identified and may even vary from person to person. The culprits are thought to include any or all of the following: high levels of the hormone human chorionic gonadotrophin (HCG); being tired; a fall in blood pressure resulting from progesterone-induced relaxation of muscles, which causes dilation of the blood vessels; less efficient digestion due to less stomach acid in the gut; an increase in oestrogen challenging the liver to break it down, so the liver works overtime; and altered senses, which means that some smells and tastes make you feel sick. (For more info see 'Pregnancy Hormones' in Week 12.)

Here are some things that may help.

⑥ Eat small, frequent snacks to avoid an empty tummy or a low blood-sugar level – keep a handbag or briefcase 'pantry' of dried fruit, dry biscuits and raw nuts, fruit or vegetables.

⑥ Have four or five smaller meals a day instead of three biggies (this can also be useful in the third trimester when your tummy is squished up).

⑥ Eat something bland *before* you get out of bed in the morning, such as dry toast or a dry biscuit, or have a small amount of fruit juice. (Some women prefer a sweet biccy. Whatever works for you.)

⑥ Have a snack just before bedtime.

⑥ Avoid the fish market or perfume counter or anything else that makes you feel queasy; this can include fatty or fried foods, cigarette smoke, coffee and alcohol.

⑥ Try a reputable herbal supplement such as raspberry leaf extract. Check the dosage and brand with your doctor, natural therapist or pharmacist.

⑥ Maintain your intake of protein (chicken soup is good) and complex carbohydrates (potato, rice and pasta).

⑥ Avoid getting tired or stressed. Head off tiredness with rests and cat naps.

⑥ Try ginger tea – infuse one to two teaspoons of grated fresh ginger (or a piece of ginger, about the size of your little finger and chopped into four or five bits) in a small teapot of boiling water for five minutes; strain; add honey or a squeeze of lemon to taste, breathing in the steam as you go.

⑥ Sniff a fresh lemon.

◎ If you've been vomiting, drink lots of water so you don't dehydrate.

◎ Try extra vitamin B6, in addition to your pregnancy supplement, if it's recommended by your doctor or natural therapist.

◎ Although some people try travel sickness bands, there's no evidence they work – and it's probably no better than a placebo (the positive effect of believing it will work). In any case, you can just press on the centre of your inside left wrist with your thumb for a while or make your own elastic band with a round button sewn onto it to do the same thing.

For some very unlucky souls the only remedy is fluids given intravenously during a short hospital stay. It's not common for vomiting to be so bad that it needs medical intervention, but if you are vomiting more than once a day for days in a row, or any aspect of your vomiting is distressing, tell your doctor straight away. The main risks are that you'll dehydrate, especially if you can't keep down fluids, or your embryo or fetus will miss out on nutrients.

Nausea is often said to be a good sign – evidence that the hormones are pumping, indicating a strong, stable pregnancy. Some people claim first trimester nausea lowers the risk of miscarriage. Others say that's utter piffle. More severe nausea is associated with a twin or multiple pregnancy, probably because the hormone levels in the bloodstream are higher.

protecting your pregnancy

Teratogens are infections, substances or environmental factors that can damage an embryo or fetus at certain stages of development – the biggest danger being in the first three months of pregnancy. (In usual tactless-doctor language, 'teratogen' is derived from the ancient Greek *teras* meaning 'monster'.) The effect of teratogens can range from impaired growth or increased risk of a miscarriage through to serious birth defects.

The impact on the developing baby depends on the teratogen – some are much more dangerous than others – and your level of exposure, as well as what stage of pregnancy you're at when exposed, and individual susceptibility, and luck. (Even if you know somebody who drank vodka like a mad thing throughout their pregnancy and had a 'normal' baby, it doesn't mean the same will apply for you.)

It's believed that not much damage is likely to be done between conception and when the egg implants itself in the wall of the uterus six to eight days later. The most vunerable time for the unborn baby is from implantation to the tenth week after conception, when organs and limbs are being formed. But some teratogens can affect major parts of the developing baby throughout the whole pregnancy, including the brain, eyes and sex organs.

illnesses that can cause a problem

All the following can interfere with an embryo, a fetus, or a baby in the last months before birth. Some of them are common but usually don't affect the developing baby; others are rare but their effect is more certain.

Cytomegalovirus   The most common infectious cause of mental retardation and congenital deafness, cytomegalovirus is a virus in the herpes group. If you've had it before you were pregnant the danger has probably passed. It's usually most dangerous to an embryo or a fetus straight after you've been infected, and even then the vast majority will suffer no effects (see 'More Info on Protecting Your Pregnancy' at the end of this chapter).

Genital herpes   An active case at the time of birth creates a risk of infection for the baby. A caesarean may be necessary to prevent this. If you have herpes your GP or midwife should closely monitor it in the latter part of the pregnancy. Some antiviral drugs taken from 36 weeks onwards can prevent an outbreak around the date the baby is due to be born.

Gonorrhoea   A sexually transmitted infection (STI), gonorrhoea can infect the baby during the birth, although the baby can then be cured with drugs.

Hepatitis C   It's believed that very few pregnant women with hep C will have babies who are infected. There are only a few case studies so far, but it is thought that babies are more likely to get hep C if their mum was exposed to it in the third trimester. There is some suggestion that transmission is more likely if the mum has HIV as well.

HIV   Pregnant women with HIV will not automatically pass it on to their babies. Estimates of transmission range from 14 to 50 percent. Retroviral drugs greatly reduce the chance of transmission. Mothers with HIV must not breastfeed, as transmission rates are much higher. (This is why formula milk for babies instead of breastfeeding is once again being promoted by health workers in Africa.)

Hyperthermia (overheating) Any illness that causes a high temperature (38.9° Celsius or more) for an extended time, especially in the first three months of pregnancy, can cause damage to an embryo or fetus.

Listeriosis This relatively rare bacterial infection is transmitted through foods (see 'What Not to Eat or Drink' in Week 2). Its symptoms include fever, headache, tiredness, aches and pains. It may cause miscarriage or stillbirth.

Rubella (German measles) Rubella can cause a high incidence of abnormalities in babies (congenital rubella syndrome includes blindness and deafness), particularly when mothers are exposed to it in the first trimester. For this reason, all British children should have been immunised against rubella as part of the routine immunisation programme, in their MMR (measles, mumps and rubella) jabs. As the opening chapter explained, before trying to get pregnant it's a good idea to have your doctor organise a blood test to check your immunity because if you have to be vaccinated you'll need to wait three months before trying to conceive. In the first trimester of pregnancy, your midwife or GP will organise a blood test to check your immunisation status.

Parvovirus ('slapped cheek') This is common in young children, causing flu-like symptoms and flushed cheeks. It can cause anaemia in the developing baby, but this is rarely a big problem.

Syphilis This now rare STI can cross the placenta and cause premature birth and stillbirth, or long-term effects in children such as dental abnormalities. It can be detected in routine pregnancy tests and safely treated in early pregnancy. It can also infect the baby during the birth, although the baby can then be cured with drugs.

Toxoplasmosis This illness can be symptomless or feel like mild flu. It's caused by a parasite commonly found in raw or undercooked meat, including game birds (all meat should be cooked to an internal temperature of at least

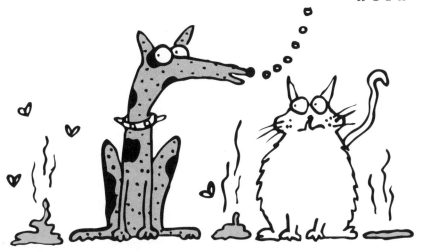

60° Celsius, and you should avoid cured meat such as parma ham and salami unless you cook them first (for example on a pizza)); unpasteurised goat's milk products; and the poo from cats. The infection can cause brain and eye damage in the developing baby, and miscarriage. The chance of transmission to the baby is highest in the third trimester, but if transmitted in the first trimester the chances are much higher that it will cause damage to the fetus, or a miscarriage.

Many people have come into contact with the parasite at some point and developed an immunity to it. However, you should take precautions in case you are not immune. Avoid cat poo. Wear gloves when gardening and to empty a litter tray. Before eating raw, garden-grown or organic produce, wash, scrub or peel it thoroughly.

Other diseases and conditions   There are many diseases and conditions that can affect your baby during pregnancy. Some of these have 'silent' symptoms so you may not be aware of a risk or problem. Tell your doctor about any high fever, rash, sweats or fluid retention (puffiness) during your pregnancy or any other symptom that worries you.

what goes in: dangerous substances

Just about everything you ingest while you're pregnant will cross the placenta in some form and affect the developing baby. This includes drugs, alcohol, chips, cheese and air. It may help while you're putting something into yourself to imagine putting it into the baby at the same time (this will remind you: chocolate biscuit okay; four cocktails noooooo).

Remember that no prescription or over-the-counter drug, herbal or natural remedy or vitamin or mineral supplement should be taken during pregnancy without consulting a doctor who knows you're pregnant. And no recreational or street drug is safe to use during pregnancy. If you haven't got 'clean' before you conceived it may not be too late, but you MUST have medical advice and help before you try because it can be even more dangerous to try to quit an addiction during pregnancy (see, for example, 'Heroin and Methadone' later). Make sure you tell your GP or midwife about any drugs you've used during pregnancy: they're not allowed to tell the police.

Alcohol   Doctors used to believe that, although an excessive amount of alcohol could cause the serious defects of fetal alcohol syndrome, a few drinks here and there were safe. Experts now agree that they can't identify a level of alcohol that wouldn't have a damaging effect on the fetus's development, so all major national and global health organisations recommend that pregnant and breastfeeding women give alcohol a complete miss. I'm often asked rather pleadingly by pregnant women to agree that one drink a day or a few times a week is fine, and it might be for some people, but it's just not possible to say definitely that this is safe. Sorry, ladies, but guaranteeing no effect means saying no grog for the duration.

Amphetamines (speed)   These drugs are associated with premature babies, baby heart problems, brain-damaged babies, drug-addicted babies and other complications.

Caffeine   As already mentioned, an intake of over two or three cups or glasses of tea, coffee, cola or an energy drink a day is associated with an increased risk of miscarriage in the first trimester and with low birth weight (see 'Eating and Supplements' in Week 2 for a suggested safe approach).

Cigarettes   Cigarette smoking stunts the growth of the fetus and damages its lungs. This has been an 'excuse' for women who keep smoking while pregnant ('It'll be an easier birth if it's a small baby'). In fact a low birth weight can put your baby's health at risk. But smoking also inhibits the growth of the placenta and is believed to be linked to miscarriage, sudden infant death syndrome (SIDS), asthma and other respiratory traumas for babies and children. If you simply can't go cold turkey, it's safer to go on nicotine patches than to keep

PAINKILLERS DURING PREGNANCY

All the active painkiller ingredients given below are sold under various brand names. Always read labels carefully and keep strictly to the recommended dose.

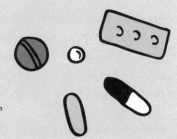

Any recurring problem that requires painkillers, such as headaches or stomach aches, should be discussed with your doctor pronto.

Aspirin   This has blood-thinning properties. Unless prescribed individually for you for a specific reason by your doctor, who knows you are pregnant, don't take aspirin if you're trying to be, might be or are pregnant.

Ibuprofen   Do not take ibuprofen if you are trying to get pregnant, might be pregnant or are pregnant. It can interfere with fetal heart development.

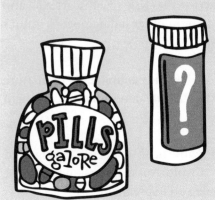

Paracetamol   This is considered safe in pregnancy at recommended doses. Although it crosses the placenta and is absorbed by an embryo or fetus, those levels are judged too small to do any damage.

Stronger painkillers should not be taken without a prescription from a doctor who knows you are pregnant.

smoking during pregnancy because the increase in your blood volume causes your body to crave more nicotine and you'll want to smoke more.

Cocaine   Even a single, one-off dose can do serious damage.

Ecstasy   There isn't much detailed research yet on the 'newer' recreational drugs – although ecstasy has been associated with increased risk of placental bleeding – but we know they're definitely not a good idea when you're pregnant.

Herbs   Many herbs, herbal supplements, herbal teas and juice-bar additives are unsafe for pregnant women and their developing babies (also see 'Herbal Teas' in Week 3). Never assume 'natural' or 'herbal' means that something is okay to take during pregnancy, and get up-to-date professional advice no matter what you're told by friends.

Heroin and methadone   These drugs can cause premature birth, low birth weight, mental problems and stillbirth. Babies share their mother's addiction and so suffer withdrawal symptoms when they are born, although this can be managed by medical staff. Prescribed methadone is preferable to heroin in pregnancy because it provides a regulated dose to the fetus. The baby must be weaned from its methadone addiction after birth. Coming off heroin suddenly while pregnant can cause miscarriage: don't stop abruptly without talking to your doctor.

LSD and other hallucinogens   LSD carries the risk of miscarriage and chromosomal damage. There is little research on other hallucinogens but it's safest to assume any amount is dangerous.

Marijuana and hashish (dope or weed)   Their use is linked to premature birth and low birth weight. There is no known 'safe' amount. Stay off them while pregnant or breastfeeding.

Vitamin A   High levels are associated with birth defects. 'Eating and Supplements' in Week 2 tells you the foods to avoid. Any acne or skin treatment containing vitamin A must be stopped while you're pregnant.

environmental hazards

If your job or workplace is unsafe for you to work in during pregnancy, you have the legal right to be given duties that don't expose you to the hazards. Avoid any of the following at home, work or the beauty salon.

Getting too hot   As with hyperthermia caused by illness, your body temperature should not be above 38.9° Celsius for an extended time. Avoid saunas, jacuzzis, body wraps and Bikram yoga. A hot bath is a problem if you keep it at a really high temperature and keep topping it up. A bath should be comfortably warm enough to get straight into, and not so hot that it makes you sweat on your forehead, or turns your skin redder. Check the temperature with your elbow (because elbows are a better judge than toes and fingers).

Poisons and pesticides   There are some potentially harmful substances at home and in the workplace and your daily life. Read labels and avoid using toxins. Definitely avoid fumy cleaning products, including oven cleaners and drycleaning solvents, most paints, lacquers, thinners, paint strippers, pesticides, herbicides, petrol, glue, many manufacturing chemicals and waste products. Beware of lead in the air in heavy traffic areas and nearby soil, in old house paint and in some water, particularly in houses with old lead pipes or lead-soldered pipes. Lead can also leach into food or drink from very old or handmade china or earthenware pottery.

People in high-risk jobs include health-care workers, farmers, gardeners, factory workers, printing or photographic processing workers, artists, chemists, hairdressers, nail artists, beauty therapists, drycleaners, cleaners, and people who work with petrol. Exposure to air pollution – such as carbon monoxide from car exhausts – may be a problem if your job involves driving in heavy traffic for much of the day, directing traffic or working at a bus station.

TELL YOUR DOCTOR STRAIGHT AWAY ABOUT ANY:

- bleeding from the vagina
- vomiting, if you can't keep down fluids
- abdominal pain
- fainting
- high temperature
- major fluid retention (puffiness)
- worries
- instruction or information they gave you that you don't fully understand
- really funny baby jokes you've heard.

There's not much info on the possible effects of hair dye, hairspray, hair removal creams, fake nail glue and nail polish remover so many pregnant women avoid them, especially in the first trimester. Obviously when you're pregnant it's also not a good idea to inject your body with Botox or any other poison. (Botox is measured in units, one of which is enough to kill a mouse – up to sixty units can be used to 'freeze' wrinkle areas.) The same goes for other cosmetic procedures that involve injected substances, such as collagen. This is not because the effect on a fetus is known (it's not), but because injected substances challenge and activate your immune system. When you're pregnant it's best not to burden it with extra duties.

Although the list of potentially harmful substances you might come into contact with is extensive, most babies turn out fine anyway. To find out whether substances or practices specific to your circumstances are harmful during pregnancy, make sure you check with your doctor, workplace health and safety officer or union. You mustn't rely on your employer as your only source of information about what's safe for you at work.

Radiation   X-rays can cause malformations in an embryo or a fetus. Tell any doctor or dentist who wants to X-ray you that you're pregnant. If you had one before you knew you were pregnant, ask your doctor about the risk to the unborn baby. It's usually not bad news. Contrary to rumour, modern computers don't leak radiation dangerous to pregnant women or a developing baby.

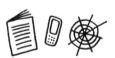

more info on **protecting your pregnancy**

talktofrank.com
   Helpline: 0800 77 66 00
   The government-funded Talk to FRANK website has a complete A–Z of drugs info. Its helpline offers confidential advice about drugs, and can help you find support services in your area.

smokefree.nhs.uk
   Smoking in pregnancy helpline: 0800 169 9 169
   The NHS's stop smoking site. From the home page, click 'Smoking & pregnancy' for information on how smoking harms your unborn baby, and how to quit. The

helpline offers further advice, and will put you in touch with the free services that are there to help you stop smoking.

nhs.uk/chq

The 'Common Health Questions' of the NHS website. Click on 'Pregnancy and childbirth'. 'Pregnancy and infections' has detailed information on various common or dangerous infections, while 'Pregnancy and lifestyle' covers smoking, alcohol and other issues such as paint fumes and jacuzzis.

tommys.org

For a detailed factsheet on toxoplasmosis, from the main page of the Tommy's charity website on pregnancy health and risks, click on 'Pregnancy information', 'Problems in pregnancy' then 'Toxoplasmosis'.

babycentre.co.uk

This large commercial pregnancy hub site has a great list of herbs that can be or definitely are dangerous during pregnancy. On the main page, type into the search box 'herb and drug safety chart'. What comes up is an alphabetical list of substances (mainly herbs) to avoid, and another list of those to use in moderation. (Always make sure by taking advice from your doctor and a herbalist trained in pregnancy.)

nimh.org.uk

The website of the National Institute of Medical Herbalists. Use the search facility on the home page to find medical herbalists near you. Click on 'About medical herbalists' for information about what medical herbalists do, how they're trained, and more.

what's going on

Your period hasn't turned up. You might feel premenstrual, with slightly swollen breasts, as well as be weeing more often and feeling queasy.

The embryo is still minuscule but starting to form into a tube shape and growing very quickly. The head and tail ends become obvious. The heart and blood vessels are only just starting to form so the embryo doesn't have its independent circulation yet. At this stage the placenta consists of lots of chorionic villi 'tentacles'. Eventually they will grow into the big, temporary organ that runs the exchange between you and your developing baby, sending in nutrients and oxygen and taking out waste products and carbon dioxide, using the vein and two arteries in the umbilical cord that connects the placenta to the baby.

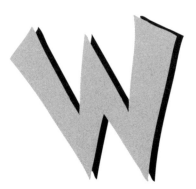

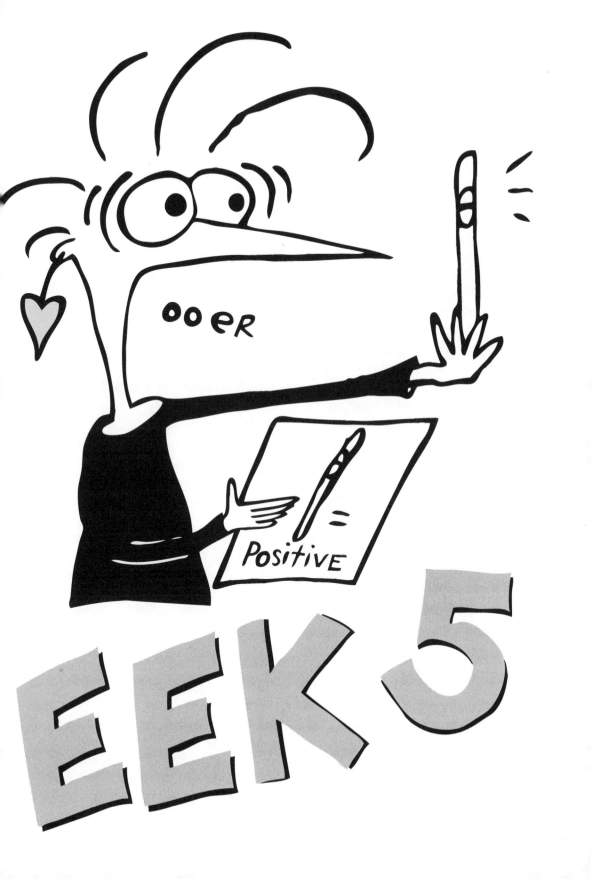

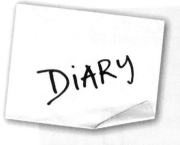
DiARy

We move house and my 33rd birthday party on Saturday is conducted amid towers of cardboard boxes full of stuff we didn't even open at the last house. My advice to anyone under 27 is don't blink or you'll be 33 before you know what happened. Kind of like Rumpelstiltskin. (Only your beard isn't usually *quite* that bad.)

People at the party keep asking, 'Kaz, do you want another drink?', and I keep saying no. Just like that. No, meaning no, I don't want a drink, which means people keep looking at me strangely. Or I say yes and then leave the drink somewhere under a tree. And it is really flash champagne too, being my birthday and everybody being nice about it.

And normally, although I've given up smoking – except other people's (oh all right, and those times when I buy a packet for a party ... yes, and those other times when ... oh shut up) – I will still have the odd puff at a social extravaganza, even one involving cardboard boxes. But this time I just don't feel like it. Begin to feel quite snappy and restless. All sort of 'It's my party and I'll pout if I want to'.

Then I get scared. I start to think: 33. Thirty-three and I don't want to party any more. It's over. It's been over since Geoff bought that mini-van. What was I thinking – that I could live in a house with a perfectly nice man who owns a mini-van and has a steady job and earns his own money and doesn't expect me to pay for everything and isn't some kind of frustrated troll of a tortured artiste?

What happened to my life? When did I get sensible? How can I escape? Maybe I should run through the streets in the nicky-noo-nar shooting out streetlights. Or I could just go to bed. I'm a wee bit on the nod and I've been squirgly again. Must be coming down with something. Need a good night's rest, probably. Nightie-night everyone. Please. Don't stop drinking on my account. I'll just zzzzzzzz.

4 a.m. Hang on a minute.

9.10 a.m. Pop down to the chemist. Need some dental floss, some cotton wool balls, some orange nail polish, naturally, and oh, what the hell, I'll take that £7.99 home pregnancy test kit on a whim.

Pregnancy tests from the chemist have obviously changed since last I was a careless idiot. You used to have to wee into some sort of container (yoghurt pot, jam jar, plastic tub with 'Sainsbury's Cottage Cheese' written on the side of it, that kind of thing), and then dip a white plastic magic wand, which was a bit like a flat biro, into it. The most useful instruction was always 'Use the midstream urine for the test'. What that meant was that you did some wee, then you stopped, if you had pelvic-floor muscles like a steel trap, and neatly did a mighty bull's-eye midstream wee into the jar, then stopped (steel trap again), removed the jar and finished the wee.

What always happened was more like sticking a thimble under a waterfall and then snatching it out again and finding that, although you had wee on your hand, the outside of the jar, your hair, the hem of your trousers and some articles in another room entirely, you'd managed to miss the jar.

Now you're supposed to hold the magic wand in one hand and – I'm sorry, but basically you just piss on it for a few seconds. This seems such an incredibly male thing to do. I almost feel like trying to write my name in the snow with my own wee. But there is no snow. Only a thin, blue line showing in the 'window', which the instructions say means you're pregnant. And I'm not talking a baby blue, a wimpy sort of a 'We think it's within the realms of possibility that you might conceivably have conceived'. No, it is almost a luminous, pulsating navy blue indicating 'YOU, madam, are *utterly* UP THE DUFF good and proper!'

I always thought I might cry a tiny tear of feminine, yet sensible joy. Instead I stare at the wall thinking 'Oh … Woo.'

Ring Geoff and tell him to come straight home after his five-a-side football, don't even have one drink, there is something I have to tell him.

'Ooohhhh,' he says, 'Woo', sounding like he knows what it might be.

I tell him at the front door. He looks pretty shocked. We just start laughing, with tears in our eyes, and then we can't stop laughing. It just seems so ridiculously UNLIKELY. Geoff says he is happy, and then talks about the finer points of five-a-side footie really fast for about 25 minutes. I think he's in shock.

'You told me it would probably take two years to get pregnant,' he says later, quietly.

'Ooops. Woo', I concur.

Geoff commences to grin for two days straight, the grin punctuated by an expression of profound bewilderment. I begin to refer to him as the bewilderbeest. Luckily he's an optimist whose most remarkable traits include a 'she'll be right' attitude to almost anything. If you told Geoff there was a hurricane coming, he'd be dead interested from a meteorological point of view.

info

early tests in pregnancy

During pregnancy you'll have regular tests to make sure that all's going well, not just a test to confirm your suspicion that you're pregnant. Here's what you need to know about the early ones and your visits to the GP, obstetrician or midwife.

confirming you're pregnant

Home pregnancy test kits bought at the chemist work the same way as a test a doctor would do on a sample of your wee. The kits test for the presence of the hormone HCG. The first wee of the day will have the greatest concentration of it.

You can do the test as early as fourteen days after conception, about when your period would be due. The results of this test are almost always accurate, especially if they're positive. A false negative result can happen if the level of HCG being produced by a pregnant body is low. So if your period doesn't start, and you still suspect you're pregnant, you can wait a few days and do the test again or go to the doctor for a blood test, which can measure HCG levels as early as one week after conception.

After a positive home test, or other signs of early pregnancy such as a missed period, tender breasts, nausea, frenzied weeing, a funny metallic

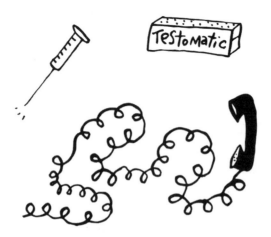

taste in your mouth, tiredness or moodiness, you should go to your GP as soon as possible, especially if you are currently on any medication. They may confirm the pregnancy with a urine or blood test, or may simply take your word for it. They will give you information about maternity services in your area and will refer you to the antenatal (meaning pre-natal or 'before the birth') team.

Depending on your medical history, you may need to see an obstetrician or hospital midwife straight away; or your first visit may be when you're about ten to twelve weeks pregnant. This first 'booking-in' appointment will most likely be with a midwife; midwives are the experts in straightforward pregnancies so if your pregnancy is relatively problem-free you may not see an obstetrician at all, until the birth.

These days, some home pregnancy tests can give a positive result up to five days before your period is due. However, the problem with being able to confirm a pregnancy so early is that it means more people are aware if their pregnancy doesn't continue. (One form of miscarriage that's fairly common happens if a fertilised egg for some reason doesn't implant properly in the first four to eight weeks – also see 'Miscarriage' in Week 6. In the 'old days' this would just have seemed like a late period.)

When the pregnancy is confirmed, an early ultrasound scan might be recommended if you have a history of repeat miscarriage, you have a medical history that might indicate a blockage in a fallopian tube, or your GP or obstetrician suspects you have an ectopic pregnancy.

ectopic pregnancy scan

An ectopic pregnancy happens when the egg implants itself outside the uterus, usually in a fallopian tube. Sadly an ectopic pregnancy can't be saved and turned into a viable pregnancy. Unless the body resolves the problem itself, or for some reason it's diagnosed early and can be sorted with drugs, an ectopic pregnancy keeps developing, and because it's outside the womb it can develop into a medical emergency requiring immediate surgery when it's diagnosed.

Risk factors include a previous ectopic pregnancy; pelvic inflammatory disease (PID); damage to or scarring of the fallopian tubes caused by infection or surgery; endometriosis; or an intra-uterine device (IUD) in place when you conceived.

Symptoms of ectopic pregnancy, which usually occur at about six weeks, may include abdominal pain, either on one side of the abdomen or more generalised, which can come and go; vaginal bleeding or spotting; dizziness, faintness, paleness and sweating; nausea and vomiting; sometimes shoulder pain; and sometimes a feeling of pressure in the bum.

Tell your doctor or obstetrician immediately about these symptoms. Early treatment improves your chances of saving the tube and maintaining fertility. (One in ten ectopic pregnancies ends in infertility.) If a fallopian tube bursts, the pain is terrible: go straight to hospital because you'll need emergency surgery. Remember, it's definitely possible to have an ectopic pregnancy even if you think you can't conceive because you're on the Pill or Minipill.

ROUTINE TESTS AND CHECKS

There are some early routine tests – meaning almost everybody has them – done by your GP or midwife or by the obstetrician if you have already been referred to one. Then as you go through the weeks of pregnancy there are further routine tests (there's lots more on these in 'Screening and Diagnostic Tests' in Week 11).

Even though serious complications and illnesses in a mum or a baby are rare, we all need to make sure everything's going smoothly. The upside of this is that we get the best information available. The downside is that we can get anxious about things that will never happen. Screening tests are recommended and offered to all pregnant women, but they're not compulsory.

Most women will have:

a blood test and a urine test at the start of pregnancy to rule out the presence of any worrying bacteria or illnesses in the mum

blood tests to identify a possible problem that could affect the pregnancy, the mother or the baby; a test might, for example, indicate a baby is at risk of an inherited disease ('Genes and Chromosomes' in Week 10 will get you up to speed on genes)

two ultrasounds during the pregnancy to check on the development of the baby and to check for abnormalities (see Week 11)

blood pressure checks, with that cuff thingie that's put on your arm and blown up, usually at each visit to a doctor, obstetrician or midwife during pregnancy; high blood pressure can be a sign of pre-eclampsia, which can cause dangerous health problems for the baby and you (see 'Pre-eclampsia' in Week 28)

● perhaps a few extra tests if your doctor or obstetrician has a suspicion that something needs checking – you might have further tests on urine or blood, or a vaginal swab.

None of these routine tests has a risk of damage to you or the baby. No test or scan is infallible, and some conditions can't be tested for.

Weeing and weighing (as opposed to weeping and wailing) Most midwives and GPs will check a sample of your wee at every visit. The main reason for this is to check for proteins which could indicate pre-eclampsia (see Week 28 for all the details on pre-eclampsia). However, most won't bother to weigh you unless there's a particular reason.

There's no ideal amount of weight to put on during pregnancy, so there's no point in everybody weighing themselves or doctors knowing how many kilos they weigh (there's more on this in 'Eating and Supplements' in Week 2). The old-fashioned idea that weight should be monitored and controlled exactly during pregnancy can lead to obsessions and eating behaviour miseries. Cake is not your enemy: obsessing about cake is the enemy.

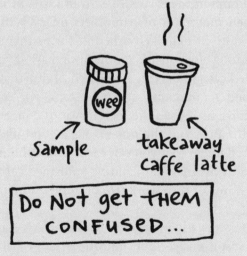

Sample   takeaway caffe latte

Do Not get them confused...

first visit to the midwife

It depends where you live in the UK, but your first medical pregnancy appointment may be at your local hospital, then all or most subsequent appointments will be with your GP or midwife, unless you need specialist care or monitoring from an obstetrician or other consultants at the hospital. In other areas, you'd skip even that first hospital appointment and only see your GP or midwife throughout. If you are referred for specialist monitoring or advice, you will be seen by a hospital-based obstetrician.

At your first – and usually longest – visit to the midwife, a comprehensive medical history will be compiled, noting details of your previous illnesses and surgery; your allergies; any prescription medications or alternative treatments you're taking; your gynaecological and obstetric history, including the pattern of your menstrual cycle; any STIs, past pregnancies, miscarriages or pregnancy terminations (abortions) you may have had; any family history of twins or genetic disorders; your lifestyle, particularly your diet, smoking, drinking, drugs, work and fitness habits; and your family's medical history, including perhaps even your mum's obstetric history. Mind you, most doctors nowadays understand that your mother's obstetric history is neither here nor there. How long your mother was in labour, whether she had nausea, what size you were as a baby – all that stuff is more than likely to be completely irrelevant to your own experience of pregnancy.

At this first appointment you'll be given loads of info and advice, and probably a small mountain of pamphlets on everything from screening tests and birth options to a likely schedule for further appointments, what to eat, and anything else you ask about. Always ask if you don't understand something (medical jargon can be hurled about that should instead be simply explained so humans can understand it). Your midwife should write all this down as if she's the secretary at the meeting, and then she'll present you with a copy of the notes – it's a good idea to stick these in a brightly coloured folder that you can easily find at home. This will become the record of your pregnancy, including your medical notes, and it should be with you at home or on a work trip or holiday and taken to any medical appointment.

Although it seems a looong way off, and at this stage you can only eye your bosoms suspiciously, your midwife will probably also start being enthusiastic about breastfeeding, and what a good idea it is and how there'll be help and services available in your area when the time comes. Take some more pamphlets and flyers for the folder. Also, she may advise you to book in early for the popular National Childbirth Trust (NCT) classes on birth and parenting a baby. (There's more on these in Week 24.)

first tests and checks

The tests and checks carried out by your midwife or doctor at your first visit will probably include:

⑥ some chat to estimate the likely delivery date

⑥ weighing you and measuring your height to see if you are under or over a healthy weight

⑥ a urine test to check for protein, glucose and any bacterial infection

⑥ a blood test to check for various things, including any diseases which could harm you or the baby, and genetic 'markers' that could indicate a risk of an inherited problem: this is just routine.

further antenatal visits

After your booking-in appointment, you will usually have antenatal check-ups with your midwife, GP or obstetrician every month or so until late in the pregnancy, after which visits become fortnightly, and then weekly. If it's your first pregnancy, you'll have about ten visits in total; if you've already had a baby it'll be only around seven visits, unless there are any complications this time round.

Take your notes to each visit. You'll probably also need to bring a wee sample which will be tested for proteins (a possible sign of high blood pressure, or other infection) or glucose (high blood sugar, which could indicate diabetes). Pharmacies sell little specimen jars with proper-sealing

RH NEGATIVE BLOOD TYPE

The early blood test may show you're among the small minority of people with a blood type called Rhesus negative. If so, your baby may still have inherited Rhesus positive blood from its father – in which case your immune system could recognise your baby's blood as an 'invader'. To prevent this causing any problems in this or future pregnancies you'll be given corrective injections after the second trimester.

screw-on lids for this purpose but do pop your sample into a plastic bag to avoid Total Handbag Disaster. At each visit the midwife or doctor should check your blood pressure, and measure your tummy to estimate the growth of the uterus. They may also weigh you (you can remind them not to tell you the number of pounds or kilos, if this is going to worry you, or you've had problems with body image). The fetal heartbeat may be monitored using an ultrasound technique or a stethoscope.

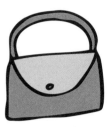

Your questions   It's easy to forget something you've been meaning to ask the obstetrician, GP or midwife. You might like to list your questions on the front page of your pregnancy notes as they occur to you and then jot down the answers during your visit, because sometimes your head's in such a whirl with all the new info that you forget to ask something or afterwards can't remember the answer. Ask if you can email any questions you have between visits, or if they have a website with frequently asked questions and answers (FAQ). If anything really worries you, politely insist on a quick visit or returned phone call or email to allay your fears.

TWINS AND MULTIPLE BIRTHS

Twins happen about once in every 80 pregnancies – although the incidence is higher if you have had IVF or other fertility treatment. Triplets (or more) are very rare unless you have had multiple embryos implanted as part of a fertility treatment. In an ordinarily conceived pregnancy, you will normally find out you have twins at your first ultrasound scan – probably at twelve weeks. Of course, if for any reason you have an earlier scan, you will find out then. Whenever you make that discovery, nothing can quite prepare you for the shock.

Your pregnancy, antenatal care and birth options will be different in many ways with a multiple birth. Nothing is quite straightforward in a twin pregnancy and you will receive more frequent antenatal check-ups, generally with an obstetrician as well as a midwife. The babies are scanned regularly to measure their growth and monitor their development. Your health will also be monitored because certain complications of pregnancy are more common with twins – pre-eclampsia, preterm labour, anaemia and, not least, sheer exhaustion.

Some mothers find the old saying of double the trouble is a very accurate way to describe a twin pregnancy. Extra tiredness, extra weight gain and more movements from the growing babies are all guaranteed. The most important advice for those carrying twins is to rest. The second is to re-think your time frame (including maternity leave). Twins are generally born early – at 37 rather than 40 weeks on average (see Week 30 for info on premmie babies). You will probably be advised to slow down towards 18–20 weeks and, if you're working, you should think about negotiating part-time hours at that stage. The work of carrying two babies is very tiring and the reality of caring for them in the first few months is so exhausting it is worth spoiling yourself whilst pregnant and taking some time off.

Your labour may also be different with a multiple birth. If the babies are lying in good positions, then there is no reason not to have labour and a normal hospital birth. But they often lie awkwardly in the last few weeks of pregnancy, in which case the safest way for them to be delivered will be by a caesarean birth.

See the Help section at the end of this book for resources on twins and multiples.

WEEK

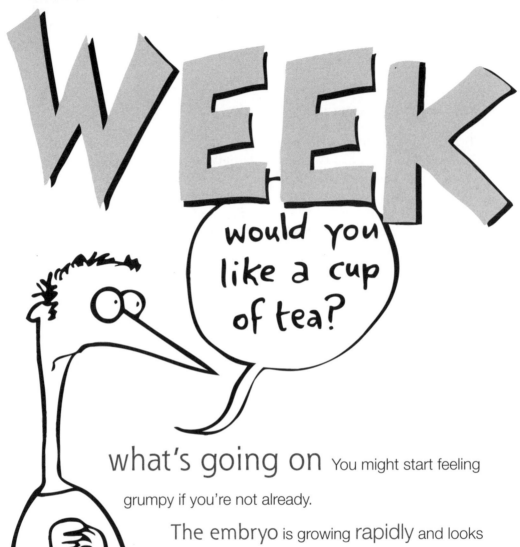

would you like a cup of tea?

what's going on
You might start feeling grumpy if you're not already.

The embryo is growing rapidly and looks like a teensy tadpole. Its tadpole tail will eventually shrink and the remnants become the baby's coccyx. In the centre of the embryo is the start of the digestive system, lungs and bladder. This is surrounded by a layer that will develop into muscles, skeleton, heart, kidneys and genitals, and this is wrapped up in what will become the skin, nervous system, ears and eyes. Tiny bumps are appearing that will grow into

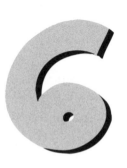

arms. The immature heart starts to beat and can be clearly seen as a pulsation on an ultrasound screen. Really, the whole thing looks like some tiny thing that might come out if you sneezed. Websites and books disagree on the size of the developing baby, partly because some measure from head to bum and some from head to feet, and partly because it's about averages not precise measurements.

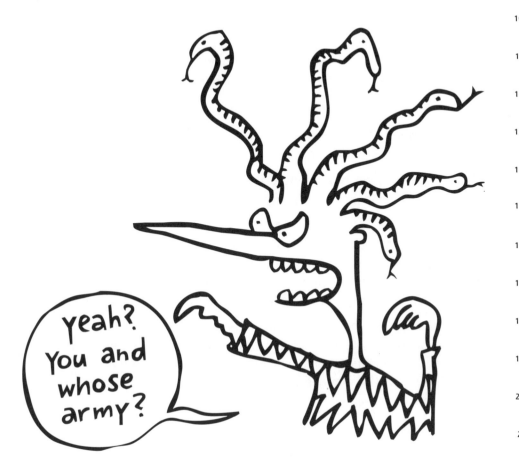

yeah?
You and
whose
army?

Average approximate embryo length this week from head to bum

cm
1
2
3
4
5
6
7
8
9
10
11
12
13
14
15
16
17
18
19
20
21

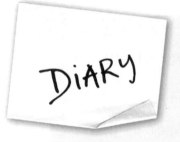
DIARY

Work is hotting up. We sign to produce two new fashion ranges for a couple of big department stores. The spicy earth colours of winter! The divine madness of spring! You know the sort of thing. Will we get it all done before the baby arrives? I can't even tell anyone I'm pregnant yet. The convention is to wait until after thirteen weeks, when they reckon the biggest risk of miscarriage is over.

We tell some close friends of Geoff's, quietly, at a wedding. They scream. I have to pretend there is a spider down my underpants to explain the kerfuffle.

I now know why horoscopes are a dead loss. You'd think they could warn you: 'This week you'll get put in the pudding club'. No, mine just said: 'Financial difficulties may arise on Tuesday. Your lucky colour is caramel'. Nobody's lucky colour is caramel. It's not even a colour, it's half a meal.

Beck says I need to get my GP to refer me to an obstetrician straight away because of my endometriosis, which can cause an ectopic pregnancy. She says an early ultrasound would check that the pregnant bit of me is where it should be – in the uterus – instead of ectopic (stuck in a fallopian tube), which can be very dangerous. My GP, Dr Sharma, is quite reassuring and refers me directly to the early pregnancy clinic at the local hospital, where he says I'll meet the midwife team who will provide most of my pregnancy care. Before I leave, he asks me to fill in a few details on the hospital referral form to take with me.

Who is your family doctor? (Dr Sharma.)

Last period? (Well, in my case about four years, but surely that's going to take too long to explain.)

Previous surgery: how many operations? (Can't remember because of all my endometriosis ops so compromise by writing 'Heaps'. That should give 'em the general idea.)

Husband's name? (Haven't got one. Well, I have got a boyfriend. Must be worse for Susanne when she reads this sort of thing on forms. I mean what is a single girl supposed to write? 'Missing In Action'? 'NA – Not Available'? 'NOYB – None Of Your Business'? Or just 'Albert Einstein'?)

Number of previous pregnancies? (One. Well, therein lies another story, but do they really want to hear about the anaesthetist who wanted to get the termination over so he could get to the footy on time? Probably not. This pregnancy business sure flicks open the clasps on your emotional baggage.)

While I'm waiting for my ultrasound appointment, I look at the posters on the wall of a fetus developing week by week. It was so long ago. I can't remember now whether I terminated at six weeks or eight weeks. So many of us women having babies in our thirties had abortions when we were younger, vowing that we would only become mothers when we could be good at it. I'm glad I waited. I didn't even know who I really was then. But I really don't want to look at that poster.

I go into a small room and lie on a flat, hard, raised couch. The ultrasound operator sits next to me at about hip level with a screen in front of him.

If I crane my neck, I can just about make out a tiny dot on the screen pulsating incredibly quickly and rhythmically. That's the embryo's heartbeat. And it's all in the right spot: the uterus. I feel incredibly relieved. Then the operator starts going all avuncular on me and saying I should realise that there might be 'wastage'. It takes me a beat or two until I realise he's warning me that it's very early days and I could have a miscarriage – only he's got a pet name for it. Geez, how sensitive.

I go to see Dr Sharma again a couple of days later. 'Everything's absolutely fine', he grins.

info

miscarriage

The miscarriage rate in women who know they're pregnant is estimated by various studies to be as high as one in five and as low as one in ten or fifteen. Many miscarriages, though, occur very early and would normally be assumed to be a period. As you get older your risk of miscarriage increases; you're also more likely to miscarry if you have miscarried in the past. (But most women who've had a miscarriage can go on to have a healthy baby.)

The vast majority of all known miscarriages happen in the first trimester. A miscarriage that happens after week 13 is called a 'late miscarriage'. Loss of a baby after about twenty weeks is usually called a '(preterm) stillbirth'. If you 'make it' to eight weeks and your doctor or midwife has heard the fetal heartbeat the risk of miscarriage drops to only one or two in 100.

You may hear a doctor refer to a miscarriage by the medical term 'abortion'. Also, when a pregnancy ends in miscarriage because the embryo

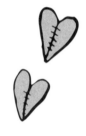

does not develop, the embryo is often called a 'blighted ovum'. These insensitive medical terms do not help your feelings at the time. Feel free to tell the doctor off for being tactless. They should learn that they're being hurtful at the worst possible time, even if to them it's just business as usual.

Vaginal bleeding is quite common in pregnancy, especially after having sex, because the cervix is 'spongier' than usual. This bleeding usually stops without causing any problems at all. But by far the most common symptom of miscarriage is bleeding from the vagina. So if bleeding happens, contact your GP, midwife or obstetrician immediately. You'll need to describe the colour, quantity and time frame of the bleeding. Light spotting may not be a cause for alarm. A heavy flow could mean you need to go straight to hospital.

After a miscarriage you may need to have a small operation to prevent infection, which makes sure the uterus is free of all the tissue that should come out. The endometrium will grow back as good as new. The operation is performed under general anaesthetic in hospital. If you miscarry before six weeks you probably won't need the op.

Don't use a tampon for any bleeding during pregnancy, and keep the pad you do use until you have spoken to your doctor or obstetrician. And don't have sex until the bleeding has been checked by them.

I know this sounds a bit gross and depressing but, if you can, keep any clots and tissue from a miscarriage in a clean plastic bag or container, so they can be examined. This can help establish whether the miscarriage is complete, and help a pathology laboratory work out what caused the miscarriage.

Possible causes of miscarriage include 'nature rejecting a problem with a pregnancy', such as fetal abnormality; exposure to certain chemicals, illnesses or medications (see 'Protecting Your Pregnancy' in Week 4); problems with the sperm, uterus, egg's implantation, mother's immune system, placenta or cervix; and hormonal imbalances.

When miscarriage occurs an 'incompetent cervix' is sometimes diagnosed. (Another charming medical term – it has not escaped attention that there's no similar medical phrase for Hopeless Penis.) It means that the cervix gets over-eager and opens too soon. This is the diagnosed reason for some miscarriages in the second trimester (week 14 until the end of week 26). It's not because you've done anything 'wrong'. Previous gynaecological surgery or laser treatments, abortions or miscarriages may possibly increase your risk of this condition – another reason to give your midwife or obstetrician your full medical history. A misbehaving cervix can be stitched closed during your next pregnancy until the baby is ready to come out.

If you've had a miscarriage, get all the information you can from your obstetrician – make sure all your questions are answered – and review the possible risk factors that could be avoided or treated in future pregnancies. If you have more than two miscarriages, you'll usually be tested for uterine problems and hormonal imbalances and have your immune system evaluated.

Miscarriage is no less distressing because it's common. Friends and family can make things worse by well-meaning but insensitive remarks, such as 'Hurry up and have another one', or 'You'll soon get over it'. It's important to allow yourself time to talk over and mourn the loss with your partner, who may grieve differently from you, causing friction. It can be really helpful to find a support group so you can talk to and hear from people who have been through it.

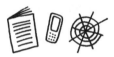

more info on **miscarriage**

Ask your GP or midwife to put you in touch with a local support group. See also 'Grief and Loss' in the Contacts and Resources chapter at the end of the book.

miscarriageassociation.org.uk
Helpline: 01924 200 799
The Miscarriage Association provides information and support for those who have suffered the loss of a child in pregnancy.
In Scotland contact Miscarriage Support (0141 552 5070, miscarriagesupport. org.uk).

Coming to Term: Uncovering the Truth About Miscarriage by Jon Cohen, Houghton Mifflin, US, 2007
An American science writer decided to investigate miscarriage after his wife's fourth one. He talks to women who've been through it and to medical experts, and covers the main reasons it happens, what can and can't be done, the truths and myths, and some encouraging news for the future.

what's going on

Your breasts may be bigger and more sensitive, and the nipples and surrounding areolae may have started to look bigger and bumpier. (The little bumps on each areola are officially called Montgomery's tubercles but who cares about Montgomery, whoever he was: 'little bumps' sounds a lot cuter.) You could have continuing nausea and need to wee a lot. Foods may taste different, and you may go off the smell of things you previously liked.

Teeny buds that will grow into legs are appearing on the embryo. Everything continues growing at a cracking pace. The heart is going strongly inside a developing chest but the lungs have only just started to form. Embryonic kidneys begin to develop and function (the finished kidneys come later). The head bulge is getting more like the right shape. The chorionic villi are becoming more and longer tentacles into the uterus. The embryo is now about the size of a pine nut (not to be confused with a pine cone!).

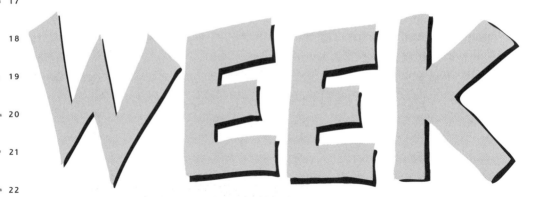

WEEK

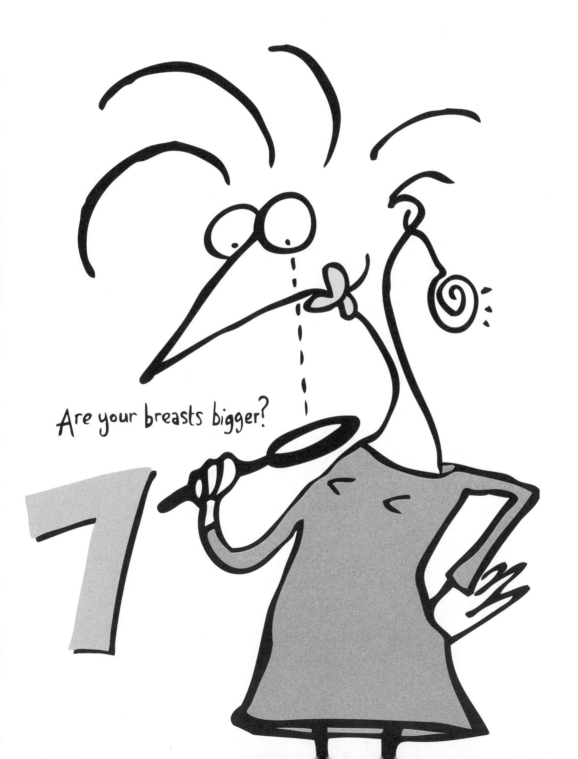

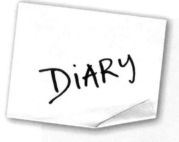
DIARY

I couldn't be less interested in sex if my private parts had been packed away in a shoe box in the back of the wardrobe. This will not do. Where is the surge of lascivious sex-kittenry the books promise and the magazines go on about?

Take the pregnancy special issue of this month's *She* magazine, and I quote: 'In the middle of your pregnancy, your libido soars. You're not too enormous but you're round enough not to be concerned about maintaining the missionary position in the quest for a flat stomach and no chins. You bounce about with abandon.' Oh bollocks.

Surely the last thing you want to be thinking about when you're having fun is whether he's noticing your double chin – and anyway what bloke is thinking anything except 'Bingo!' with a grown-up girlie on top of him? – so, apart from a few pointers on that kind of palaver, I'd just like to know where these magazine writers get off, telling us how we're going to feel. As if everybody is the same as them – that is, wanders around saying things like 'Beige is the new black, essentials this summer include platform pantyliners with a daisy motif, and in the middle of your pregnancy you'll be a bonking fool.' Well, apparently some women do go mad for it when pregnant. And some men find pregnancy makes their partners EMG (Even More Gorgeous).

I've been reflecting on the ultrasound operator last week using the appalling word 'wastage' to warn me about a possible miscarriage. It must be his regular spiel to everybody. Anyway, it has reminded us again not to tell anyone in case something goes wrong. So we've only told Debbie, Tania, Susanne coz she's already pregnant, Beck because, let's face it, she is my medical adviser and I'll probably need a bit of advice, Liz and John, Jo and Anton, Pete, Jayesh, Kate, Rhiannon and Ari, Graham and Haryun. Less than 100 people, anyway.

Apart from that, I might have to tell some people at work so they don't think I've lost my mind. I go around with this permanent off-the-air expression, which actually indicates I'm talkin' sales figures but thinkin', 'Creature inside me! Creature inside me! Size of a Tic Tac. I feel seasick right now and I have to pretend I don't! Bleeeeuuurghhh! I beg your pardon, I appear to have thrown up on your shoes', or simply 'I know something YOU don't know.'

We don't want to tell everyone we're 'expecting' and then have to say, 'Oh we lost it', as if we'd been a bit careless in the Safeway car park and left the little bundle in the returned trolleys section by mistake. I heard that one in ten pregnancies ends in miscarriage.

'Oh no, that's not right', says Beck.

'Thank God I've got you to calm my fears with proper medical facts, Beck', I say.

'I think it's one in five', she explains helpfully.

So much of pregnancy seems to be about odds. It automatically turns you into a gambler. The statistics mean everything and nothing at the same time. One in five is high, even if some of those are miscarriages you wouldn't know about because they would be just like having a period. And if you do have a miscarriage, your own personal chance was 100 percent. And if you don't have a miscarriage, your individual risk was zero percent. But you can't help brooding on 'one in five' and every other percentage risk they tell you about.

We go to a birthday do at Geoff's mum's – we don't tell. The next night Geoff has a work dinner do that is full of pregnant gardening associates. Geoff wants to tell everyone and has to be sternly restrained.

Poor Geoff. He's got a seasick, exhausted girlfriend who'd rather stick peas up her nose than have sex, and he's going to be a daddy. I think we're both feeling kind of like it's all been a theory and now it's really going to happen. Well actually, it still feels a bit theoretical. Maybe I'm in denial.

I know intellectually that I'm pregnant, but it just doesn't feel real. I can't tell by looking, and I don't suddenly feel like knitting bootees or protecting my offspring with the ferocity of a lioness. I have no more idea about raising a child than I did six weeks ago. No sudden illuminated shaft has split the heavens asunder, pierced the top of my noggin and said in a very deep voice, 'You are going to be a mother.' Just as well, really. I'd probably wet my pants.

I am very grumpy indeed. Geoff has read somewhere that newborn babies look like their father so the father will stick around. I reply that all newborn babies look like Winston Churchill, and what's that got to do with anything? Geoff wonders why hormones would make you grumpy when surely nature intends you to keep the man happy, to protect you. I refrain from saying that being grumpy is a perfectly bloody natural reaction, and furthermore it is no doubt serving the important purpose of teaching you that if the bloke runs off with a sailor, or proves to be a complete flop at hunter-gathering, you can do it all yourself.

After all, most women with one child and a husband feel like they have two children and anyway why is there a mess in that corner and I believe you forgot to put the rubbish out again and WHERE'S MY BLOODY DINNER?

info

tiredness

One of the symptoms of the first trimester can be an incredibly draining exhaustion – which you can't even complain about because most people don't know that you're pregnant.

Here's the weird thing: in the past, if you've been really tired, you have probably pushed through it. With first trimester pregnancy tiredness, you find yourself following your feet up the hall and getting into bed. You have turned into a robot. Welcome to reality: your body is now running you, rather than the other way around.

First trimester tiredness is FULL ON. Don't feel guilty about going to bed at unusual times otherwise you may get more nausea from the extreme fatigue.

A lot of women who go out to work full-time spend the first trimester coming home from their job, going straight to bed, waking up and demanding dinner from their partner or flatmate or calling in a takeaway for themselves, and then going back to bed.

Most women start to feel perkier and less nauseated by week 14 (but the tiredness comes back in the third trimester).

Here are some of the reasons why you may be so tired:

⑥ the high levels of progesterone in your system during the first trimester can have a sedative effect

⑥ your metabolic rate increases 10–25 percent to support the developing fetus, and a whole lot of other parts are working overtime, such as your heart

⑥ all that extra night-time weeing means you're not getting the deepest, most restful part of sleep

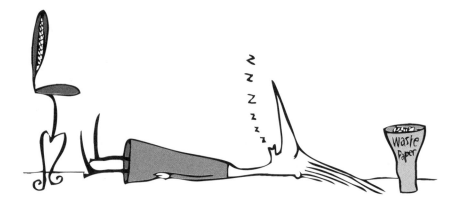

WHO TO TELL? WHEN TO TELL?

Some people spread their good news immediately. This means they've got support from the get-go. Others wait until the end of the first trimester to publicly announce their pregnancy, when the greatest risk of miscarriage is over. This allows them time to adjust to the idea of being pregnant and to share feelings in private. It also delays the moment when relatives go berserk and can't shut up about it. Once they know, your mother, mother-in-law, father and father-in-law (not to mention acquaintances) will descend with advice, horror stories, theories and judgements about your plans to return to work or not return to work. Even totally positive expressions of joy from your extended family can be overwhelming.

Parents often choose not to tell their toddler until the pregnancy is visible (Mum's tum is bigger) because for a little'un it can seem like an eternity until something interesting happens. (Well, actually, you don't have to be a toddler.)

Work Exactly when you want to tell your employer will depend on your relationship with them and your position within the organisation, but they should hear the news from you and not on the office grapevine. Your employer should be advised in writing that you are pregnant and when you plan to start your maternity leave. You will probably need to include a doctor's certificate confirming your due date. You might want to give as much notice as possible so your employer can consider how best to cover your job while you are on leave. Many women hide their pregnancy for as long as they can because of possible discrimination. Before you tell your employer, find out your leave rights (see 'Work Entitlements' in the first chapter, Getting Ready).

⊚ your body is putting the development of the fetus first – you are making eyelids and bones and sex organs and lungs and a placenta and stuff so for heaven's sake who WOULDN'T need to lie down with all that going on?

⊚ just being nauseated (see 'Nausea' in Week 4) can make you feel exhausted.

Some ways to combat tiredness are:

⊚ win the lottery; quit work; sleep all the time; get a cleaner, a masseur and, oh, hang the expense, a personal chef like Oprah's; live in a posh hotel

⑥ give in to it, don't fight it – your body will win this round anyway

⑥ find a storeroom or sickroom where you can nap if work commitments mean long days at the office (if all else fails you could always just Lie Down under your desk) – and don't forget to eat lunch at your desk if you use the lunch hour for a kip

⑥ nap when you get home if you work away from home

⑥ nap when you can if you work at home

⑥ meet friends for lunch or on the weekends at your place rather than risking an exhausting late night staying sober while everyone else is legless

⑥ keep one day, or at least an afternoon, on the weekend completely free; and don't be ashamed in any way if you want to spend All Weekend in bed for the first three months

⑥ if you have a partner or flatmate who has not been pulling their weight in the housework department, renegotiate so they see that doing the tasks/ chores is about rights and responsibilities rather than about 'helping' you or doing you a favour; alternatively, get used to mess – or both

⑥ if you already have little children, give them away to relatives. Sorry. No. Try to nap or at least lie down when they do. If you have only one rule, have this one: your toddlers and preschoolers must have their afternoon nap, even if it turns into 'quiet time'. Make them safe and be utterly uncompromising – the nap is not negotiable.

weeing all the time

Weeing all the time is a very common symptom of pregnancy in the first thirteen weeks or so. It's not that you're over-excited, it's just that your uterus is taking up more space, putting pressure on the neighbouring organs, including your bladder. Even more congestion is caused by the extra blood vessels and blood flow developing in the pelvis to sustain the placenta and carry the added weight.

It may be less of a problem in the second trimester because the uterus 'pops' outwards at the front, making the pelvis temporarily less crowded. But the constant weeing usually comes back in the third trimester when there's a serious space shortage – at which stage it can feel as if your baby is kicking your bladder, or grabbing it, or generally tossing it around and headbutting it.

You still need to drink lots of water during the day to avoid dehydration, but you can try drinking less in the evenings in an attempt to reduce the number of trips to the toilet during the night. (Experienced mums will grimly inform you that getting up to wee all night long is good training for the interrupted sleep caused by night feeding once the baby is born. I say try not to do it until you have to.)

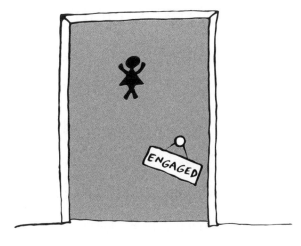

If you get a burning or stinging sensation when you wee a lot, mention it to your doctor. You may have a urinary tract infection, which may need treating with antibiotics. Cranberry juice can also help.

worries

This is a common time to go into a bit of an 'Oh my God' spin. Questions you might be asking yourself include:

⑥ How can I give up my independence?

⑥ How dare my partner not realise how scary this is?

⑥ How dare my partner … [fill in the blank here]?

⑥ Do I really want a child?

⑥ My family life was awful – what if it's the same again?

⑥ Because I was abused will I be able to break the cycle?

⑥ Did I mention I don't even like kids?

Talk to a counsellor if these thoughts are dominating you (your GP can refer you to one). But usually these tumultuous worries will lessen in intensity, and the 'mental chatter' will settle down. (And be comforted that if you're one of the people who recognises that their childhood was unhappy or abusive you have taken the most crucial first step to breaking that pattern: talking to a counsellor and learning new parenting skills really can help.)

what's going on You are

continuing to wee more often because your

bladder is being crowded by the uterus.

A lot of fancy hormonal footwork is going on

to keep building the placenta. You might feel nauseated

AND constipated: jackpot! You may be starting to feel

tired: your body has a lot to do that is normally not on the

agenda. Your hair may be getting thicker, and downstairs

there may be more vaginal mucus than normal.

Your embryo has become that classic curled

shape, the big fat head with a tail (not a very attractive

shape at this point, and similar to a prawn from space,

sure, but we all have to start somewhere). It's still SO

tiny – roughly the size of a peanut – but it's about a million

times bigger than the fertilised cell that started moving and

shaking six weeks ago. The external bits of the ears now

start to be visible, and the tiny hands are webbed.

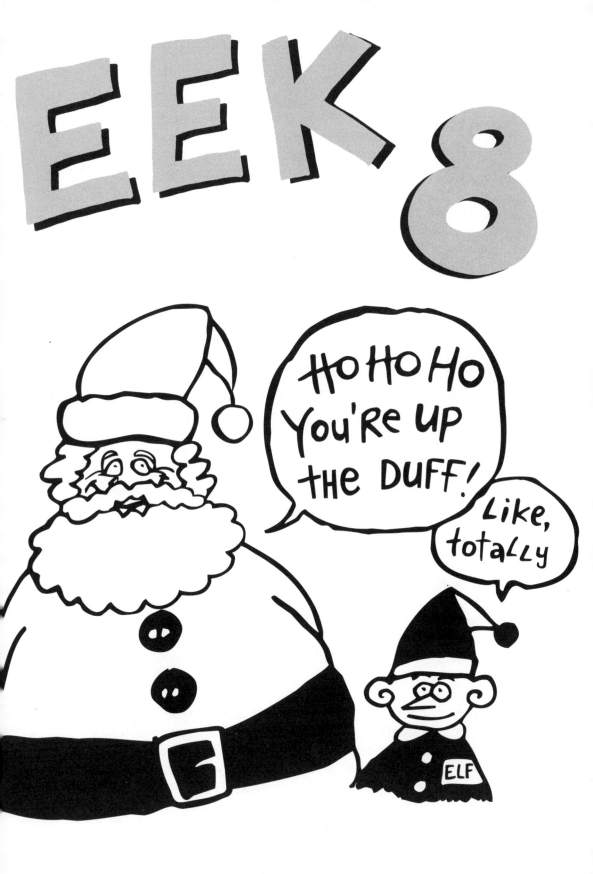

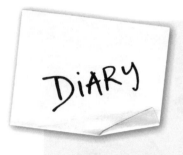

I am having strange, vivid dreams. Last night I dreamt that American author Gore Vidal came to afternoon tea and I gave him a Toffee Crisp on a silver plate and he said, 'How perfectly charming.' I was completely furious that Geoff woke me up at that precise moment to kiss me goodbye as he went to work.

'But I just gave Gore Vidal a Toffee Crisp!' I said accusingly.

'Yes, dear', he replied, which was probably about the only thing he could have said.

I also dreamt I went to a funfair on the Isle of Wight with a well-known model who had too much luggage to fit in the helicopter. In the end it didn't matter as our turn on the Ferris wheel was interrupted by a tornado.

Christmas Day. We spend it pretty quietly, knowing that in the twinkling of an inkling we'll be agonising over whether to come clean about Santa and how to try to teach a rapacious toddler about the spirituality of giving rather than receiving. (Fat chance.)

I've bought Aunt Julie a pair of silk slippers and a flash handbag. She's bought Geoff and me a sandwich toaster. Uncle Mike (we've got him a phone with satellite navigation) presents us with a book that looks like it came from the Oxfam shop, which he doesn't bother to wrap because wrapping paper destroys the environment. Instead he sticky-tapes a homemade card to the front of it. And when I say a homemade card, I mean a bit of cardboard from the inside of his girlfriend's packet of tights. (Re-use, recycle, read my lips: my Uncle Mike has become a real eco-cheapskate.)

Uncle Mike's new girlfriend is 25 years younger than him and has purple dreadlocks and is a total fruitcake. I suspect she drinks hemlock. Her name, allegedly, is Aurelia. We are already calling her 'Oh Really' behind her back.

You can't choose your family, I guess. I wonder how our baby will turn out. Maybe just like Mike. Or just like Mum, but I wouldn't know because I can't remember her. At least I have some photos. Will I have more respect for what she went through, or for the way Aunt Julie and Uncle Mike raised me? Will our child inherit Aunt Julie's instinctive morbid dreads? Or Aurelia's purple dreads? Or be influenced by Uncle Mike's habit of saving rubber bands, rolling them into balls and then trying to sell them to Jehovah's Witnesses who come to the door?

Bloody nausea. Queasy isn't the word for it. I am nauseous all the time and desperate for it to stop. Whoever called it 'morning sickness' was a complete maniac. (I keep involuntarily singing 'Get it in the morning, get it in the evening, get it at suppertime'.) Beck thinks it's just too much oestrogen in my system and my liver is having trouble clearing it out.

Aurelia would probably say if I was a Pisces I would accept my pregnancy and wouldn't get 'morning sick' and that it's all in my mind. At least I've got a mind, I could tell her.

'The HCG hormone almost certainly has something to do with it, but we don't really know what causes it', Dr Sharma said when I asked him about it during my first visit. Nor did he offer any fix, quick or otherwise.

Why do the pregnancy books just say, 'Eat dry crackers before you get out of bed in the morning'? I mean, that's not very informative, is it? They might as well say: 'Sacrifice a chicken and study its entrails. An interestingly shaped spleen means you will continue to have nausea until the thirteenth week.'

Beck says, 'Don't worry, nausea means the baby is hanging on in there. If it stopped suddenly THAT would be a worry because it could mean a miscarriage.'

Nausea stops suddenly for a whole day. Oh my God.

Nausea starts again. Thank God.

Bloody nausea.

I'm also weeing all the time. In some circles this is regarded suspiciously, and one person even starts a rumour that I have such a severe cocaine problem I have to go to the toilet three times during a dinner party. In other circles you get smug looks from mothers who think they're onto you. And one of the models at work asked if I was bulimic and suggested I try laxatives instead. Crikey.

Geoff and I take a long walk on the beach and decide we don't want to have a baby with Down's syndrome because it's not fair to have a child who might need constant medical intervention yet mightn't understand why. And we can't take care of our child forever: one day we'll be gone. We decide that we would terminate if we had to. Geoff says the decision is ultimately mine and he'll support it. I know that many would disagree with our reasons and decision: they'd say people with Down's syndrome lead full and happy lives, and that termination is wrong. I reckon it's a really personal, difficult decision, and the 'right' answer may be different for different people. It's all very tricky. Beck advises that if it comes to that, we could always say there was a miscarriage so other people who knew about the pregnancy didn't judge our decision to terminate. Sounds like a good idea. The result of all this is we decide I should have a test that estimates the risk of giving birth to a baby with Down's syndrome.

We've chosen an interim name so we don't have to say 'it' all the time. Cellsie – as in bunch of cells – is what we're calling the embryo-baby-offspring-thingie inside me. We'll have to come up with something else before nursery school but it'll do for the moment.

info

cravings

You know how you sometimes crave chocolate or pasta, or maybe red meat, when you're premenstrual? Pregnancy cravings can be similar, and doctors don't know how to explain them all. Most pregnant women get a craze for one sort of food or another for a short period – usually ice cream or something sugary. You can go through stages, craving steamed veggies, then chocolate, then tropical fruit. You can also go right off a food that used to be a favourite. This can include strong-smelling foods and green leafy vegetables that are the slightest bit 'slimy'; it's probably a hard-wired aversion to things that have gone 'off'. This may also explain why some women crave crunchy things (including ice) – maybe the lizard part of our brain thinks crunchy means fresh.

It's okay to indulge any cravings, but make sure you know what your body's saying. Some people who're pregnant get odd cravings (called pica) for dirt or washing powder (no, don't eat those), which probably means they need iron. Try a steak instead. You want a cheeseburger a day? Maybe you need more carbs – try some mashed potato. On the other hand, maybe you really want a cheeseburger. As long as the food you crave is itself safe, meaning not a high bacteria risk (see 'Protecting Your Pregnancy' in Week 4), go for it.

You might get a funny taste in your mouth that seems kind of metallic. This is thought to be due to the high level of various hormones in your blood, which can change the taste of your saliva.

constipation

High progesterone levels are relaxing the muscles in your digestive tract, causing intestinal activity to slow down. This means your poo is going on a slower journey than usual, so it loses water and can become hard, causing constipation. (In the third trimester you may experience even worse constipation as your ginormous uterus squashes the bowel.)

Here are some ways to avoid constipation.

◎ Drink at least two litres of water, spaced out across the day; you might find some warm water is less of a shock to the body first thing in the morning, as long as it doesn't make you feel nauseated.

⑥ Eat plenty of natural fibre – fresh and lightly cooked root vegetables, fruit, wholegrain breads, high-fibre cereals, such as porridge, and brown rice. Choose whole foods instead of processed foods and pre-prepared breakfast cereals whenever possible. If this is a bulkier load of fibre than your body is used to, have smaller meals more often while you adjust. Remember that the more fibre you eat, the more you need to drink.

⑥ Getting sugar into your bowel using, say, melon or prunes can help.

⑥ If chemical iron supplements are causing constipation, talk to your doctor or natural therapist about a herbal alternative.

⑥ Get plenty of exercise.

⑥ Constipation can also come with the added discomfort of bloating and farting. This should disappear

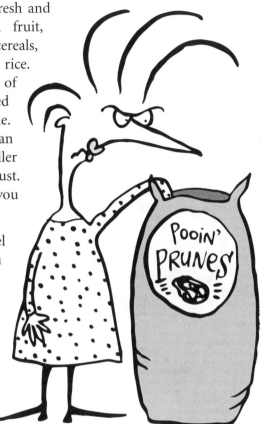

when the constipation goes. Too much unprocessed bran, and sometimes too much raw food, which is hard to digest, can cause bloating. Lightly steamed veggies are easier to absorb than hard, completely raw ones.

⑥ Don't take any laxative preparation without discussing it first with your doctor – some laxatives, including those that contain senna, can produce violent expulsive actions, causing painful contractions of the bowel, which in turn can upset the uterus next door.

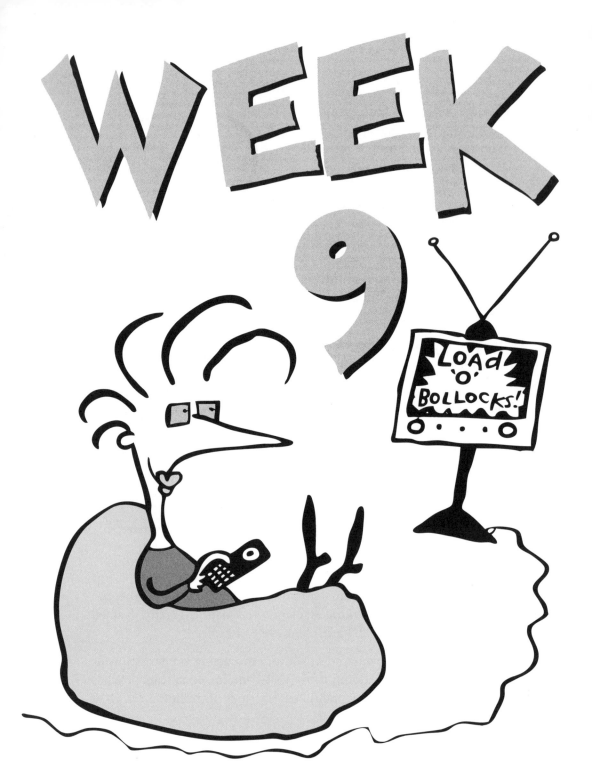

what's going on

Your stomach may not be at all preggie-looking yet. As it grows, your centre of gravity will change and you will become, well, a person with the grace of a hippopotamus rather than a fruit bat. So this is the time to attend to any handy-type problems around the house – loose carpeting, tricky steps, bits of bathroom that get slippery or dangerous or awkward to manoeuvre around. And if there's something you need to get at regularly that involves standing on stepladders or a chair, lower it for the duration.

The embryo's eyelids appear, and its body elongates but its head is as big as its body. The internal sex organs are starting to develop into boy and girl bits, but you can't tell the sex from the outside yet. The ends of the limbs are looking a bit more like hands and feet but you still couldn't play 'This little piggy went to market' unless you changed the words to 'This little webby bit ... '. To continue our food comparison, the embryo is now as big as an olive.

Average approximate embryo length this week from head to bum

cm
1
2
3
4
5
6
7
8
9
10
11
12
13
14
15
16
17
18
19
20
21
22

DIARY

Apparently the government will give us some money for having a baby: some people are saying that's why women get pregnant now – for the cash. Could this be a chance for a get-rich scheme? Could I have one a year? 'Oi! You, yes, the bus driver! Want to have unprotected sex?' Maybe not.

And as for all those ratbags who complain about paying for single mothers, I've been paying for everyone else's children and their hospital care and their education and their roads even though I've been a childless, unlicensed, non-driving taxpayer for almost fifteen years. So you can all bugger off. I'd rather my money helped single mothers than paid for another MP's expenses.

Where was I? Oh yes.

Even though it still seems miles off, I have to make plans for the actual (it's hard to say this out loud), um, you know … birth. I went for a booking-in appointment with the midwife team at the hospital and we discussed my options for antenatal care, the tests available, and the delivery options – which basically came down to hospital or home birth. I'd heard about places called birth centres, which seem a bit like Wendy-house hospital extensions, with subdued lighting, and a midwife-only team looking after your needs. However, the nearest one to us could be a white-knuckle ride in bad traffic, so I've plumped for a regular delivery in the local hospital.

A home birth seemed attractive for a brief moment of fantasy, but even with a couple of midwives in attendance – well, I'm just too neurotic. I'll take the twenty-first-century technology, I said to the midwives. It's still twentieth-century round here, they replied. But there you go. The midwives also asked if I had private health insurance (no luck). Seems like you sometimes get a few options thrown in if you do, like a private room and executivey food after the delivery. Oh well.

I picked up a pamphlet advertising the services of independent midwives at Beck's clinic. You could tell they were very modern because the mother on the front cover, holding her minutes-old baby, had a very charming tattoo on her arm.

I have informed Beck she will have to be my private midwife and I refuse to get a tattoo. Beck has agreed to this cunning plan, and now I have to square it with the midwives that I can have her as an extra birthing partner at the delivery. It feels like being a kid and asking if a friend can stay over. Still, best to check. We don't want any punch-ups on the day.

All this stuff arrives from the hospital, which I'm supposed to read and fill in. There's a hospital admittance form that has on it 'Diagnosis: confinement'. Confinement?! It's a word out of a Jane Austen novel, or some 1950s sitcom, when pregnant bellies were hidden indoors for the last few months so nobody had to be reminded that pregnant women HAVE HAD SEX. Confined, for Christ's sake. It's a wonder the form doesn't say 'BYO handcuffs'.

The list of things we're instructed to bring to the hospital on Cellsie's birth day is more mystifying the longer I look at it. 'Underclothes including underpants and maternity bras.' Well, what other kinds of underclothes are there? Do people usually take flounced petticoats and lace teddies? 'One to two packets of nursing pads.' Oh dear. Not a clue what they are. Surely nurses can look after their own needs? 'Two packets of super-adhesive sanitary pads (maternity sanitary pads such as Always).' Oh my giddy aunt, who names these things? If I thought having a period would go on always, as in forever, I'd be ready to start shooting out street lights with a handy blunderbuss.

Then there's a whole list of baby stuff they want you to bring, for which we'll need to use Geoff's van. 'Four babygros.' Four? What's going to happen to the other three? Does the baby shred them during tantrums? Do they all go on at once? How cold can the kid get? 'Baby hat, and bootees or socks, and mittens (optional).' Well, I'm glad it's all optional. Because to be honest it hadn't previously occurred to me that a person less than a week old should have a hat and gloves. Stockings, maybe, but let's not go overboard. The kid can develop its own sense of elegant matching accessories when it leaves home and can afford to buy its own formal wear.

Under 'What to bring for partner' there is a most unsatisfactorily short list. 'Men's night attire please if staying overnight e.g. tracksuits, pyjamas, dressing gown.' (I asked about this, and apparently most of the midwives have seen willies before, but an elderly cleaner at the hospital copped an eyeful of a bloke's leopard-skin posing pouch early one morning and took immediate retirement.)

As Geoff has none of the recommended items except trackie bottoms this could be a bit of a problem. And anyway, why assume the partner is male? Why should a lesbian partner be forced into 'men's night attire'? It's downright unnatural. And the list of what a partner should bring to the hospital should include: enormous boxes of chocolates, latest magazines, new and attractive clothes, tickets to Paris (springtime) etc. Diamonds would be acceptable. And a boat with a bowling alley. What am I saying? By the time I give birth we'll have £2.50 between us.

The upshot of reading all this material from the hospital is that you get wildly ahead of yourself. You've still got months and months to go and you're wondering what to pack. Not to mention a few decisions about ambience.

For delivery, the hospital suggests 'relaxation music'. Not a good start. Relaxation music always makes me very tense. Comedian Mark Little once pointed out it sounded like dolphins playing the piano. Besides, if you gave birth to Enya music, the quietly contemplative ambience might be somewhat offset by the fact that you are screaming the place down and something huge is coming out of your vagina and at least two people you don't even know are watching. And anyway, if we can subliminally remember birth, why would you want the poor child to forever associate pain, screaming and fluorescent lights with Enya's latest hits?

Further suggestions include 'camera'. Oh for God's sake, if I want a photo of myself red in the face, grimacing and drooling and shouting I can take a happy snap next time I'm pissed at a party. Also 'essential oils, glucose lollies, large T-shirt or old nightie, socks, toiletries, book or magazine etc., T-shirts and shorts or swimwear for partner if desired'. I have never imagined labour as a scenario in which I am lying back reading while Geoff does a few laps. It is all very confusing. And at what exact point during labour would one read a book? 'The baby's head is crowning!' 'Don't bother me now, Mr Darcy's just asked Lizzie to marry him.'

info

choosing your childbirth place and team

Even though it seems such a long way off, it's time to start finding out what sort of birth facilities are available to you and thinking about where you'd like to have your baby and who you'd like to help you through the labour. And so begins the search for your birth team and a decision about birth alternatives.

Remember that the choice you have about where to have your baby and how you are cared for will depend to some extent on where you live and what is available in your area. But it is still a choice – yours. There are various options so it's worth getting informed and thinking through what you want.

The three main choices of place for childbirth are home, a birth centre and a hospital. However, some birth options are only available if you have what is called a 'low-risk' pregnancy. Your pregnancy is considered 'high-risk' if, for example, you're going to have a multiple birth, you have a pre-existing condition such as diabetes, you develop a complication during pregnancy such as pre-eclampsia or a baby in the 'breech' position, or you're aged 40 or older.

Birth choices are contentious terrain. Some people argue that because birth can become a medical emergency very quickly, it is crucial to have your baby in a birth centre or hospital – ideally one that can provide an atmosphere you'll feel comfy in, but with specialists and equipment on call. Meanwhile, home birth advocates say that most medical emergencies develop with plenty of warning, and home is a much better (and healthier) place to give birth if you have an uncomplicated pregnancy. Most women look for a safe balance between a comfortable environment and the best care available.

Before you make your own choice, have a good read of this section, discuss the local options with your GP or midwife, and try to talk to other mothers who have had a baby recently, or to your local branch of the NCT (see box in Week 24). You may also like to have a squiz at '"Natural Childbirth" vs Medical Intervention' in Week 31.

hello fatty

KISS ME

fig (A): OBStetRiciaNs to Avoid

home births

If you fancy a home birth, the earlier you start to research your options the better. Mention it to your midwife, or midwife team, early on. The Royal College of Obstetricians officially supports home births for women who are assessed by a senior obstetrician and midwives as having an 'uncomplicated pregnancy', taking into account any relevant medical factors.

This is called a 'low-risk' pregnancy, and is usually applied to healthy women in their twenties or early thirties, especially if they've had a straightforward pregnancy and birth before. Teenagers and older mothers have a statistically higher risk of complications during birth. An uncomplicated pregnancy is no guarantee of an easy birth, but it contributes to a 'low risk'.

If you're given an assessment of low risk, and you request a home birth, it will be scheduled by your midwives. However, because two midwives must attend the birth, if staffing levels don't permit that when you are in labour, you may be re-directed to the hospital. While having two midwives is considered 'best practice', some independent midwives are confident in attending home births alone. (This doesn't come cheap: see the box on private maternity care coming up.)

About three percent of births in England and Wales happen at home. Many more women would like a home birth but choose to be in a more medical environment just in case, or are dissuaded by medical staff who assess them to be a higher risk.

Although up to half of women who planned a home birth end up giving birth in hospital, in most cases the decision is made before labour begins, perhaps because of a complication in their pregnancy, or a lack of available midwives.

The benefits of an uncomplicated home birth are obvious and it's no wonder it's an attractive option for many women. In an ideal world every birth would be like this, without problems, in a comfortable, familiar environment with two medically trained attendants.

Pain relief   Your options for pain relief are much smaller when at home, but if your uncomplicated run continues, anecdotal evidence says you'll be calmer and probably won't need as much. You can't have an epidural because it must be given by an anaesthetist. You may be offered other general painkilling drugs – ask your midwives beforehand what they'll have on hand, and see more on pain relief in Week 32.

Complications and intervention   Advocates of home birth say its calmer atmosphere and philosophy will dictate less need for interventions such as a forceps delivery or an episiotomy (cut at the entrance to the vagina). But many doctors and some midwives dispute these claims, insisting that complications can occur, without warning, that are irrelevant to whether you're at home. These include a drop or irregularity in heartbeart that indicates 'fetal distress', meaning that birth should happen within 30 minutes to avoid possible brain damage to the baby, and the need for an episiotomy or forceps delivery because the timing of the labour is not able to be controlled, or because bub has a big head and shoulders.

Amid the hopeless muddle of available UK statistics, many of them outdated and based on small studies (most without 'control' groups), it seems possible to tentatively say that because most women approved to have a home birth are 'low risk', they tend to do really well. It's in the case of an unforeseen emergency that hospital is the best place to be. The most common reasons for women to be transferred by ambulance in labour are because labour has slowed or stopped, more pain relief is necessary, or there's 'fetal distress'. At the time, the transfer may be a sensible precaution rather than a frightening emergency.

Midwives at home can monitor a baby's heartbeat, and give drugs to reduce the risk of post-partum haemorrhage (when the mother doesn't stop bleeding after the birth), but they have no other specialised equipment or surgical skills. Ambulances and paramedics are also not equipped for any possibility. In a very small minority of births, there may be a need for hospital-only equipment, such as resuscitation equipment, blood transfusions, or immediate access to general anaesthetic and staff prepared for an emergency caesarean.

Many midwives don't like mentioning these possibilities, and I understand that they can sound very scary, and in most cases are extremely unlikely. But I believe that just as women have the right to plan a home birth, they also have a right to know that the worst-case scenario is a lot less worst-case if you are already in hospital. Many midwives say that if a woman needed a blood transfusion, or her baby needed to be delivered very quickly because of 'fetal distress' she would be taken to hospital by ambulance, but time can be critical. The availability of ambulances and journey time from your home to the local hospital may be a consideration: even in an urban setting, from the phone call to being on the operating table will, in reality, probably be at least half an hour.

Ask your midwife to talk frankly with you about the risks and don't rely solely on what you read on websites or in books advocating home birth, as they tend to focus on the positives. And while there is always the possibility of serious complications, remember that they happen to a minority of women and their babies. Don't assume that they'll happen to you.

When plans change   If you do want a home birth but it doesn't work out that way, it's important to remember it's not your fault. Home birth advocates agree that the most important thing is your health, and the safety of the baby. (See Week 31 for lots more on the 'natural birth' vs medical intervention debate.)

birth centres

Birth centres (aka maternity homes or midwife-led units) are often seen as the result of hospitals responding to public demand – as a safer option than giving birth on the bed at home and a more pleasant and natural option than giving birth on a trolley under bright lights in a room that smells like industrial-strength Dettol.

But there's much more to a birth room than a double bed and a potted plant, and you can't assume that an inviting-looking birth centre necessarily means an absence of hospital attitudes. If you are looking at a birth centre with a view to having a more 'natural' birth you should ask about the likelihood of interventions such as rupture of the membranes, fetal monitoring and vaginal examinations during labour, as well as the rate of transfer to the hospital/ obstetric delivery suite for caesareans and other procedures. And find out how crowded the birth centre usually is – mothers in labour could be 'bumped' to a hospital ward if the centre is full. (That way at least you are prepared for the possibility.)

Birth centres may be part of a regular maternity hospital or be a separate unit a few miles from the main hospital. These units are for low-risk care where it looks as if everything is going to be straightforward. In the event of an emergency during labour you may need to be transferred to the main hospital; if the unit is part of the main hospital, then of course emergency facilities are close at hand.

If you have your baby in a birth centre you probably won't be able to have an epidural, but the centre may offer other facilities not available at your local hospital, such as water births and complementary therapies. At a birth centre, your baby can be delivered by your community midwife, by your GP, or by a hospital midwife. The care in the unit tends to be more personal since you will usually be looked after by people you are familiar with. The length of time you will remain in the unit after the birth depends on how well you and your baby are. If you were transferred during labour to the main maternity unit you may find yourself back at the birth centre for a period of rest and recuperation with all the familiar faces around you again before going home.

hospitals

At a hospital birth you'll be attended by whichever midwives and obstetricians are on duty. However, it's important to know that few obstetricians are able to attend an entire birth. They usually pop in and out during labour and are really present only at the end, for the birth, unless something unusual is happening. So your other support people and in particular the midwife team (remember that they operate in shifts) are likely to be just as important.

Large NHS hospitals, because they train staff, often have top specialists available if they are needed and will almost always have anaesthetists on call, which is a big help if surgery is needed quickly or epidural pain relief is required. These hospitals will also sometimes have various students observing at the birth – student midwives, trainee obstetricians and the like. If too many extra bodies in the room gives you the irrits you can tell them to go away.

The labour itself is almost always in a private room, then you're transferred to a ward with other new mums and their babies. Depending on how you and your baby are getting on, you may be able to go home in a matter of hours, or may stay in the hospital for a few days.

If you have decided to have a hospital birth there may be several choices in your area and it might be possible to visit them before making your mind up. Many hospitals have tours especially for parents who are in the early part of pregnancy and wish to look around. When you see the hospital do not be put off by the surroundings and interior decor. Remember it is the people who make the hospital what it is. The attitude of the obstetricians and the midwives towards you and your baby's birth is an important factor in making the experience a rewarding one. Once you have decided on the hospital, ask your GP to write you a letter of referral.

any questions?

Some questions you might like to ask when choosing your place of birth include:

⑥ Would I go to the hospital antenatal clinic for all or just some of my antenatal appointments?

⑥ Does the hospital run antenatal classes?

⑥ Does the hospital offer team midwifery, domino care or case holding schemes (see below)?

⑥ What are my chances of knowing the midwife when I am in labour?

⑥ What are the policies on pain relief, different labour positions, electronic fetal monitoring, episiotomy and forceps delivery?

⑥ Are fathers, relatives or friends welcome in the delivery room?

⑥ Does the hospital encourage women to move around in labour and find their own position for the birth?

⑥ What services are provided for sick babies?

⑥ What is the normal length of stay?

⑥ How do you feel about following my special wishes for the labour? (We'll get on to birth plans in Week 31…)

your antenatal care and birth team

The majority of NHS maternity care is well organised, in defiance of threadbare surroundings and occasionally alarming shortages of staff. Most antenatal care is carried out by midwives, as they are the specialists in normal pregnancy. Should a complication arise you would be referred to the obstetrician. Hospital midwife departments all strive to provide continuity of care throughout your pregnancy, birth and postnatal period. But there is quite a variation in the styles of how they do it. Here are the main ones:

Shared care Shared care is the most common style of hospital care. You see the local community midwife and your GP during your pregnancy and have a hospital midwife attending you at the birth. You may have one or two visits to the hospital obstetrician during the course of your pregnancy. After the birth the same local community midwife would visit you at your home – NHS midwifery care continues for 10 to 28 days after the birth. Ideally this system aims for you to see someone you've come to trust throughout your pregnancy and in the first few weeks after the birth.

Team midwifery, case holding and domino schemes Some hospitals have gone a step further and introduced team midwifery. You are offered care from a team of midwives throughout your pregnancy, labour, and postnatal period. The team of familiar faces should be able to offer you more personalised care and make the whole experience around the time of birth more rewarding.

The two other schemes that aim to offer continuity of care are referred to as 'case holding' or 'domino care'. There are regional variations and these may not be offered in all hospitals. The idea is that the midwife who you have been seeing during your antenatal period attends you at the birth. She may visit you at home during labour, go to hospital with you for the birth, and then see you at home in those first postnatal weeks.

High-risk care If you are having a pregnancy that is described as 'high-risk', you and your baby/babies will need extra attention throughout your pregnancy and during your hospital stay. You may need to see your consultant obstetrician on a more regular basis and possibly other specialists within the hospital. You may still receive shared care and get to know your local midwife but it is unlikely that you will be offered midwifery-only care. You will probably need to have your baby in a hospital.

Your relationship with your GP, midwife and obstetrician is intimate, and dependent on trust, mutual respect and free communication. You'll come to depend on your midwife (or midwives), in particular, over a number of months, from the early days of your pregnancy until the birth and beyond. You will be entrusting them with your life and your child's life. In an ideal situation they will be equal partners with you in the process.

Tell your obstetrician and midwife what sort of birth experience you are hoping for and what sort of patient you are. Say, for example, that you like to have clear explanations given to you about why things are done; or will be needing extra reassurance because your last pregnancy ended in a miscarriage; or want to continue with your alternative health care as well as seeing the obstetrician or midwives.

Wherever you are during your antenatal check-ups – in a doctor's office, a community health clinic, an NHS hospital or a birth centre – it is your right to refuse to allow students to attend consultations or procedures, but remember it is only by attending and participating that they can learn.

PRIVATE MATERNITY CARE

If you can afford it, or you have an insurance policy that covers it, you could book for private obstetric care and see the consultant throughout your pregnancy; they would agree to be present at the birth and may even deliver the baby. Most obstetricians will attend private patients in an NHS hospital, which will help to keep costs down. Or you could go for broke and book into a private maternity hospital, if there is one in your area. However, you should be aware that, as with a birth on the NHS, the obstetrician is unlikely to be in attendance for the whole birth.

Another possibility is hiring an independent, 'freelance' midwife – not a hospital employee – who advises you before the birth, stays with you during the birth, and helps you afterwards with breastfeeding and other issues. (An independent midwife is likely to cost between £1000 and £4000, depending on the care you require.) Having a private midwife gives you the comfort of a chosen and familiar adviser through your pregnancy (including any consultations with an obstetrician) and they will (if all goes well) personally deliver your baby. However, births being the unpredictable things that they are, there is no absolute guarantee of your midwife being available when you go into labour: private midwives tend to work in small groups and provide back-up for each other, so be sure you are comfortable with all members of the team.

Independent midwives can attend home or hospital births. If you are planning on a hospital birth, make sure that the hospital will accept your midwife as your primary carer during the labour (that is, the person who delivers your baby, with the doctor). For legal reasons, all hospitals will insist on the independent midwife having an honorary contract with them. If the hospital does accept the private midwife, then they will be part of a 'shared care' team with your GP and obstetrician, or your hospital.

To find an independent midwife in your area, see under 'Midwives' in the Help section at the back of the book.

Always take your time during visits, perhaps bringing a list of questions from home. If you feel intimidated, patronised or confused by, or at odds with, an obstetrician or midwife, change to somebody else. It may be possible to access fact sheets on the hospital's website, and many offer a telephone helpline to answer questions arising between appointments. Ask about these services.

birth partners and other support people

Birth partner   If you have a partner you'll probably want to have them at the birth. But if your partner isn't keen it may be better to choose somebody who'll be more useful and supportive at the time. Other common support people are sisters and friends. More rarely parents are involved, especially mothers. Don't forget that if you have a long labour it's better for everyone that your support person gets rest breaks or even a bit of shut-eye. They won't have your endorphins, and you don't want them fainting at the wrong moment. (Whatever a right moment is.)

Many people want a record of the event in photos or on video: some even want it shown live on the internet. It can be hard for somebody to be in charge of support, lollies and multimedia at the same time.

Some people invite a cast of thousands, only to regret it later. Don't forget that the people who are actively involved need room to do their work. Some midwives and doctors believe that the more people in the room the longer the birth. Most women don't want to be distracted by visitors or worried about how their small children are coping with what can be a pretty heavy scene for them, let alone whether their lipstick is on straight. (Some birthing places won't even let you wear lipstick – somebody alert *Vogue!*)

Doulas   Some birth centres, as well as some hospitals, allow you to bring a support person to the birth, such as a 'doula' (a medically unqualified birth attendant) or an independent midwife (see box opposite). 'Doula' is the ancient Greek word for head female slave, but the modern idea is that they provide one-on-one support in the antenatal months preparing for birth, during labour and perhaps afterwards. There has been a huge increase in the number of doulas available for hire, and training courses have been set up to accredit doulas. These are so far unregulated. At the time of writing anybody could watch a mail-order 'training video' and call themselves a doula.

If you'd like a doula, getting a recommendation from a like-minded soul is probably better than trying to steer yourself through the tangle of internet ads. You should then check references from several previous clients. Doulas can provide continuity of care and advice about your new baby in those crucial first weeks when you can feel at a bit of a loss. Costs are agreed between the parties but usually run to several hundred pounds.

Some independent midwives who have had nursing training and wide midwifery experience also perform this role for a similar fee.

Many doulas and independent midwives available for private hire will happily attend any kind of birth. Others have very strong ideas about the importance of a 'natural birth' and even suggest that the presence of a doula will guarantee you one (some websites make unsubstantiated claims about doulas lowering the rates of caesareans, episiotomies and painkillers during births). These attendants can become so focused on helping a woman to insist on a natural birth that they can come into opposition with medical advice. As you can imagine, conflict in a difficult birth situation can be very distressing.

Hospital and birth centre policies allow only medical staff to be in control of a birth. A doula or other birth attendant can only give you support: you need to know that in the event of a disagreement they will be automatically overruled by the qualified staff.

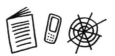

more info on **choosing your childbirth place and team**

nhs.uk

Type 'maternity services' into the search engine, then click 'choosing your maternity service'. At the bottom of the page, enter your postcode and select 'compare services' to get a clearly presented table comparing the different aspects of hospitals and maternity units in your area on a whole range of criteria.

birthchoiceuk.com

Provides a huge quantity of stats about different hospitals around the country – from caesarean rates to women's views about their care and birth experience. Click on 'Maternity statistics' in the left-hand panel. Or click on 'Checklist' for a page that guides you through the whole decision-making process, from deciding on the type of birth you want to finding the right place for that to happen.

Also see 'More Info on "Natural Childbirth" vs Medical Intervention' in Week 31 for info about home births. Some extreme home birth advocates suggest 'freebirthing' as an option – giving birth at home without a medically trained attendant such as a midwife or doctor. This is otherwise universally recognised as too dangerous for you and your baby.

1

2

3

4

5

6

7

8

9

10

11

12

13

14

15

16

17

18

19

20

21

22

Average approximate fetus length this week from head to bum

what's going on
You're hungry. Eat. Your body is doing a lot of work making a person (or two) and you need more fuel than usual.

The embryo becomes a fetus this week. Very few organs are actually working yet, but they're in the right spot. The head is still big in proportion to the rest of the fetus. The nostrils and tear ducts are finished off. (If anybody asks why you're tired, just say you've been building a brain all night long.) Around about now the little tail will 'disappear' as the rest of the fetus grows. The limbs get longer; the arms can bend; hands and feet can touch each other; and toes and fingers lose their webbing and become fully separated. This week's nutty report: the fetus is about the size of a brazil nut. Weight: about 8 grams.

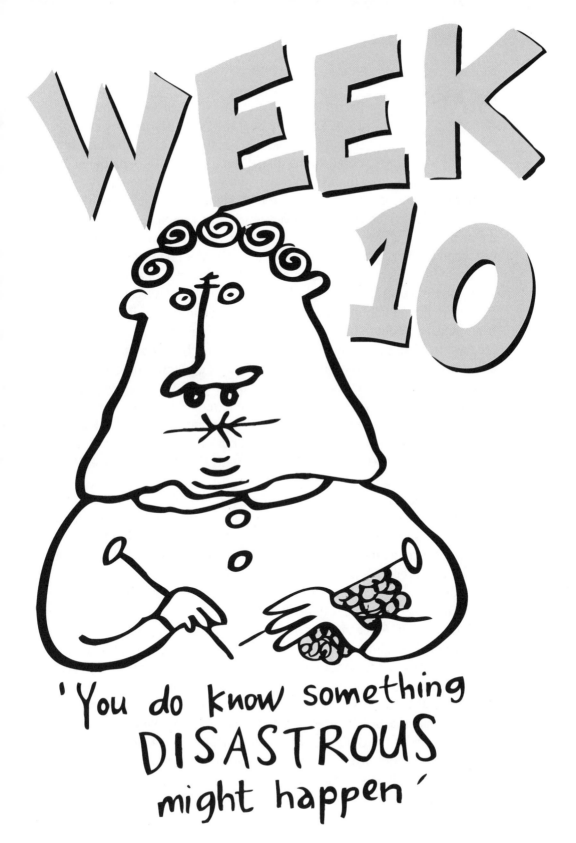

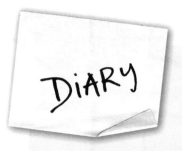

For some reason my sense of smell has become really acute. I can only wear men's aftershaves. Any even slightly girlie, florally scents make me go bleuuuergh. God help me if I get stuck in a lift at a department store.

We're getting closer to the magic, don't-have-to-be-so-scared-about-miscarriage point, so we decide to tell everybody we haven't told. Geoff's parents are thrilled, and send us a lovely email from Pembrokeshire, where they are on assignment investigating rare fungus up some mountain. Aunt Julie is very happy, I think, but it's hard to tell. Aunt Julie cries no matter what happens.

Uncle Mike seems seriously avuncular about the idea of a grand-niece or -nephew. He makes the same joke he does every two months about being glad we're not getting married so he doesn't have to pay for it. 'Oh, we've been thinking about that', Geoff deadpans, which gives him a quick jolt. Meanwhile, Mike's girlfriend Aurelia shrieks, throws herself off her stilettos and onto Geoff, gets coral-coloured lipstick in his eyebrows and ears (she's thorough), and expresses the opinion that a few good thumps never hurt anyone and she hopes we won't be the type to mollycoddle the little bastard. I'm tempted to reassure her that we'll start whacking the living daylights out of it as soon as we see its head coming out, but I find it harder than usual to be jocular about child abuse in my present state. Guess it's those pesky 'baby hormones' the books blame everything on.

Aurelia demands that Uncle Mike take her down to the pub to celebrate. Uncle Mike departs, saying he's very happy for us but he's never changed a nappy in his life and he doesn't intend to start now, bugger it. I think everyone has made their position clear. Five minutes later Uncle Mike comes back to get Aurelia's gold Glo-mesh cigarette case.

'Your mother would have loved this', he whispers. I get tears in my eyes. I've always missed her, but I think I'll feel it more when the baby comes.

Geoff's cousin Annie, mother of six, which is a truly appalling prospect, the one who has spent years asking me when I was going to get pregnant and then, when told to knock it off, asked everyone else in the family every time she saw them, is continuing to be insufferable. She announces loudly and frequently, 'I *knew* you were pregnant!', and has taken to poking me in the stomach and squeezing me on the arm as if I'm a Shetland pony she's buying for one of her children. 'Mmm', she says each time. 'Yes, you're definitely pregnant!' 'No, I just said I was for something to do, you idiot', I feel like saying. Or 'Yes, I had an inkling. I feel pregnant, the tests show I'm pregnant and the doctor says I'm pregnant. But still, thanks for the heads-up.'

Other immediate reactions to 'I'm pregnant' have included:
'You'll never get rid of them!' (60-year-old woman)
'That's wonderful!' (all the nice people I know)
'Your life is over!' (Miss Francine, my beauty therapiste)
Complete silence and choking sound. (my boss)
One of my clients buying the latest range wants me to commit to a fashion conference in Cannes, in September. Cellsie will be four weeks old. 'It will only be for a day and a half', he says. 'You'll be dying to get out and about by then, and reclaim your identity. I mean, I know when we had kids it satisfied my creative urges for a while, but then you really need to reclaim your own space.' Lordy. What a dork.

Aunt Julie has her own take on pregnancy advice. She has been depressed since 1957, but carries about her the air of a wounded martyr delivering vital messages to the Front. Unfortunately now she knows I'm pregnant she has decided the Front is me and the messages must be as tragic as possible. She always has a horrendous story to tell, usually about some dreadful thing that has happened to a small child: left on the beach, flung from a train, attacked by feral guinea pigs – you name it, Aunt Julie can tell you the long version.

'I'm not congratulating Geoff yet, dear,' she announces on the doorstep instead of saying hello, 'in case something goes wrong.'

Tact and optimism are strangers to our Julie. After a few other pleasantries (babies who have been abused, small children murdered by their estranged parents, children with three legs because their mothers drank too much in pregnancy), she bursts into tears and tells me about some friend's daughter who went into early labour after carrying a toddler in a buggy up the stairs in the Tube when the escalators had broken down. 'Promise me', she sobs, looking at me accusingly, 'You're not lifting anything, are you?'

Aunt Julie eventually leaves, temporarily reassured, after pressing some packets of herbs into my hands, neatly labelled with their names. 'Make yourself some tea with these, dear, they're very natural', she confides.

Not bloody likely. After she goes I ring Beck for the herb inside story, and sure enough, one of the herbs is an abortifacient, which means it could abort or deform a developing fetus. Now I have to ring Aunt Julie and tell her to stop being an amateur herbalist around the joint before somebody comes out in hives, loses their hair or snuffs it. (What is it about pregnancy that brings out the amateur doctor or herbalist in people?)

'Your Aunt Julie', says Geoff that night, 'is mad. It probably runs in the family.'
'I prefer to blame everything on hormones', I shout.

info

genes and chromosomes

At conception the egg and sperm join to make a single cell. This one cell, combining 23 chromosomes supplied by Mum (in the egg) and 23 from Dad (in the sperm), contains the entire genetic plan for your child. At that moment, your baby's genetic destiny is decided: what sex it will be, how tall it will be, whether it'll be a naturally good singer, what its skin colour will be, whether its hair will be curly, and maybe what kind of illnesses it will be prone to.

Even though its genetic inheritance comes equally from both parents, a baby will not be an exact 50:50 mix of both parents' characteristics. It may end up with red hair that has 'skipped' a generation, or with a skin that's far more like Dad's than Mum's, or vice versa. Your child may look not much like either parent, but more like long-lost Great-Aunt Agatha (who had a moustache). Some families have genes that always seem to win out, such as distinctive ears. But the son of a footy champion may have inherited his mum's footy genes instead of his dad's. Which genes you inherit from your parents are a matter of random luck.

Your baby will eventually have trillions of cells. Your baby's (and everybody else's) genetic code is stored in a chemical called DNA (deoxyribonucleic acid) that's found in 46 chromosomes inside each of these cells. The DNA contains more than 20,000 genes, which lay the groundwork for your child's unique development. (If you have identical twins the genes will be the same, but the kids will still have their own experiences and develop different personalities

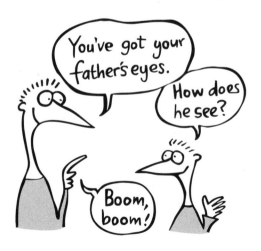

and skills.) Although the DNA blueprint is normally packaged in those 46 chromosomes within a cell, in rare cases there's a chromosome missing, or an extra one, and that can cause change or imbalance in the genetic code.

problems with genes and chromosomes

A 'genetic disorder' – rare in the overall population – is a condition caused by a change in the genetic code. A change can be inherited, or it can occur in the fetus's DNA for the first time.

About four in 100 newborns will have something that's classified as a birth defect. Some abnormalities are heartbreaking and serious, causing a baby to die before it's born or very soon afterwards. But many 'defects' are minor (such as an extra toe, which can be easily removed) and don't cause problems. There are conflicting studies on whether IVF babies are very slightly more likely to have birth defects (perhaps a rise of 2 percent). Research is continuing.

'Dominant disorders' are the most common type of inherited genetic disorder. They are caused by a single strong gene change that can be passed on from parent to child for many generations in a family. An example is Huntington's disease, which usually lies dormant until adolescence or adulthood, when it can cause psychiatric symptoms including the early onset of dementia. Parents who are at risk of having a child with a dominant disorder may have the condition themselves or know of it in their family history. Occasionally a dominant gene change happens in the DNA of a fetus without any family history of the condition (these conditions have to start somewhere).

Some inherited genetic disorders are 'recessive': they happen when both parents carry a change in the gene code. The gene change may not affect either of the parents, and they may not even know they have it, because they also have a second, 'spare' copy of the normal gene; but when a fetus inherits a double dose of the gene change it is affected. An example is cystic fibrosis, which causes chronic lung disease and food absorption problems.

Haemophilia, a bleeding disorder, is a rare hereditary condition linked to the X (female) chromosome, and only causes symptoms after birth if the baby is a boy.

Some inherited genetic disorders are linked to geographic regions or ethnic groups. These include the blood disorder sickle-cell anaemia, which is more likely to be associated with people of African descent, and thalassaemia (more likely in people of Mediterranean, Middle Eastern or Asian family ancestry). The life expectancy of people with these problems is hugely improved compared with years ago, and treatments are available to alleviate many symptoms. (If people in your family have one of these disorders you may find that older members are not aware of these health advances and will tell you unnecessarily worrying stories that are really about how things were in the past.)

If you or your partner has a family history of an inherited genetic disorder, you can be referred to a genetic counsellor for a risk assessment. See the box coming up soon called 'Genetic Counselling'.

In England, Scotland and Wales, screening in the first trimester, which includes a blood test and ultrasound, may be able to identify some specific genetic problems in your fetus. (Genetic screening is not offered on the NHS in Northern Ireland, because it is illegal to terminate a pregnancy except to preserve the life of the mother; if you want the tests you will need to have them at a private clinic.) This can then be confirmed by a diagnostic test, if you choose to take it. The routine tests can't check for every possible genetic problem, but you may be able to request other specific tests if there's a family history of something you're worried about.

down's syndrome

Down's syndrome, also known as trisomy 21, is probably the most well-known chromosomal condition. It's not caused by recessive genes; it's the result of a cell division accident that causes a fetus to inherit three copies of chromosome 21 instead of the usual two.

A child with Down's syndrome will have an intellectual disability (this used to be called 'mentally retarded', a term that is now considered outdated and offensive, but still pops up in some medical conversations and on various websites). He or she will usually have a characteristic appearance that includes distinctive eyes and shorter arms and legs among other things, will be physically slower and less dexterous than other kids, and may also suffer from a large range of medical problems, such as heart defects, that may need corrective surgery. As they grow into adults, people with Down's syndrome are more likely (because of the condition, not lifestyle) to suffer from obesity, heart disease, diabetes and early-onset Alzheimer's disease. Many will be incapable of independent living. Some children with Down's syndrome also have psychiatric or behavioural problems into their teenage years. Most families with Down's syndrome children say their kids are characterised by a gentle and winning nature and a great capacity for affection.

The older you get the more likely you are to be carrying a fetus with Down's syndrome, although about half of all pregnancies with Down's syndrome happen in women under 37, because women under this age make up the majority of the child-bearing population. Here is an approximate calculation of the likelihood according to age, based on UK medical figures:

20-year-old women – one in 1450 pregnancies
29-year-old women – one in 1050 pregnancies
35-year-old women – one in 350 pregnancies
40-year-old women – one in 85 pregnancies
43-year-old women – one in 45 pregnancies

deciding whether to terminate a pregnancy

If Down's syndrome or any other serious disorder is diagnosed early enough most people decide to terminate their pregnancy. Termination is legal in England, Scotland and Wales, with conditions about timing and other details (see 'Termination of Pregnancy' in the Contacts and Resources chapter at the end of the book). If you're living in Northern Ireland and decide on a termination you'll have to travel to a private clinic in another part of the UK or abroad for this. Almost all terminations happen in the first fourteen weeks.

Termination may not be the right decision for you. People who are sure they wouldn't choose it usually decide not to have the relevant tests. Others want the tests so that they can prepare, mentally and otherwise, for a child with special needs. They may also want to know because a pregnancy that involves a fetus with a genetic disorder may have a higher risk of ending in miscarriage or of the baby dying soon after birth.

Some people feel sure they can make a happy family with their child and they are confident they can arrange for the child's ongoing care, even after they are gone. Some have religious objections to pregnancy termination for any reason.

Others feel they will be unable to cope with, or do not want their child to have to deal with, the medical problems associated with a serious genetic condition: the quality of life for a child with Down's syndrome, for example, is hard to predict because the extent of mental disability and physical and other problems isn't known until after birth. Some people, especially those who are in their late thirties or forties, acknowledge they won't always be able to care for a child who grows into an adult and do not want to pass that responsibility to their other children. Some women who anticipate being a sole parent, or who have no family support, feel especially concerned about the future.

The diagnosis of a serious fetal genetic disorder is very confronting. Decisions are entirely personal: they must be made by the individuals

GENETIC COUNSELLING

Genetic counsellors can give you an accurate picture of the likely risk of having a baby with a hereditary disorder, narrowing down your chances in the lottery of life. Depending on the condition, if both parents carry the gene their statistical chances of having a baby with that condition could be, say, one in four, or one in twelve or more. Counsellors can tell you if you and your partner carry a recessive gene that could cause a certain disorder, and very often reassure you that the chances of a problem are very low. If you've already had a child with a disorder, genetic counsellors may be able to predict your chances of it happening again.

The information genetic counsellors use can include blood tests, an examination of both families' medical history, and genetic analysis based on the known risks of passing on individual disorders. If you don't have access to the man's family history because you don't know who he is or he is uncooperative, you can still have your own risk assessed.

Your GP, obstetrician or midwife can refer you to a genetic counsellor for any of the following reasons (but referral is not automatic so if you've got any worries ask for one):

- you or your partner or a member of either family was born with a congenital abnormality
- you or your partner has a family history of inherited physical or psychiatric disease (although psychiatric problems are not automatically passed on from parents – and in fact the risk can be extremely low)
- blood tests have shown that one partner or both carries a genetic disorder (these tests usually have to be requested)
- you've had several miscarriages (a genetic disorder can cause a miscarriage, but is not always the reason for miscarriage)
- you've already had a baby with a chromosomal or genetic problem
- you've had a baby who died before or shortly after the birth, especially if the baby was not normally formed
- you've had a diagnostic test that confirmed a chromosomal abnormality in the fetus
- you and your partner are related (cousins, for example).

concerned, who will make the decision that is right for them. The decision to terminate is never easy. Neither is it easy to decide to transform your and your other children's lives with the addition of a child who will always have special needs and take much of the family's energy and attention. Many parents in this situation feel that they have only two lousy options. Whichever one they take, their decision is not open to the judgements of others.

Many people who do decide to terminate opt for privacy, telling people they 'lost their baby', or referring to a 'miscarriage', rather than explaining further. Everyone who makes this decision is sad about it and may continue to grieve, even if they are sure it was the right thing for them.

Regardless of what you decided, please, if you are feeling guilty or self-blaming, or you're feeling inconsolable or confused, talk to a counsellor. Your doctor can refer you. Sometimes these feelings are based on incorrect information, which can include the false belief that the genetic problem was caused by something you did wrong, or that pregnancy termination will automatically damage your ability to get pregnant again.

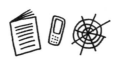

more info on genetic issues

Make sure your info is up to date, and that you consult the newest edition of a book, pamphlet or fact sheet or a frequently updated website. There is new medical info in this area all the time. It's also important to see the 'More Info on Screening and Diagnostic Tests' in the next chapter, Week 11. You may want to talk to a professional counsellor: ask your GP for a referral or see 'Grief and Loss' in the Contacts and Resources chapter at the end of the book.

downs-syndrome.org.uk
The website of this national charity takes a positive but honest attitude to living with Down's syndrome. Click 'Resources' then 'Publications' for downloadable booklets on a range of topics, including advice for expectant parents and information about the educational and health difficulties a child with Down's syndrome is likely to face. For support groups, click 'Contact us' then 'Local support groups'.
Helpline: 0845 230 0372

Average approximate fetus length this week from head to bum

1

2

3

4

5

6

7

8

9

10

11

12

13

14

15

16

17

18

19

20

21

22

what's going on Nausea should start to

settle down from now on. Hurrah.

Outside influences, such as certain drugs and

chemicals, could have damaged the fetus while it was still

forming; the dangers are still there after week 10, but are no

longer so acute. (This does not mean you can get on

the vodka.) The placenta is continuing to get bigger,

keeping pace with what the fetus needs. The

completely formed heart is pumping away.

The ear and hearing structures are nearly

finished and ready to grow. Your fetus is

looking a lot more like a tiny human

with a big head, short limbs and not much

clothes sense. (In fact about now the head

is almost half the size of the whole fetus.)

Weight: about 10 grams.

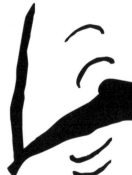

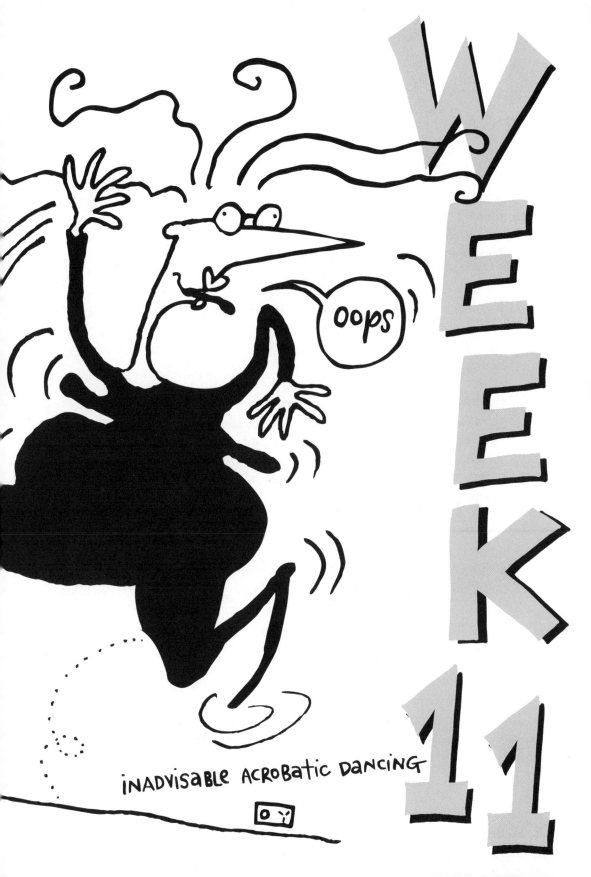

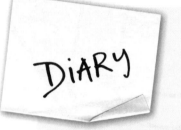

DiARY

I've been lent a lot of baby-care books for the duration. One is Aunt Julie's decrepit second-hand copy of child-raising 'expert' Dr Spock from approximately the Jurassic Period, which she immediately borrowed after Mum died to work out what she and Uncle Mike should do with this small creature (me) suddenly on their doorstep.

I fancied a look at some pregnancy and childcare books, but I discovered most of them are absolutely shocking. For one thing, they're always banging on about husbands as if every pregnant woman had to have one. Mind you it's not just insulting to the single mother-to-be. The blokes don't come out of it well either. One book actually recommends that you teach 'your husband' to make his own breakfast before you go to hospital: say, by week 32 to be sure. If a bloke doesn't know how to make his own breakfast, I say you're better off without him.

It's kind of comforting that even the experts disagree – this means you don't have to get worried if you're not at exactly the stage a book reckons you should be. On almost every major yardstick I'm not. And quite frankly I don't expect to have a multiple orgasm the first time I breastfeed.

Even some of the good books have the most absurd photographs to enliven their pages. Under the section on nutrition or appetite there is usually a photograph of a woman with a plate of food, in case you have forgotten what a plate of food looks like.

And I don't wish to be rude, but I'd like all the people who have done illustrations for pregnancy books rounded up and killed. They can't be allowed to go on. Who ARE all these women in the illustrations, pale-as-pastry, frumpy, with disgusting haircuts, wearing duvet covers? And who are these husbands looking manfully into the distance with gigantic sideburns? They are the line-drawing equivalents of knitting-pattern photos from the 1970s. With captions like 'A new father can bottlefeed a baby'. Yes, and given half a chance he can tie his own shoelaces, and all.

One book has four filthy drawings of bright pink couples 'making love' during pregnancy, in different positions. In the first position they look bored. In the second position they look like they've had a lobotomy. In the third they look really smug, and in number four, I don't know how this is quite conveyed, but I'm pretty sure they were singing 'Michael Row the Boat Ashore'.

Another book, called *A Child Is Born*, has graphic photos of the fetus in the uterus. It's disgusting. Geoff reads it every night. He's fascinated by the pictures. They make me want to projectile vomit.

'Look, that's what Cellsie looks like now.'

I scream and hide under the sheets. 'That looks like a prawn made of snot!'

'But it's amazing. Look at this one – this is what it'll be like next week.'

Great. A portion of especially dumb plankton, with eyes like ball bearings. I cannot relate to this. It is a greater test of maternal instincts than anyone should have to undergo. Nobody could love a snot prawn. How can I bond with a crustacean?

There really is too much information in these books, and yet not enough. For example, 'Acrobatic dancing is, of course, unwise at any stage during pregnancy'. How acrobatic? Are we talking those circus girls who can put their head up their own bum? Do we refer here to the sort of wafty, Stevie-Nicks-type hippie dancing while waving shawls? Which is surely ultimately more offensive and therefore more dangerous than the lesser-known acrobatic dancing. Perhaps it means chandelier work.

And personally I cannot take anybody seriously who uses the word 'brassiere' in a complete sentence. Especially if the sentence is 'The advantage of having a well-made and properly fitted brassiere cannot be emphasised too strongly'. Certainly not, Mrs Shelf-Bosom. Emphasise away, and mind you don't take my eye out.

One of the books, by Miriam Stoppard, has an entire section devoted to how to wear make-up during pregnancy (on your face, I presume). Anyway, there are handy hints such as how to cover up dark circles under the eyes, and camouflage puffiness by shading a little brown blusher subtly beneath the jawbone and on either side of the neck. Look, this might work if you are standing still, being professionally lit and photographed, but if you're walking around like a normal human being no amount of brown blusher on your neck is going to disguise the fact that you're a bit puffy.

You would be better off constantly introducing yourself to people by saying 'Hello, I'm a bit puffy. It's because I'm up the duff and a big fat baby is going to come out of my vagina', and getting on with things. I can guarantee nobody will mention any puffiness after that. Not to your face anyway. Here's a great pregnancy make-up hint: 'To draw attention away from your jawline, try using a blusher at the temples so that your eyes become the focus'. Or, say, wear a hat with a rotating stuffed zebra leg on it.

info

screening and diagnostic tests

Screening tests are offered to all pregnant women to check that their fetus is growing and developing normally. Most women choose to have the tests – and the vast majority are given the all-clear – although some don't because they would never consider termination. (And note that screening for Down's syndrome is not offered on the NHS in Northern Ireland, because you wouldn't be allowed to have a termination there if Down's syndrome was diagnosed.) The combined results of an ultrasound and a blood test will give you the risk factor of carrying a fetus with Down's syndrome (explained in 'Genes and Chromosomes' in the previous chapter, Week 10). The tests can't show every current or possible future problem (for example, there's no test for autism).

If there's something in your first routine screening results that shows you have a higher risk of a problem, your doctor may recommend you have another, more invasive test, which should be able to give you a definite yes or no diagnosis.

Having the screening and diagnostic tests at the right time is crucial because they must be done at very specific points in the fetus's development. To get the timing right you need to identify the first day of the last period you had as the beginning of the first week of your pregnancy, and count from there. Ask your doctor or midwife if you're confused. Some hospitals offer an early dating scan at eight weeks or soon after: if you have one of these, that will confirm your dates.

It can be stressful waiting for results, even though by far the most likely outcome is that everything's fine. If you do get a result that's worrying or unexpected, you'll be offered help so that you have as many options as possible when deciding what to do next.

REMINDER: BOOK YOUR SCREENING TESTS NOW

You should already have an appointment for your nuchal scan (see opposite), which needs to happen between the start of next week and the end of week 14. If you haven't, call your GP or midwife now and make sure you get booked in. Check whether you need a separate appointment for the blood test. This chapter explains why the timing of these screening tests is crucial.

ORDER OF ROUTINE SCREENING TESTS

FIRST TRIMESTER
From start of week 12 to end of week 14 but ideally right at the start of week 13 – 'combined test' for Down's syndrome (nuchal scan and blood test)

SECOND TRIMESTER
From start of week 16 to end of week 21 – blood test (only if you missed the 'combined test' above)
From start of week 19 to end of week 21 – anomaly scan

All these tests are fully explained in this chapter.

first trimester screening

Nuchal scan The 'nuchal scan' (or 'nuchal translucency scan') is the first part of the Down's syndrome screening test. You may hear it referred to as the first trimester ultrasound, but that makes it seem as if it can be done at any time within that period. In fact it needs to be done during weeks 12 to 14. For best results, the scan should be right at the start of week 13 or as close as you can get it.

The ultrasound operator's main task is to check the width of the 'nuchal translucency', a layer of fluid on the back of the neck of every fetus, which is only measurable during weeks 12 to 14, with the best view usually at the start of week 13. If this feature is much wider or thicker than normal, it indicates an increased risk of Down's syndrome.

If you've not already had a separate scan to confirm your dates, this ultrasound will also be the first opportunity to check whether you're carrying more than one fetus, and if your 'due date' needs to be revised (the box coming up has all the info on what happens at ultrasounds).

Blood test This is also called the 'maternal serum screening'. The test is done at the time of your nuchal scan. They just take a small sample from a vein in your arm.

Combined first trimester screening results The results of the blood test and nuchal scan will be combined with your age to

HAVING AN ULTRASOUND

An ultrasound scan doesn't hurt you or the fetus. It's a way of seeing what's going on inside your uterus without going in there. Ultrasound operators (technically known as sonographers) measure various lengths and sizes at the precise times that give them the best view of the developmental characteristics they want to check (that is, at the start of week 13 for the nuchal scan, and weeks 19–21 for the anomaly scan in the second trimester).

Who does it? Your ultrasound will be done by a sonographer who is trained and experienced in pregnancy scanning (rather than one who usually does general ultrasound scans on, say, footballers' knees).

How is it done? The sonographer pulses sound rays into your uterus, which bounce back when they run into something solid (such as the fetus) and this is used to create an image on a computer or TV-like screen. The ultrasound is done while you're lying down. The sonographer puts some lubricating jelly on your tum and then moves a device around on your skin. It's as if your tummy is the mouse mat for a computer, and the sonographer is using the mouse.

Some ultrasounds (especially early ones) are done vaginally: the sonographer inserts a probe (*such* a charming name) about the size of a large pen, with a bulb-shape on the end, into your vagina and points it up towards the uterus. It doesn't hurt, but while your knees are akimbo it's probably not something you'd want the neighbours to get a glimpse of.

What will you see? At times the sonographer will freeze the image on the screen to make a measurement or observation, and will usually tell you what they're seeing and what it means. Ask them any specific questions you have.

As well as checking the 'nuchal translucency' (see the previous page), the nuchal scan is often the happy moment when you first see your fetus. At this stage sonographers can see general rather than subtle things because the fetus is still so little. They can't give you a 100 percent all-clear but will probably say things like 'Everything's looking nice and normal'.

Depending on the fetus's position, a skilled sonographer should be able to have a go at guessing the gender. So if you don't want them to blurt out 'I'm 80 to 85 percent certain this one's grown a willy' or 'It's a girlie!', tell them before the test that you don't want to know yet. And if you do want to know remember that it's only a good guess, never a certainty. At week 13 boys and girls have a similar-looking bit that will develop into either a penis or a clitoris; it points up in boys and down in girls but can be hard to see. So don't let Nanna knit seventeen pink jumpers yet.

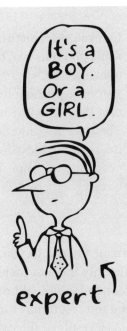

It can be a bit spooky seeing your fetus at week 13. You will probably be able to see a tiny heart beating, a see-through brain inside a skull, and the fishbone lines of a spine. A front-on view of the face shows big eye sockets and a gaunt face like a classic Hollywood alien. Remember that the image on the screen probably isn't life-size – it's likely to be greatly enlarged. Ask the sonographer to show you how big the fetus really is.

By the time of the anomaly scan in the second trimester, the sonographer will be able to see much more detail because your wee fetus has grown so much in the roughly seven weeks between scans. Again, they will be checking 'bits': they need to see bones (because they're checking the spine for neural tube defects), images of the baby at various close-up angles, including the face and heart, and where the placenta is. Because the sonographer is measuring and checking for specific things you may not get a good view of the baby as a whole. And if you do, it will still look more fetusy than babyish. All the same, it's probably fun to have another sneak peek into the womb and to say hi to your little alien. Remind your sonographer if you don't want to know the sex.

Who else can go? Because an ultrasound is a medical procedure that can involve lower-half nudity and a vaginal probe, with the rare possibility of unwelcome news, you may like to reconsider having a guest list. It's usually best to take just your partner or main support person, not a bunch of rellies who are excited about 'seeing the baby' (and who may not be aware that medical ultrasounds are not the documentary-style videos of near-term babies they've seen on the telly). If you're pressured, stand firm and promise pictures later. ▶

Can you get a picture? In most cases the sonographer will be able to give you a photo to take home with you, for a small fee. Remember to ask when booking.

Some private ultrasound clinics offer very expensive '3D' or '4D' scans of a baby (4D just means a moving picture), usually at around 29 weeks. These are for entertainment value only – don't expect any useful medical information. Most doctors are reluctant to have patients undertake a medical procedure for a non-medical reason. It's also possible that the fetus may not be in a good position for the photo or video, but you'll still have to pay.

calculate the risk of your fetus having Down's syndrome. This is the best way to identify the vast majority of high-risk cases. It does not specifically check for anything else, although a skilled ultrasound operator and a suspicious blood test result may turn up other problems.

As a result of the calculation, 3 percent of parents are told they have an 'increased risk' of carrying a fetus with Down's syndrome. Even if you're told this, by far the most likely outcome is still that your fetus doesn't have Down's syndrome. And somebody with a 'low-risk' assessment – for example, a young woman with an estimated risk of one in 1000 – could still be carrying a fetus with Down's syndrome because she could be that one in 1000.

Because most people who are told they have an increased risk want a firm yes or no answer to 'Does my fetus have Down's syndrome?' they choose to go on to have a diagnostic test to get a definite answer.

diagnostic tests: chorionic villus sampling and amniocentesis

We'll call them CVS and 'amnio' for short. These are diagnostic tests for chromosomal defects including Down's syndrome and – if they are being looked out for because of a genetic history – some rare serious disorders and disabilities, including cystic fibrosis. If Down's syndrome is ruled out by one of these tests there may be another reason why an increased nuchal translucency has been seen at your nuchal scan, which you may need to have investigated. (The box opposite explains what happens during each test.)

Either CVS or amnio is usually offered if:

◎ you've been told you have an increased risk of having a child with Down's syndrome, most often because of the combined result of the nuchal scan and blood test

◎ there's a known genetic condition in one of the families.

HAVING CVS OR AMNIO

Both procedures involve using a syringe to take some of the fetus's own genetic material – not from the baby itself, but by drawing out cells from the placenta (if it's CVS) or the amniotic fluid (in the case of amniocentesis). These cells are then sent for analysis. Results can take a couple of weeks, but DNA tests are now available on the NHS that give a result in a day or two.

Who does it? These tests are done by specialist obstetricians. Their level of experience is very important. I know everyone has to learn somehow, but if I were having one of these tests I would want to know that the doctor had already done hundreds.

What happens? For the procedure you lie down and the specialist uses an ultrasound to see the position of the fetus in the uterus. A needle is pushed through your tummy into the uterus, where it takes up a sample from the amniotic fluid or the placenta. (CVS can also be done through the vagina.) Just so you're prepared: amniotic fluid is yellow. The needle does not touch the fetus, as both can be seen on the ultrasound screen by the doctor during the procedure.

What happens afterwards? Having these medical procedures can be stressful. If you have preschool-aged kids somebody else needs to look after them for the day of the procedure. You will need to take special care of yourself afterwards, and avoid strenuous activity for a couple of days – it's a good excuse to lie on the couch, waving the remote, for a day or two.

The upside of the tests is that they're very accurate because they sample the fetus's own DNA, so you get a definite result. One downside is that both procedures carry a small increased risk of you miscarrying (about one in 100 for CVS and one in 200 for amnio, above the general miscarriage risk). Another drawback is that neither test can check for every possible problem. All women who undergo these tests are offered information and genetic counselling, at which partners are also welcome.

CVS should usually be done between week 11 and week 13 and shouldn't be done before week 10, to minimise possible damage to the fetus. Amnio should wait until after week 15 to avoid the procedure taking too much, or causing a leak, of the amniotic fluid needed to cushion the fetus. (These invasive tests will become obsolete when researchers figure out how to get the fetus's DNA information just by testing its mother's blood sample or cells from the cervix taken in a smear test. A one-off blood test is being researched, but it is not yet ready or available.)

The tests are probably not for you if you're certain you wouldn't terminate a pregnancy under any circumstances; if you don't want to be warned about a special-needs child on the way; or if you don't want to increase your risk of miscarriage by even a very small margin in order to get a definitive diagnosis.

second trimester screening

Weeks 16–21 blood test You don't need this second trimester maternal serum screening if you had the 'combined test' in your first trimester. Most women who have it didn't know they were pregnant until later on, or got their dates wrong, and so missed the window of opportunity for the 'combined test'. Blood for this test must be taken between the start of week 16 and the end of week 21. The test screens for Down's syndrome, some other chromosomal problems, and neural tube defects including spina bifida.

Anomaly scan Although this ultrasound scan can be taken any time during weeks 19 to 21, bang on the start of week 20 is often recommended. It's said that good images are taken in week 19 if a woman is slim, or week 21 for a larger lady.

The scan checks on the fetus's progress and for any developmental abnormalities. Finding a problem that is correctable after birth (such as a cleft lip) means parents have time to prepare themselves and organise the treatment. Finding a very serious problem at this stage can mean, for some people, a late-term pregnancy termination. Such problems are very rare.

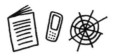

more info on **screening and diagnostic tests**

fetalanomaly.screening.nhs.uk

The website of the NHS Fetal Anomaly Screening Programme. Click on 'Explanation of the tests' for online information about ultrasounds, maternal serum screening, amniocentesis and CVS, or 'Information leaflets' for more detailed information in downloadable booklet form.

arc-uk.org

Helpline: 020 7631 0285

ARC (Antenatal Results and Choices) is a charity dedicated to supporting parents through the antenatal testing process with information and impartial advice about the tests and your options if a problem is detected. Click on 'Tests explained' for what to expect and how to interpret your result. Under 'Need help' there are pages of advice on both termination and continuing your pregnancy, as well as details of support networks and organisations related to specific conditions.

Also see the 'More Info on Genetic Issues' section at the end of the previous chapter, Week 10.

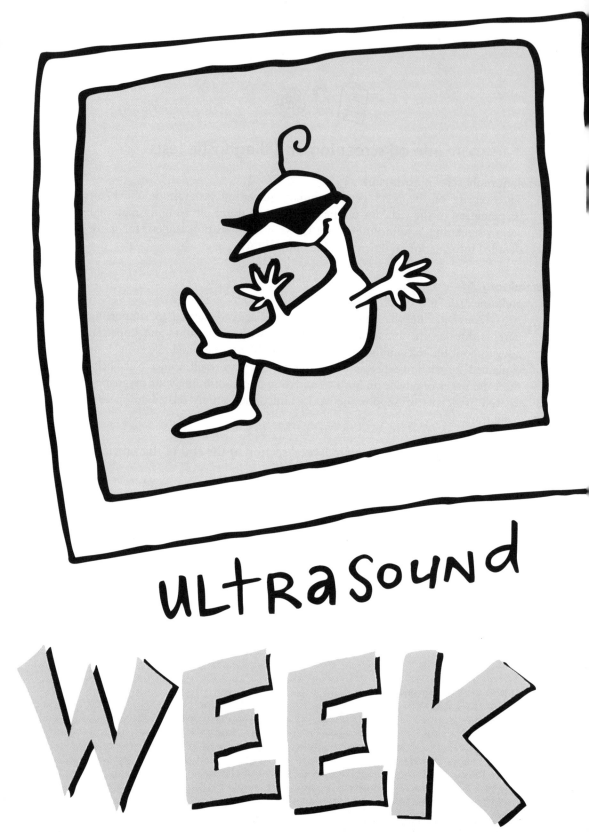

ultrasound
WEEK

what's going on You may be feeling very tired – after all, you're not just a fascinating, sophisticated minx any more, you're a walking host organ. Inside, your fetus looks more like a baby but with the head still bent forward. The face has a human profile and the jaw hides twenty developing tooth buds. Muscles are growing and increasing the movement of the fetus, but you still can't feel it because it has plenty of room to slosh about in the amniotic fluid without touching the sides. As it has been doing since week 5, the placenta is routinely sending oxygen and nutrients down the vein of the umbilical cord, and taking away waste such as fetal wee, which travels up the two arteries in the cord. Weight: about 18 grams.

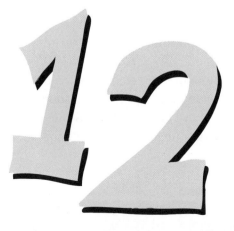

I'm not sure but I think some of my wrinkles – sorry, I mean character lines – are less obvious. This is because fluid retention is puffing them out – take that, cosmetic companies!

Most of my daily thoughts consist only of the following mantra: 'I have no interest in food, I cannot cook, I must lie down, I need to watch crap on television, would you get a load of Oprah's hairdo. Help me. I can't get off the sofa.' It's all just too, too exhausting. If only I was the sort of person with four servants and a heart-shaped box of chocolates and a four-poster bed with a quilted-satin duvet cover, it would probably all look quite glamorous. I could have a negligee and a peignoir, and other French words for jarmies.

I go for the nuchal scan. This is an ultrasound scan that checks for a thickening at the back of the baby's neck, which is an indicator of Down's syndrome. Geoff comes for a look. The sonographer, Tania, specialises in pregnancy ultrasound, which is comforting. I'm glad she looks at fetussy things most of the time, and not footballers' knees. She pokes around to get Cellsie in the right position by pushing hard on my tummy, and I really don't feel good about this.

There's Cellsie on the screen, waving its wee bits.

'There's your baby', says Tania.

'It's not, it's a Christmas beetle', I retort, looking at an insecty shape stuck on its back and wiggling a lot of little legs in the air.

'Look, it's waving', she says, pointing out a head, two arms and two legs.

The head seems to turn towards us, showing black, almond-shaped eyes in a triangle face, like something out of an alien movie.

'Oh fuck, that's too weird', I say and nobody answers.

It occurs to me that you're not supposed to say fuck during an ultrasound. Repeat after me: Mummies ought not to say fuck. Sigh. So much to learn.

The creature on the screen looks like any sort of fetus. It could grow into a lizard, or a lap-dance club owner, or something equally hideous. And even though inside me it's actually only about five centimetres long, on the screen it looks as long as an adult hand. This is very disconcerting. Makes it seem more advanced and less human at the same time.

Suddenly the heartbeat monitor at the bottom of the screen shows an up-and-downie, mountain-shaped graph running along merrily – and the sound! Like a Latin techno beat! The fastest heartbeat I have ever heard. Looking closer, we can see the heart actually beating inside the lizardy thing. I begin to feel quite fond of it.

'That's not my heartbeat is it?' I ask. 'Because if it is, I think I'm having a heart attack.'

Tania says a fetus's heartbeat is so fast because its brain hasn't developed enough yet to slow it down. She says it's quite normal. Everything is normal. Size, normal. Shape, normal. All bits present so far. Normal. Normal, normal, normal.

Normal? I want to sneer. I've spent my whole life running away from normal. I don't DO normal. I refuse to live in the suburbs. I want to be special, I want to be interesting, I want ... Okay, it's kind of reassuring that everything's normal. I'll admit it. You don't want to hear an ultrasound operator saying 'What the...?', 'That can't BE!' or 'Holy catfish! I've never seen that before. Do you mind if I call some friends to come over and have a look?'

Tania explains that her report will be combined with my week 11 blood test to give an official result on the Down's syndrome question, but everything looks good and we shouldn't worry.

We leave, and I surprise myself by bursting into tears. For some reason I feel great indignation at Cellsie being unceremoniously poked into a better position. I guess the baby must be starting to feel more real. I didn't expect to feel protective of my little space prawn.

I have started to wrestle with constipation: I decide to adopt Beck's secret seed-breakfast method. Every time I get constipated I get at least one spot, probably two. But after a day or two of crushed mixed seeds on my muesli, I'm running like a train again and zit-free.

info

pregnancy hormones

Every time you mention a symptom of pregnancy – from bigger breasts to being grumpy, to wanting an ice cream, to feeling unspecific morbid dread, to wanting to stand on the roof and shriek – somebody will say in tones of enormously ponderous knowledge, 'It's the pregnancy hormones.' Well, what exactly are the pregnancy hormones, and which ones do what? After all, it's not as if those medical professors sit around at university and in hospital

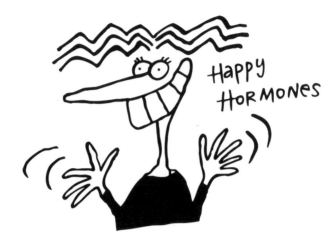

meeting rooms going, 'Ooh, you know, pet, pregnancy hormones, whatever they're called.' At least I hope not. Many of the pregnancy hormones are produced by the placenta, the organ inside the uterus that sustains the developing baby through the umbilical cord. This is kind of a neat trick as the placenta comes out just after your baby does, right when you won't need those hormones any more.

◎ **Endorphins**, which mimic the effects of morphine and help blunt perceptions of pain and stress, are hormones produced by the brain up until and during childbirth. After the birth the levels drop sharply. This has been implicated in the temporary 'baby blues' most new mothers experience, and the more lasting feelings of depression that sometimes follow as your 'happy hormones' are switched off.

◎ **Human chorionic gonadotrophin (HCG)**, the 'thin blue line' hormone, triggers a 'positive' result in pregnancy wee tests. A high level during the first three months is one of the suspected reasons for nausea. HCG stimulates the ovaries to produce more progesterone, which in turn shuts down the monthly period department for the duration of the pregnancy.

◎ **Human placental lactogen (HPL)** is the name for the 'Oh my God, look at these bazoombas' hormones needed for milk production – prolactin, oestrogen and progesterone. HPL is responsible for enlarging the breasts and for the secretion of colostrum, the 'pre-milk' or 'practising milk' which may leak from your nipples from about the fifth month (or not) and is produced for the first few days after the birth.

◎ **Melanocyte-stimulating hormone (MSH)** is the 'colouring-in' hormone. In the later months of pregnancy, high levels of MSH can make your nipples darken, and can cause dark patches on your face and a dark vertical line down the middle of your tummy called the linea nigra (Latin for 'black line').

◎ **Progesterone**, one of the big two girlie hormones, affects every aspect of pregnancy. It's produced by the ovaries when you're not pregnant, but eventually the placenta takes over the task during pregnancy. It relaxes smooth muscle: in the uterus so it's less likely to contract and cause miscarriage, and in the bladder, intestines, bowel and veins so they're more flexible as they're squashed by the growing uterus. It increases your body temperature and breathing rate, causes dilated blood vessels, which can reduce blood pressure and make you feel faint and nauseated, and helps produce breast milk. Immediately after the birth, the level drops and continues to drop for a number of days.

◎ **Oestrogen**, the other major girlie hormone (or, more correctly, group of oestrogens), is also produced by the ovaries and then the placenta during pregnancy. Oestrogen helps make everything in the reproductive department behave as it should throughout the pregnancy, including the breasts (enlarging nipples and developing milk glands), the uterus (strengthening it) and body tissue (softening it). Many believe that excess oestrogen causes nausea in the first three months. As with progesterone, the relatively high level of oestrogen drops immediately after the birth, and continues to drop in the days that follow.

◎ **Oxytocin** is the squeezer hormone: it stimulates the practice (Braxton Hicks) contractions of the uterus and the contractions of childbirth. Injections of this hormone can be used to induce labour and to expel the placenta.

◎ **Relaxin**, the 'hang loose' pregnancy hormone, makes ligaments and tissues soften up and become more elastic, which provides the increased flexibility in the joints of the pelvis and back needed for labour. It may also contribute to the 'waddle' of later pregnancy. (The other contributing factor being that you've turned into a giant wombat.)

WEEK 13

what's going on Soon your tummy may start to 'show' – 'pop out' – and everyone will begin noticing. Any nausea will probably stop or begin to trail off about now.

Down in fetusland, reflexes for sucking, swallowing and breathing have begun. The amniotic sac surrounding the fetus is full of 100 millilitres of amniotic fluid – a fully appointed unit with lots of room still to bob around in. The ears are finished but can't hear yet. The lungs, liver, kidneys and digestive bits are still maturing. The head has been growing more slowly than the body since week 11. By the end of this week all those organs and limbs in place are ready to grow and be fine-tuned. But the fetus can't survive on its own because the organs wouldn't function well enough. Weight: about 30 grams.

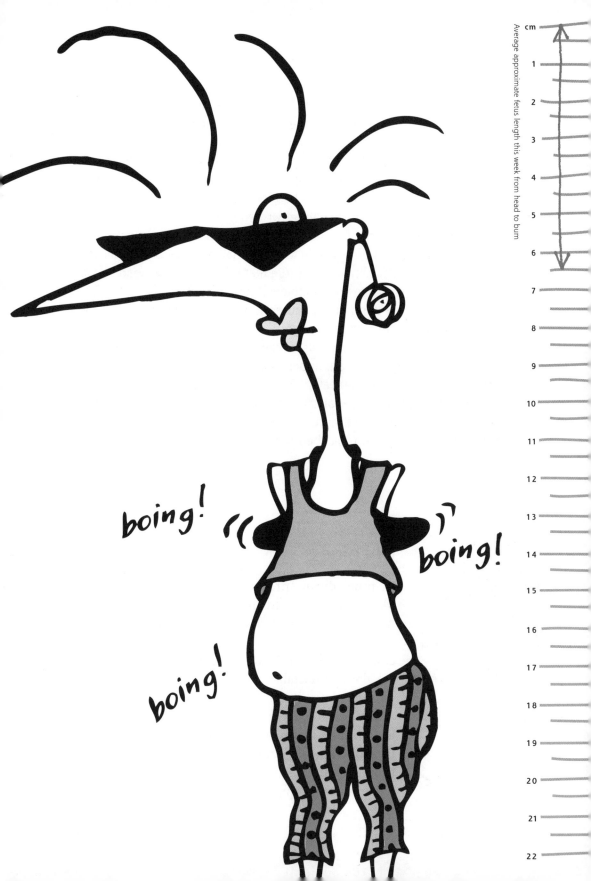

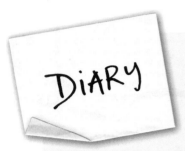

I am soooo grumpy. All I want is an extensive personal staff to clean the house, fluff the pillows, cook my dinner and suck up to me. I have injured myself by sneezing in the middle of a yoga stretch. It felt like I tore through muscles or ligaments on each side of my tummy, down low near the hip bones. Bloody exercise: it's bad for you.

And there is far too much palaver written these days about balanced meals for the pregnant woman. A perfectly nutritious and attractive meal can be had by eating three pieces of Vegemite toast and half a packet of milk chocolate in seven seconds flat. Although it is true that I'd probably be dead if I wasn't taking my pregnancy vitamin and mineral supplement thingy.

It's the weirdest thing being nauseous and getting no fun out of food, but still feeding your face relentlessly.

My gums keep bleeding. This is obviously some sort of design fault. Again, many of the books are hopeless, presuming the 'mother-to-be' has the brain of the average anteater: 'The baby hormones may be making your gums bleed. Take special care with dental hygiene.' I always lose consciousness at about the word 'hygiene'. Beck suggests a bit more vitamin C and that seems to help. Maybe I just had scurvy.

info

weepiness

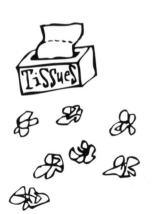

At times during pregnancy you can feel ecstatic, elated, like a fertile winged mythical love goddess (well, okay, maybe not), contented, confident, optimistic and relaxed. But you can also feel depressed, terrified, worried, tense, crabby, moody and like a blundering water buffalo. Tears are almost inevitable.

Sometimes it can seem that you're on a hair-trigger. Anything can suddenly set you off: sad movies or news stories about things that happen to babies or mothers. The rest of the world goes on despite your pregnancy, and with a bit of bad luck yours might coincide with a relationship break-up, other personal complications, or a death in the family.

Even without extra stress, you can feel miserable, especially during the first trimester when your hormones seem to be stuck on the spin-cycle. Maybe you recognise some of the symptoms from PMS (premenstrual syndrome). About 10 percent of women have mild to moderate depression while pregnant.

Your moodiness might be manifested by you being cranky and overcritical; or flying into a rage or panic about something that isn't really so important; or crying for no specific reason. Or when you see a puppy.

Thinking about pregnancy and becoming a parent can bring up unresolved issues you may have with your own mother and father, or sadness or anger about your own childhood. And it's natural to feel ambivalent about being pregnant, worry about many aspects of pregnancy and parenting, and grieve for a lifestyle lost. Some of these feelings were mentioned in Week 7, but let's play another round of Scary Questions (and Reassuring Answers – which is much more fun). Your continuing pregnancy worries can include (but are not strictly limited to) the following.

Will my baby be born healthy and 'normal'? (Very probably.)

Do I deserve a healthy baby? (Oooh, yes.)

How will I juggle parenting and career? (You won't know until you get there, but you can talk to people who do it and see if any of their strategies might suit you.)

How will I cope with childbirth? (The best way you can.)

Sleep deprivation? (Get all the sleep you can now.)

Breastfeeding? (There's lots of help available, and in the end it isn't compulsory.)

Curtailed freedom? (There are compensations. But yes. Life ain't perfect.)

And loss of autonomy? (It will pass in about twenty years or so.)

Will I have 'maternal instincts'? (Being a good parent is about being kind, patient and ready to learn, not about 'instincts'.)

Will I bond with my baby? (Probably, and if you don't there is lots of help available.)

How will my relationship with my partner be affected? (You'll probably both be sleep-deprived and grumpy for a while. Express your fears and keep talking.)

How will my partner cope with the demands of parenting? (Don't know, but there's lots of help available.)

Will my baby suffer from me being a single parent? (Children need a stable, loving environment. You can do that.)

Will I ever recognise my body again? (Yes, and you should stop looking at photos of famous actresses and models who have had children. They also have 47 nannies, personal trainers and teeming hordes of hair and make-up artists.)

How will I/we cope with a reduced income and increasing expenses? (Have a strategy: see the financial info in the first chapter of this book, Getting Ready.)

Aaarghh! (Fair enough.)

Why wouldn't you have the occasional wave of panic when you remember any or all of the above worries, plus the fact that your life is about to be transformed, and there's no going back?

Maybe you just need a good cry every now and then or to share your feelings with your partner or a friend. If a particular issue is really getting you down, or if you feel depressed most of the time, it might help to get some professional counselling. It's better to sort things out now than when you have a real, live, non-theoretical baby on your hands.

Here's the bit everyone bangs on about, but only because it's true: if you're feeling shocking, don't guzzle alcohol and caffeine and stuff your face with junk food. Eat a healthy diet, and get yourself some exercise, fresh air and plenty of rest.

Partners and friends, who are always on the lookout for a way to help you, should be ordered to cheer you up. And you need to hang out with some cheerful parents.

the way people react to the news

Most people will be thrilled for you and say 'Congratulations!' with a big smile. But you could be surprised by a couple of reactions to your pregnancy that you just didn't see coming.

Do try to be sensitive when telling somebody you know is having trouble conceiving (see the box below for advice on how to handle this). If anyone else says negative or rude things, it comes from their own experience or their own personality, their own fears or their own problems with body image, babies, their mother, whatever. Every time you hear something discouraging ('Your life is over') or ludicrous ('Childbirth doesn't hurt at all'), just say to yourself, 'It's not about me, it's about them.'

TELLING FRIENDS WITH PREGNANCY TROUBLES

You may have a friend who wants to be pregnant but it's not possible for them right now. They may be having trouble conceiving, have had a miscarriage or several miscarriages, or they may be going through IVF treatment. You may even have a friend whose baby died. The news that you are pregnant will be bittersweet for them. Here are a few hints that might make it easier.

  Tell your friend about your pregnancy privately, perhaps in her home when nobody else is around. Although she will be happy for you, she may have a cry because your pregnancy reminds her so much of what she wants for herself. Don't tell other friends about her situation if she wants to maintain privacy.

  Let your friend know that you will answer any questions about your pregnancy, but that you'll try not to talk to her about it all the time, and she has your full permission to tell you to shut right up if you get obsessed with baby business.

  It might be a good idea to arrange that your friend first visits you and your new baby at home, away from the hospital, when you won't have other visitors. Don't insist that she hold the baby, or discourage her. Don't be alarmed if she cries when holding the baby. She will find her own way to deal with it in her own time.

  Don't, for heaven's sake, tell her to 'just relax' and she'll get pregnant, or insist she try some folk remedy you've read about, or suggest that she do whatever you did. She may already know about an infertility support group or counsellor. Often available in both city and rural areas, these services can usually be contacted through GPs, family planning centres and hospitals.

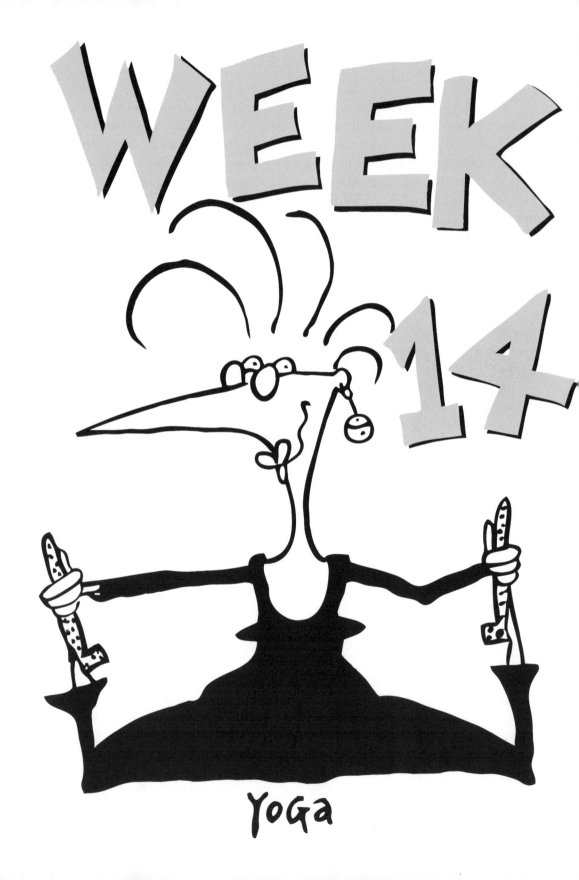

what's going on You're into the second

trimester. You're probably starting to feel a bit more

energetic. With a bit of luck the nausea should be gone

or almost gone. You may get that dark line from your navel

to your pubic hair, called the linea nigra because doctors

think 'black line' sounds soooo much more sophisticated in

Latin. On white skin it's not a black line: it varies from a pale,

shadowy pink to a browny colour. On dark skin it can look

darker, or not be visible at all. You will almost certainly have a

'bump'. According to the fruit-metaphor brigade your uterus is

the size of a large grapefruit.

By now the bones are forming in the arms, legs, rib

cage and skull. It's the start of your baby's skeleton. Weight:

about 45 grams.

Average approximate fetus length this week from head to bum

cm
1
2
3
4
5
6
7
8
9
10
11
12
13
14
15
16
17
18
19
20
21
22

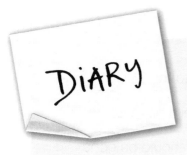

I've stopped being grumpy and started being weepy. I'm trying to regard this as progress. I'm getting more forgetful: this might be pregnancy hormones, or just having more to think about. So much for the alleged energy surge of the second trimester that everyone goes on about … I feel a little better by the end of the week. At least the nausea's gone and only pays a surprise visit now and again.

I investigate my sneezing/yoga injury. There is a muscle called the psoas that extends from the lower back to the front groin and I have injured mine waving my legs in the air. My chiropractor, a reassuringly sensible woman of the world, gives me an extremely gentle exercise to do three times a day and says a walk of ten minutes or so at a time is plenty until it gets better. She can't feel around because the fetus is in the way, and she says that since everything is changing in the pelvis healing the muscle isn't going to be top priority for my body.

I decide that my ill-fated attempts at yoga are simply folly. If you're not already a yoga enthusiast you can end up injuring yourself. On the other hand, if you are the sort of person who ties themself up into a pretzel every Wednesday night, if you stretch every day and can climb up your own left leg, well, there's no problem. But if you start yoga cold in pregnancy, you can do more harm than good. I should have taken instruction from an exercise person who is trained in pregnancy – I suspect that a lot of people who work in gyms or conduct yoga classes say they know about pregnancy exercise, but don't really.

Beck asks whether I've had any puffiness. Nobody mentioned puffiness. There had better not be any puffiness. I'm against it. I've got enough to deal with, thank you very much.

The fact that I feel like I weigh about 56,795 kilos is beginning to depress me. Beck says I will have to exercise from week 20 on, but I shouldn't do too much exercise before then because my system would be not so much shocked as horrified.

'But what about the people who swim five kilometres a day and hike around Borneo when they're pregnant?' I ask.

'They are not your type', she replies.

She's right.

I buy a swag of pregnancy magazines at the newsagent, call in sick, and take to the couch. Some of them seem pretty reliant on giveaways. I remind myself that a whizzbang product being given away is probably not in the magazine because it's necessarily the best or safest thing. It's there because its manufacturers get a free plug and a picture of their stuff in the mag.

One magazine actually gives away baby walkers even though an article in the same issue says they are not recommended for kids because they can slow real walking progress, lead to tippy-toe walking and cause spinal and neck problems.

Others are very focused on image, 'training' (exercise) and diet, with pages of suggested menus. All those models in the pictures seem to go through pregnancy a size eight with a melon up their micro-mini frock. How appalling of me not to look like a whippet in a wig and cook up some Tuscan, three-course, delicious, low-fat, gourmet meal every two minutes.

One mag claims to have 'Amazing facts about pregnancy and birth'. And they're right. They *are* amazing. 'A child born feet first will have the power of healing later in life.' This is such amazing piffle it makes you doubt some of the rest, such as 'The heaviest baby born to a healthy mother weighed 10.2 kilograms (more than 22 pounds)'.

info

second trimester hassles

This is often the most comfortable trimester of the pregnancy. For most women, nausea stops or decreases, energy levels are up and mood swings moderate. However, in this trimester, you may need to deal with one or more of the following.

sore, bleeding gums

Your gums may develop gingivitis, becoming sore, puffy, inflamed, and prone to bleeding, especially when you brush your teeth. This is caused by the increased progesterone and oestrogen in your blood, which makes gums softer and increases the blood pressure in the capillaries at the point where gums and teeth meet. This makes gums more susceptible to damage from food and being bumped by your toothbrush.

Try daily flossing, frequent brushing with a soft toothbrush (after each snack or meal if possible) and at least one dental visit during pregnancy for a professional cleaning job. Make sure the dentist knows you're pregnant so you're not given an X-ray or dangerous medication. 'Local' dental anaesthetics are safe during pregnancy.

Proper levels of calcium, vitamin C and other nutrients in a pregnancy supplement will also help. Also, avoid eating toffee-like stuff or sticky date puddingy things that can get stuck in nooks and crannies and encourage infection.

congested nose

Something else you may share with the pregnancy sisterhood is a blocked, congested nose or one that is runnier than usual. You may also get nosebleeds (this can go on until you've given birth). These schnoz problems are the result of the same hormonal effect that creates gum problems, which causes an increased blood supply, softening and swelling of the mucous membranes inside the nostrils, increased mucus production and easier bleeding. This means colds and upper respiratory tract infections can take longer than usual to clear up.

Bleeding can be triggered by unrestrained honking (overstrenuous nose blowing) or even by a dry atmosphere, which can harden mucus and make it more likely to cause damage to mucous membranes when you blow your nose. Try to avoid allergens. Humidifying the atmosphere and making yourself steam inhalations can help relieve the symptoms. You can also rub some emollient cream inside each nostril at bedtime.

To stop your nose bleeding apply gentle pressure on the affected side of the nose while leaning your head forward. Frequent or heavy nose bleeding should be mentioned to your doctor. Don't use any nose drops or sprays without checking first with your doctor. And ... er ... hate to sound like your granny, but don't pick your nose.

vaginal secretions

I realise this is hardly dinner party conversation, but you'll be pleased to know that all those extra-wet knickers are actually normal. Your vagina is producing more mucus and I think it's time we had a better term. Like lady's lotion. God. Sorry. Maybe not.

It's caused by the combined effect again of progesterone and oestrogen: the softer, more swollen mucous membranes of pregnancy produce more secretions. (Unpoetically, the medical description is 'an increase of normal mucoid discharge', which sounds like something a special-effects technician would say on the set of a critter movie.)

This normal discharge, called leucorrhoea if you want to get technical, should be clear or milky white. There can be rather a lot of it, and it's likely to increase as the pregnancy progresses.

To help with the hassle of vaginal secretions in overdrive:

⊚ avoid tight undies or trousers

⊚ wear undies and trousers made from natural fabrics such as cotton or wool – avoid nylon and polyester

⊚ wear panty-liners and change them frequently during the day

⊚ don't use tampons when you're pregnant because there is a higher risk of vaginal infection

⊚ if it's easy, take a couple of changes of underpants with you in your handbag (and if you think you need a bigger handbag to leave the house now, just wait until you have a baby!).

Increased blood flow to the genitals can mean a more sensitive than usual clitoris. (Another reason to stay away from tight undies or trousers. Or not.)

infections

If your vaginal discharge is yellowish or greenish or has an unhealthy smell, you have probably got an infection, which will need to be treated. An imbalance of friendly and unfriendly bacteria and high oestrogen levels in the vagina can make you more prone than usual to thrush, also known as candida, which may need to be treated by a doctor who knows you're pregnant. Symptoms include a lumpy white discharge and an itching and burning feeling.

If you are having thrush problems, remember to be careful to wipe front to back after going to the toilet. This is because thrush can hang out in the bowel and be transferred to your vagina. It is linked to a high-yeast diet, so try avoiding refined sugars, and eat lots of yoghurt with live *Lactobacillus acidophilus* cultures. Yoghurt can also be applied inside the vagina.

Air the nether regions when possible. You may do this by running around in the nuddy and waving your legs in the air, or by doing things like wearing no clothes or a nightie to bed instead of pyjamas. If you're lucky enough to have warm weather, wear a sarong or skirt with no undies when you can.

Average approximate fetus length this week from head to bum

1
2
3
4
5
6
7
8
9
10
11
12
13
14
15
16
17
18
19
20
21
22

what's going on Your heart is doing a

lot more than it used to and has a lot more blood to

pump. (Contrary to old ludicrous persons' tales, your heart

doesn't actually get bigger.) Nausea might come back

if you let yourself get too tired or hungry. You may

be looking even more divine than usual as your hair isn't

falling out at the rate it normally does, so it looks thicker,

your skin looks plumped out and the extra blood in your

system is giving you what they call the 'glow'.

The fetal fingernails are developing, and the

facial features are clearly defined. The fetus may suck

its thumb. (All together now: awwwww!) The skin

formed is still very thin, so if there was a tiny camera in

there transmitting pictures you could see blood vessels

underneath. The fetus begins to put on weight more

rapidly about this time. Starting soon

the arms and legs will begin to be more

co-ordinated when moving – imagine

languid fetal aerobics.

Weight: about 80 grams.

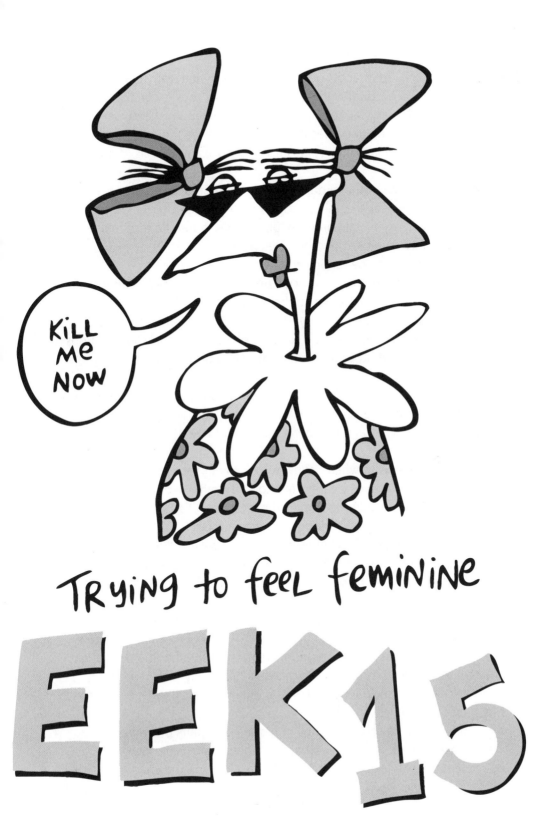

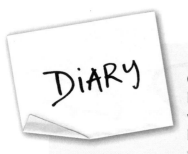

DiARY

Geoff and I go for a tour of the maternity ward at the hospital we're booked into. Our tour is conducted by a very capable midwife called Helen. In the nursery, we look at babies in plastic boxes with the tops cut off. I mean, they're posh plastic boxes on wheels, not home-made or anything.

Because they are in the middle of being renovated, the delivery suites and private rooms look like tacky country motel rooms after being trashed by a desultory heavy metal band. Awful, hideous, floral, flouncy bedspreads I couldn't possibly give birth on. I tell Helen so.

'They like things to be feminine', she says.

'Helen', I point out, 'if you're squatting down with a baby coming out of your fanny, I reckon you'd know you're a woman.'

Some random realities: Sunday. Valentine's Day. We realise we've forgotten our anniversary nearly a month before. Start eating lemon drops all the time. Drag myself around. Leg hurting. The bottom half of me is a milk-white sea of cellulite.

I'm starting to have the feeling that there's no going back. Getting to bed far too late, then not sleeping, then waking early and can't get back to sleep, then finally sleeping in and being late for work. I think I may have jet lag, without any jetting.

Nausea gone except when I allow myself to get tired and hungry. Weeing all night long. The idea of wearing my normal clothes – e.g. anything with a ZIP or WAIST – is totally laughable. The books say 'You won't be showing yet'. Showing? I'm not just showing! I'm showing OFF!

Searching for maternity clothes in the shops is like wading through the rejects of every other season. A few years ago it was orange and lime-green clothes for women – so now it must be orange and lime-green maternity wear. Cack!

As a clothes designer I know people try to reduce costs by cutting things thinner rather than wider, and shorter rather than longer, but in this case it seems pretty damn mingy. You don't want to be in a hobble skirt when you're already going to be waddling, surely? And why is there nothing between mini- and maxi-length? It's as if only strippers and Queen Victoria buy maternity clothes.

I end up buying sensible items in black – two pairs of trousers, one T-shirt, one jumper, a frock, two pairs of tights – and hand over the equivalent of the Mexican national debt. You'd think they had emeralds sewn into the hems. And that's in the normal maternity shop. The posh maternity shop has shiny polyester jackets that aren't meant to be shiny for £120 and various other rich-lady outfits. I look like the *Titanic* in all of them.

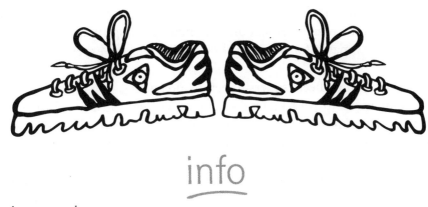

info

being active

You don't have to be really fit to have a baby. Moderate exercise during pregnancy is good for you and your offspring. When we say moderate exercise, we do not mean flinging yourself about like a non-pregnant person with a gym obsession and a desire to run a marathon before lunch. Sensible exercise is good for circulation, relaxation and energy levels, and helps to stop constipation, cramps and backache.

If you're not fit before pregnancy, this is not the time to adopt a strenuous exercise regime. Try low-impact things such as walking, gentle yoga and stretching, swimming, dancing, antenatal exercise classes and aquarobics. Look for gyms, swimming and recreation centres or physiotherapy clinics that run exercise classes designed for pregnancy and have instructors with a special qualification in pregnancy exercise; at the very least make sure your instructor knows you're pregnant. Check with your midwife or antenatal clinic that the activity you're doing or about to do is safe for you. But don't feel you need to pay for any special pregnancy exercise classes: walking and swimming are free or cheap.

Many instructors are not aware of the special risks of pregnancy. The extra release of the hormone relaxin, which makes your ligaments and joints more stretchy, can make you more prone to injury. Sit-ups and other strenuous abdominal exercises are generally a bad idea during pregnancy because they can cause a separation of muscles in your stomach, creating a hernia-like effect.

Yoga can help you become aware of how comfortably you are standing, sitting or lying down. Its breathing and meditation practices can relax you during pregnancy and labour. Special antenatal yoga classes can help with many of the discomforts of pregnancy, as well as improving the body's suppleness and strength for labour. The mind-body-spirit approach of yoga can be a good match for the mind-body-spirit-altering experience of being pregnant.

Even if you've been super-fit before pregnancy, you'll need to apply some limitations to your regime. Consult your gym or fitness professional as soon as you know you're pregnant to get some expert advice on exercise modifications, and choose a slower-pace, lighter-impact class and hand weights not exceeding half a kilo.

If you have played sport regularly before pregnancy you can usually continue until the third trimester, unless it's a sport that can cause impact injuries, such as football (contesting for the ball), trick rollerblading (falls), water polo (being kicked, accidentally or otherwise), kickboxing (duh), and tennis (rabid opponents prone to attacking you with a racquet).

Other activities not recommended during pregnancy include horse riding, any kind of skiing, backpacking, and lifting heavy weights and other heavy manual work. Jogging, running and other athletics can be too stressful on joints, breasts and baby, so check your exercise programme with your doctor. Cycling, for example, might be fine early on but a bit wobbly as you get way bigger towards the end.

You shouldn't exercise while pregnant if you have a history of medical conditions such as recurrent miscarriages, placenta praevia, 'incompetent cervix', pre-eclampsia or heart disease. Other conditions, including diabetes, thyroid disease and anaemia, may sometimes mean exercise is not recommended.

when exercising

⑥ Wear supportive footwear and a properly fitted sports bra.

⑥ Drink plenty of water before, during and after, and make sure you have some healthy snacks handy.

⑥ Remember your centre of gravity is changing, which will affect your balance and co-ordination, so take it easy.

⑥ Listen to and trust your body – stop if any activity makes you feel uncomfortable, overtired, hot, dizzy, faint or crampy.

⑥ Don't worry if your heart rate is higher during pregnancy even when you're not exercising. It doesn't mean you are losing fitness; it simply reflects your increased rate of circulation.

⑥ Don't get overheated for prolonged periods – this can be damaging to the fetus, particularly during the first trimester.

⑥ Exercise intensity should be measured during work-outs; a fetal heart rate stays normal when exercise intensity is moderate and your heart rate doesn't exceed 140 beats per minute (bpm), whereas if your heart rate reaches 180 bpm this can cause fetal distress and a lowered fetal heart rate. You can wear one of those pulse monitor thingies (that's the technical term) to check your heart rate.

⑥ You can walk until you are slightly puffing or reach 140 bpm, then keep this up for 15–20 minutes. Puffing work-outs should be only every second day and depend on your fitness level.

⑥ Strictly limit exercises that involve lying flat on your back to a maximum of two to three minutes from the beginning of the second trimester, and omit them altogether after twenty weeks. The weight of the uterus can compress the inferior cava vena, the vein that carries blood back to your heart from your lower parts, ultimately resulting in a reduced blood flow to your head and to the baby. So if you feel dizzy or faint while on your back, turn onto your left side and rest.

⑥ Don't forget to exercise your pelvic-floor muscles (see the box at the end of this chapter). These muscles are like a hammock or sling that sits underneath all your inside organs. Doing the exercises will mean faster pelvic-floor recovery after delivery, and will help prevent accidental weeing after childbirth (also known as stress incontinence) when you sneeze, cough or laugh.

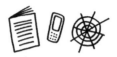

more info on **being active**

Anybody doing yoga during pregnancy needs a specialist instructor or advice from somebody who understands the needs of the pregnant body, and how you can protect yourself from injury or discomfort. Make sure you tell any class teacher that you are pregnant. If you're already experienced in yoga, but can't find a class that caters to pregnant women, you might find the following books and DVDs helpful. However, there is always a danger when learning from a book or a DVD that bad habits or wrong postures can be adopted. If you're at all unsure, or completely inexperienced, consider a couple of lessons in the basics from a qualified instructor experienced with pregnant clients.

Yoga for Pregnancy, Birth and Beyond by Françoise Barbira Freedman, Dorling Kindersley, UK, 2004

> If you use a book for instruction on yoga during pregnancy, make sure it's one like this that's specifically intended for pregnant women, not a general yoga book. This has lots of short step-by-step sequences for each trimester and also for after the birth, clearly illustrated with DK's trademark photography.

Pregnancy Health Yoga with Tara Lee, Earth Warrior Productions, 2008

> This DVD covers breathing and physical stretches and exercises as well as a visualisation and relaxation practice by Dr Gowri Motha, and a 20-minute bit showing some yoga treatments for common pregnancy problems such as pelvic pain.

wsf.org.uk

> Your local council, or the Women's Sport and Fitness Foundation (website above), will have lists of team sports in your area that you may be able to get involved in when you are settled in with your baby. It's a way to get an hour to yourself here and there, feel good, be healthier and meet people. It's a luxury available only to those who have childcare help, of course. Toddlers are fun but they sure get in the way during hockey.

mwsf.org.uk

> The Muslim Women's Sport Foundation can help you find a football, badminton, basketball or other team from local to international level that fits your religious requirements regarding dress and women-only teams.

PELVIC-FLOOR EXERCISES

Different midwives and obstetricians have different guidelines, but here's what a US obstetrics department that studied techniques for improving bladder control found worked best:

1 lie down if possible – the muscles don't work as hard if you're standing up
2 squeeze your pelvic-floor muscles for a count of four, then relax them for a count of four
3 build up to doing this for five minutes twice a day – but keep breathing!
4 and keep doing them – it can take up to three months to build better bladder control, but exercise does make a difference.

To check that you're exercising the right muscles Only your vaginal muscles should be working: you shouldn't be also tensing your buttocks or your abdominal or thigh muscles. Although one means of identifying the muscles is to wee and then try to stop halfway through, it's not a good idea to practise pelvic-floor exercises that way: once is enough. A better way to check is to put a finger in (ahem) your vagina and squeeze: if you're exercising correctly you should feel the muscles tightening around your finger.

what's going on

It is possible you might feel the movements of the fetus as 'butterflies' in your belly from now on, especially if you know what to pay attention to, but you also mightn't feel them for weeks.

You now have about 180 millilitres of amniotic fluid. Your uterus is kind of like a balloon full of yellowish water. All the joints of the fetus are working and the fingers and toes are all there and waving about. Toenails are just starting to form. The head still looks kind of oversized but the rest of the body is catching up. The downy fetal hair called lanugo has started to grow on the body. (Lanugo means fine wool in some ancient language.) There are various opinions about what the lanugo might be for: it might help keep the fetus warm, or it might be an underfelt for the gooey stuff that eventually covers the baby. Or maybe the fetus is just trying to develop a fashion instinct. Weight: about 110 grams.

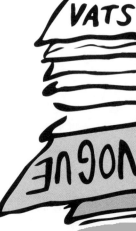

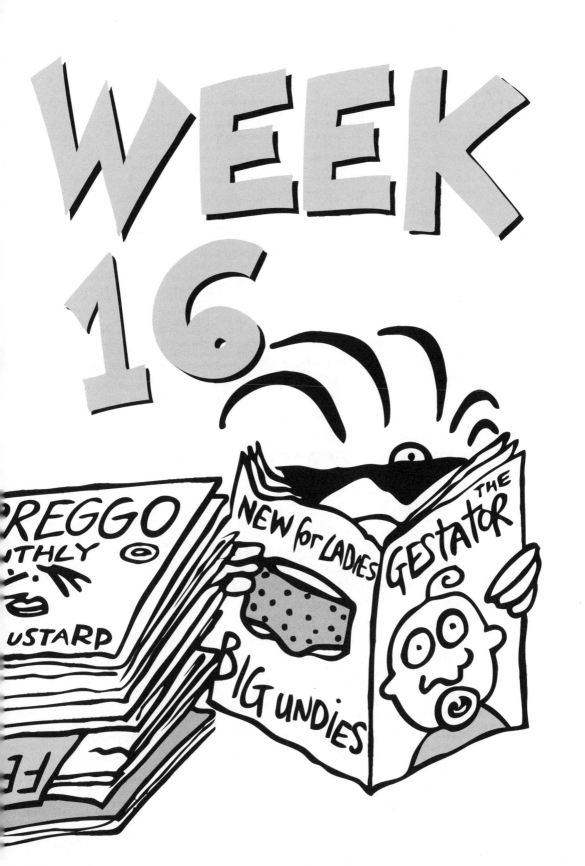

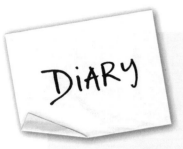

DiARY

Another appointment with Dr Sharma, so he can check out the ultrasound results, and me. In the waiting room the woman next to me has a small child she speaks to in a Very Loud Voice. She is Extremely Annoying. The child looks at pictures in a book.

'Here's Daddy', he says, pointing to a man.

'That's not *our* daddy', she bellows, cheerfully.

Our daddy! 'Madam', I feel like saying, 'he is the child's daddy. He is not your daddy.' I ponder the whole spooky idea of calling your sexual partner mummy or daddy.

I sit there remembering my weekend of feeling weepy, hideous, fat, disgusting, spotty and vilely repellent in every degree, and getting really freaked out about the sea of cellulite. So far I've been Sneezy, Sleepy, Dopey and Grumpy. I'm hoping for the full complement of the Seven Dwarfs before the confinement. There wasn't a Weepy, sadly. Or a Crappy. Or a Dippy. Spotty never got a look in. Or, indeed, a Fatty. Can't think why.

Once I've made it into his room, I try this out on Dr Sharma, who says I could be Happy. I feel like saying you can be Doc, Doc. When it comes to the crunch I suspect I'm going to be Shrieky, or at least the Evil Queen. Then he tells me somebody has already made the Seven Dwarfs joke in a book he can't remember the name of. Great. So now I'm Plagiary as well.

I further distinguish myself by whipping off my trousers and undies when he just wants to feel my tummy and 'measure the fundus'.

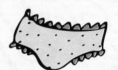

The man obviously thinks I'm some kind of crazed exhibitionist who enjoys lying on couches naked from the waist down except for boots, with her ankles somewhere near the light fittings.

Well, maybe I am. What's it to you?

I wonder what a fundus is? Oh. It's the top of the uterus.

He gives the old tummy a bit of a poke and a feel (this is called 'palpation' apparently) and seems pleased with the progress.

'It's definitely growing.'

Despite the obviousness of this banality I am absurdly pleased. He smiles.

'Everything's going as well as could be expected. Couldn't be better.' I beam. Oh hurrah. I feel like I've received a gold star and an elephant stamp on my homework.

He puts a little instrument on my stomach and it amplifies the baby's heartbeat. It makes me grin.

'It sounds groovy', I say. 'Kind of swishy.'

'I always think it sounds like Rolf Harris', he says. 'That wobble board thingy. Anything else worrying you?'

'Yes. I am 78 kilos.'

'That's okay.'

'Am I putting on too much weight?'

'No, and you can't diet.'

'Yes, I know. I was just wondering whether I should hire a wheelbarrow to get around in.'

'You'll be having most of your pregnancy care, from now on, with the hospital midwives', Dr Sharma goes on. 'But I'm on hand if any worries come up along the way.'

This is the opening I need to 'fess up about the booze. I've been brooding about it ever since reading the first of those pregnancy manuals. 'Well, there is something', I stumble. 'I had some reeeeally alcoholic punch that tasted like herbicide at a party when I was already pregnant'.

'How much?' asks Dr Sharma.

'Only one glass. Erm. And a cigarette.'

'No one can tell for sure, but it's almost certainly totally fine.'

Phew.

More good news: Dr Sharma says my combined blood test and ultrasound result says I don't have a high risk of having a Down's syndrome child. Relief! Burst into tears.

Dr Sharma takes the tears in his stride: I remind myself that lots of pregnant women have a low tear threshold so he's probably used to this. He asks if there's anything else I want to talk about. I have written down three questions: can Beck be an extra birth partner? (Yes – Dr Sharma says it's very cool to have an experienced birth partner along to the 'party', as long as she understands she won't be the boss of everything.) Is the hospital set up for any emergency, and will it be equipped to perform a caesarean if it's needed? (Yes and yes.) And what books does he recommend? (Janet Balaskas's *New Active Birth*. He's a bit of a New Man, my Dr Sharma.)

info

'fess up to being pregnant

You're slower, you're more tired, you're more scatty, especially in the first three months, and apparently you've got it to look forward to again in the last three months. (That leaves these middle three months in which everyone tells you you're looking divine, just glowin' up a storm.) Tell people you're tired. Let them help. And let them make allowances. Forgot to pay the phone bill? It's because you're pregnant. Have to sit down on the floor during a meeting and put your feet on a chair and show everyone your undies? Because you're pregnant. Had to buy a new pair of red shoes? Pregnant. See? It's easy.

the pursed-lip brigade

Not married? Married but wearing tight clothes? Planning to go back to work before the baby turns seventeen? Somewhere, somehow, someone will disapprove of you. Get used to it, and learn to shrug it off. If you stay home with the baby, some idiots will start asking, 'What do you DO all day?', as if you're just sitting at home watching Oprah and eating Mars Bars (ahem). If you're at work, people will ask 'You haven't put your baby in child care/hired a nanny, have you?', as if it were the same as asking 'You haven't tied it up and popped it in a tree for the day, have you?'. Apply the same logic as you do for unsolicited advice: it's not about you, it's about them. Some people just love to judge others.

stuff you didn't know before

⑥ Breast milk comes out of the nipple like water comes out of a sprinkler – there are heaps of little holes, not just one. And one breast may produce heaps more milk than the other.

⑥ What the inside of your navel looks like.

⑥ You *can* want to throw up and eat at the same time.

⑥ You *can* go and wee all the time and still retain fluid.

⑥ Sleep deprivation starts well before the birth.

stuff that other people don't know

It makes people be nicer to you when they know:

⑥ you are carrying 25 percent more blood than you usually do

⑥ in the second half of the pregnancy the baby whacks you in the internal organs all the time, and it's not always a cute little whack – sometimes it's really uncomfortable, sometimes it actually hurts

⑥ your feet swell with fluid retention to twice their usual size (well, that's what it feels like)

⑥ you can't get the required amount of deep sleep because you have to wee all night – it's the equivalent of someone waking you up every couple of hours.

So tell everybody.

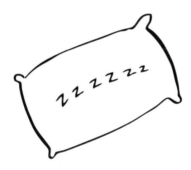

WEEK 17

what's going on

You may be sweating, spitting and running like a tap at the nose as well as having those pesky vaginal secretions. Basically you're a leaking bag of various fluids. I'm sorry, but there it is. Find room in your handbag among the lipsticks, spanners and panty-liners for tissues, spare deodorant, spare undies, a couple of wet-wipes, maybe a beach towel. (It's really not that bad.)

By now the baby's sex organs are completely formed. The fetal kidneys produce lots of urine: the fetus wees about every 40–45 minutes (at least you don't have to change nappies yet). Icky though it may sound, the fetus takes in some of this wee when it swallows mouthfuls of amniotic fluid. But most of the fetal waste products go through the placental membrane and into your circulation, where it's dealt with by your body's usual functions.

Weight: about 150 grams.

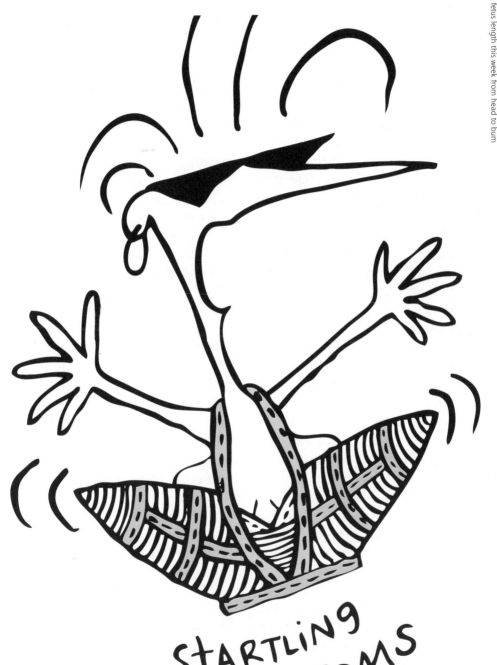

STARTLING
BOSOMS

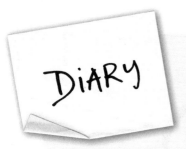

My bosoms are getting bigger, and none of my bras are comfy, even the bigger ones I bought. My bosoms used to stick out straight from my body, practically in opposite directions from each other. They were known as East and West. Now they're kind of bigger and lower slung, meaning there's a bit underneath where it gets sweaty. And all these little skin tags have grown there as well. Thank God I finally found a book that said this was perfectly normal.

Sports crop-tops seemed the best, but now they feel like elastic-bandage boob-tubes three sizes too small. If I'm sitting around at home I don't wear a bra at all. No doubt this means I'll end up having bosoms shaped like tube socks that I can tie in a knot behind my neck when they get in the way. Don't care. Those areas around my nipples I can never pronounce have started to go brown and are getting bumps on them.

Farewell, my strawberries-and-cream nipples, my horizontal, pointy bosoms! Will you now both be called South forever? Why don't I have a photo of you?! Was my youth so misspent that I never even posed for nude photographs? What was I thinking!

The bath in the new house is of such a ludicrous design by some kind of deranged handyman that before I can get in it I have to crawl over about half a metre of tiles or take a huge, dangerous step on one leg. (Well, obviously, otherwise it would be a jump, not a step. I'm losing my mind.) And given that there isn't enough room in the bathroom to swing a cat – actually there isn't even enough room to *shout* at a cat – it won't do. The whole thing is a disaster waiting to happen for a woman whose centre of gravity is changing every day.

I call Piotr the plumber to come and fix it. Piotr, of course, finds that the bathroom floor is practically rotted through as well and that there's some other piping-style disaster, which means the job turns out to be five times bigger.

One of the reasons I feel like I'm going mad is sleep deprivation. It never occurred to me that this would happen BEFORE the little mite arrived. One of the books says this is because I'm sleeping like a baby – not much deep sleep but plenty of REM sleep. That stands for Rapidly Enraged Mother-to-be.

Call me dense, but it's only just hit me I'm not one person who's pregnant – I mean, I am – but I'm also two people. No. I'm not two people but there are two people – a big one and a little one – sharing the same body. Well. That's a bit spooky.

Apparently many people at this stage of pregnancy find that they can have a few sips of wine or beer occasionally without a violent reaction. Geoff poured a thimbleful of what he described as 'a very smooth cab sauv' for me to try, but it tasted like meths and I spat it out.

He's reading bits of a book for wannabe fathers, which argues that men shouldn't be expected to be at the birth because they can't fix the pain, and if they prefer, they can plant a tree or invent a new dance instead, to celebrate the birth. I'm afraid Geoff is the sort of bloke who thinks this is a load of old cobblers, and the way that book is being hurled about it won't last the evening. I don't think he's the making-up-a-dance type.

info

breasts

Ah, bosoms. On the one hand there are the people who go 'Phwoaaarrr' and, on the other, people who worship them as sacred life-giving vessels of compulsorily acquired nourishment. Blimey. Get a grip. They're just bosoms.

Probably one of the first pregnancy changes you noticed was your breasts getting larger and more tender. They'll keep growing, but extreme sensitivity usually settles down after the first trimester. From here on, the hormones oestrogen, progesterone and prolactin stimulate more growth and the production of some pre-milk stuff called colostrum.

Each breast contains about twenty segments or lobes; each of these is made up of grapelike bunches of glands called alveoli; and each of these is lined with milk-producing cells. During pregnancy your bosoms get bigger because not only do your dormant milk-producing cells and ducts enlarge, your body also grows new ones to help out. (Your original breast size bears no relation to whether there'll be enough milk for the baby.)

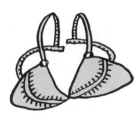
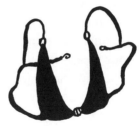

changes

Breast changes are usually more extreme in a first pregnancy. Your breasts may feel tender, tingling, warm, full, heavy, painfully sensitive or lumpy. You may even have some stabbing pain.

You'll be able to see more veins, often blue, close to the skin's surface, carrying the extra blood supply to the area. They're especially noticeable if you have fair skin.

The nipples and areolae (the areas around the nipples) become larger and darker, particularly if your natural skin tone is dark. Most nipples and areolae go a shade of brown, even if they have been pink before. This can happen gradually to the entire area, or in patches.

Each areola is dotted with sebaceous (oil-producing) glands called Montgomery's tubercles (those little bumps), which secrete a fluid that keeps the nipples supple. The glands become more prominent during pregnancy, so you get a bumpier effect.

You may have a small amount of colostrum – a thin, yellowish liquid – leaking from your nipples towards the end of pregnancy, and even earlier on, but not everyone does. This can cause wet patches, but can be soaked up and hidden by breast pads, otherwise known as nursing pads; you can buy these in the baby section of the chemist or supermarket. Actual milk production won't start until after the baby arrives.

Inverted nipples If you have flat or inverted nipples get a midwife to have a look at them at this stage of pregnancy so they can talk you through a few tricks to try for breastfeeding.

Breast surgery Almost everyone who's had breast enlargement or reduction surgery will need to supplement their breast milk with formula. Some bubs won't be able to breastfeed at all.

bras

Wearing a well-fitted supporting bra during pregnancy is recommended. You often need to increase your bra measurement and cup by at least one size. The increase might even be more, depending on the overall weight gain and whatever your breasts feel like doing. (For example, you might go from 34B to 36C.) You can buy bras to fit your changing size, even though it might mean buying a new size a couple of times during the pregnancy. You don't need a maternity bra (with front fasteners that make for easy bosom access) or new size while your present bra fits well, is comfortable and gives you enough support.

Good features of a maternity bra include wide straps, a wide band of fabric under the breast and a high cotton content. Anything that digs into the skin is even more intolerable than usual, so make sure you get a comfy fit.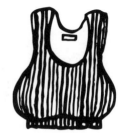

Maternity bras often fasten at the front between the cups; or where the straps meet the cups at the front; or they don't fasten at all, but rather stretch so you can just pop a bosom out the bottom to breastfeed. Whatever suits you best. If you started with big bosoms, you'll probably need more support than the stretchy crop-top style.

lumps
Stay alert before, during and after pregnancy for breast lumps. Always get any lump checked by a doctor ASAP – that means in the next few days – and never assume it's just something to do with hormones or breastfeeding.

afterwards
Don't be sucked in by cosmetic surgery hype that breasts are 'deformed' by breastfeeding and need to be 'enlarged' with sacs of plastic and saline. Sharky cosmetic surgeons don't really care about your bosoms, they just want your money. And there are many possible hideous side effects, including rupture, pain, scarring, lost nipple sensation and inability to breastfeed again.

Likewise, beware the faffy marketing techniques of the cosmetics companies trying to sell you 'bust firming' lotion and 'breast cream' and 'body treatment' moisturisers. (Often the names are in French or pseudo-French.) They will not prevent your breasts from changing shape or sagging. These creams don't affect the tissues inside the breast, and many are a shockingly expensive waste of time. A cheap moisturiser that smells nice is just as good at keeping the surface of your skin moist, and just as likely to keep your breasts firm – that is, not at all.

Often these creams and oils have ingredients that feel tingly or make the skin seem tighter – the same tightening feeling can be achieved by putting egg white on your breasts and waiting for it to dry. Don't be fooled – there's no lasting effect on your bosomry and certainly these creams are no match for Mrs Gravity once she's decided to make her presence felt.

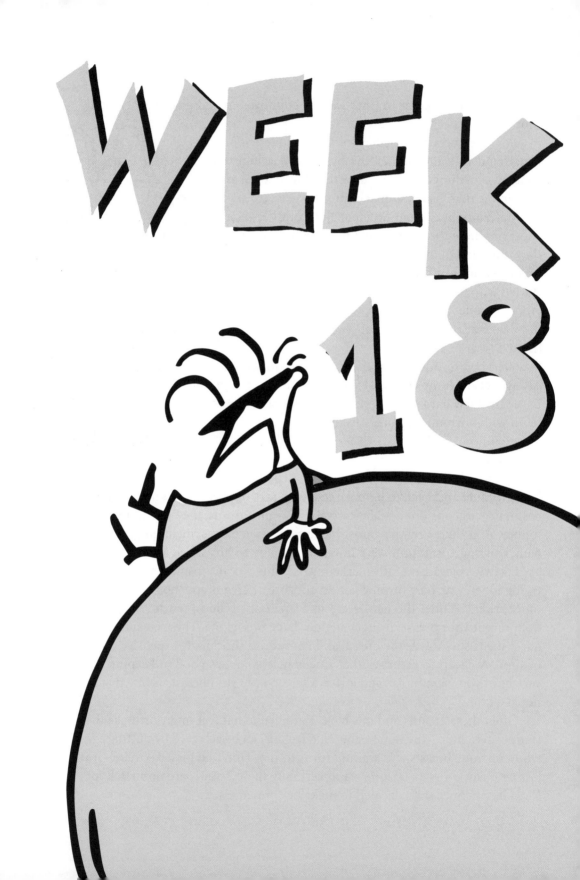

what's going on

You'll find many pregnancy books tell you that this is the week you'll start to feel a first baby move around. Don't hold your breath: you might not feel it move for weeks yet, and that doesn't mean there's anything wrong. Babies mostly move when you're resting at night: basically after 8 p.m. and before 8 a.m. When you move around during the day you rock the baby to sleep. Use pillows to support your growing tummy while you sleep.

According to some pregnancy experts, this week the fetus can make facial expressions. Oh yeah? Like what? Astonishment? 'Euwww yuk, that amniotic fluid tastes bad'? Anyway, the fetus is definitely able to move around a lot, swing on the umbilical cord (well, that's what it looks like) and bite its own fingers or do the hokey-cokey if it feels like it. There is lanugo hair all over the body, and blood cells start to form in the bone marrow.

Tastebuds are forming.

Weight: about 200 grams.

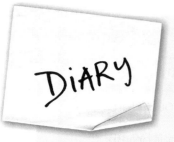

DiARY

I pop along to a group physio lesson at the local hospital. It is mostly couples, except me (Geoff is watching the footy at home), and exactly the sort of thing I hate – name tags and a whiteboard and splitting into two groups to workshop questions such as 'What does fitness mean to you?' and 'Will exercise help?'. (Duh, I think. 'Course it will.)

I am very annoyed to discover that mad exercising in the last few weeks of pregnancy will not actually guarantee a short labour. This seems to be another major design fault of this whole caper, along with painful childbirth.

A 'student' called Anthea, wearing a black velvet Alice band on her long blonde hair and shoes that cost more than all the rest of the clothes in the room added together, tells the class smugly that she is still going to the gym every day and doing a special programme of exercises and weights. She looks bloody shocking – has a grey pallor and is scarily thin for someone who is up the duff. Kate, the physio, asks her if her gym instructor is fully qualified in antenatal fitness. No, Anthea says, rather patronisingly, explaining that it's a very superior sort of gym and they do know she's pregnant and IT'S FRIGHTFULLY EXPENSIVE.

Later in the class when Kate explains an abdominal muscle injury that causes bits of your organs to poke through in a line under the skin of your tummy in a characteristic shape, Anthea squeals in recognition, 'Oh my GOD, I've got that!', and goes a bit quiet for the rest of the class. One imagines the very superior gym is about to receive a call from her rather frightfully expensive lawyer.

We practise (a) sitting on giant inflatable balls to strengthen our squatting muscles and straighten our backs, (b) sprawling on beanbags, and (c) a relaxation technique that I fail at miserably. Not for me relaxing in a hospital room full of strangers lying on nylon carpet with the fluorescent lights temporarily off, thank you. We are informed about the importance of pelvic-floor exercises and I just know I'm not going to do them. I've tried. I did six in a row one Saturday and got bored. We all pass around a plastic pelvis and stare at it as if it might suddenly have something to tell us.

Here's what I learn in group physio:

✳ The average female pelvis is ludicrously small for what's expected of it.

✳ Pelvic-floor exercises exercise the pelvic floor (hello). (The pelvic floor is the trampoliney bit that is stretched under all the pelvic organs.) The main jobs of the pelvic floor are to stop all your organs from falling out of your fanny (well, they wouldn't really, but it would all get a bit saggy in there); contracting around the holes to prevent unscheduled leaking, especially during coughing or sneezing (that is, it's a continence accessory); and allowing your vagina to contract rhythmically if you are in any way interested in sex, which is hard to imagine.

⚹ How to exercise the pelvic-floor muscles without anybody noticing. My favourite instruction was 'Your buttocks should not be moving'. I often think that.

⚹ They now say to squeeze your pelvic-floor muscles for a count of four and then release them for a count of four, twice a day for five minutes but building up to longer sessions. I am bored already.

⚹ It is difficult to have a mid-class snack while the physio is explaining to a young woman how to poo properly. (Tragically I walked away, so I'll never know.)

⚹ Nap when you can, even for 15 minutes.

⚹ Bend and rotate your arms backwards like you're doing a chicken dance, when you can. Also put your feet up when you can and, if you can't, flex them back and forth. Both of these will keep your muscles flexible and help your circulation.

⚹ Don't hunch over your stomach. Sit backwards on a chair, with a pillow between you and the back and your legs to each side, or sit on a giant inflatable ball, which you can buy from midwives, gyms and giant-inflatable-ball shops.

⚹ If you have to pick something up, use the lunge position (bend at the knee, one leg in front, keeping your back straight). If you vacuum, hold the cord behind your back with one hand, which automatically keeps your back straight. When you're at the sink, stand on one leg and put the other foot on the shelf under the sink, as long as the shelf is low enough for you to feel comfortable. Anthea says what are we thinking of, we should all hire a housekeeper. (I suggest we could dress her in a long, black frock and call her Mrs Danvers.)

✳ A diagram of a uterus looks like a bagpipe with a tent rope on it.

✳ Being fit may not ensure an easy labour, but it will mean a better labour and recovery than you would have had if you were unfit.

✳ Because the relaxin hormone goes into overdrive during pregnancy and slackens all the ligaments, joints and muscles, don't overstretch or bounce on stretches.

✳ Don't go into spas, hot tubs or saunas or get a body wrap at a salon. Your temperature can be raised to dangerous levels for the fetus without you realising.

✳ Don't get really hot and then jump in a cold pool, or otherwise shock your system with sudden temperature changes. (Anthea says she'll tell her pool man to regulate the temperature. Everyone rolls their eyes. 'I did mean public pools, but okay', says Kate.)

Kate says that's all we need to know and ends the class early, possibly to avoid the urge to throttle Anthea.

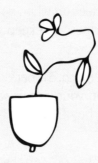

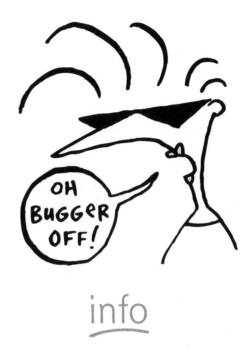

info

repelling unwanted advice and comments

When people give you that firm advice – 'You *must* have a nanny', 'You *must* always look after the baby yourself', '*Men* can't look after babies', 'You *must* use disposable nappies' – remember it's about them, not you. They're usually just telling you what THEY did and insisting that you do the same, maybe partly because that's all they know and partly because if you do it the same way it will make them feel better. Don't forget: your experience will be different from everybody else's. Listen, but don't automatically follow their advice.

It starts as soon as you tell people you're pregnant, and continues throughout parenting life. Having babies is such a universal experience that everyone has opinions and advice to share, whether you want to hear them or not.

You'll hear things about whether you can tell if you're having a girl or boy based on how sick you are, how much your baby moves or what shape your tummy is; why you should only see an obstetrician or only listen to midwives; why you should/shouldn't use pain-relief drugs during childbirth; how to avoid an episiotomy/caesarean/cracked nipples; why you must/mustn't breastfeed; why you should always use/never bother with cloth nappies; how to make your baby sleep through the night (pick it up/

ignore it/give it a stiff gin); how to avoid nappy rash; why you must go straight back/never go back to work; what sort of child care is best; what sort of schooling is best; what to do when your child is arrested in its mid-thirties. The list seems infinite.

Some advice will be useful and compatible with your own ideas, and some won't. Read books you like the philosophical feel of, and choose a couple of friends to listen to. In the end you'll find that having to deal with your own, real baby will provide the best information.

Another mind-boggling thing is that people want to touch your tummy, and sometimes they don't even ask if it's okay. This is easier to cope with than the advice. You can say 'I'd rather you didn't', or grab hands that are heading towards your belly.

at work or social gatherings

Sometimes people, even in a meeting at work, will bang on about anything to do with pregnancy, including cervical mucus, in front of anyone at all. (Make sure this isn't you.) You can learn to get out of these mortifying situations by saying pleasantly and firmly 'Let's stick to the agenda, shall we?' Even if it's a lie, you can always try 'Oh, I've got a rule – no pregnancy talk at work/parties/whatever', then gently disengage and move away. You can go to the loo and come back if you think someone will have changed the subject in the meantime.

strangers

Advice can be worse in your first pregnancy because people assume you want their opinion, and you have no ammunition to defend yourself against it. You can give strangers a distant smile and no verbal response. A lot of pregnancy/baby chit-chat when you're out and about is from people who are just looking to pass the time of day or strike up a conversation. These ones are easily dealt with: 'Gosh, is that the time? Must fly', or 'Thanks! Bye now!'

friends

Advice from friends is usually offered with good intentions, and they can give you some invaluable insights and short cuts. Store away anything that seems useful and ignore anything you don't like the sound of. Alternatively, you can always tell friends you'll come to them if you have any questions, or that you're sick of everybody giving you advice and could they please shut right up before you slap them.

the older generation

Take with a pinch of salt any of the pregnancy and baby-care advice from previous generations, which is likely to have a long-expired use-by date. Unfortunately, while many members of the older generation, including grandparents, have moved with the times, others have fixed ideas about how things should be done (the way they did them). It's worth having a tactful chat early on about how you see their role in relation to the baby. Without putting too fine a point on it, they need to understand that, as far as the baby goes, you're the boss. Here are some of the outdated notions you may have to firmly explain are not acceptable.

bad advice

BEFORE THE BABY ARRIVES

'Eat lots of liver.' (No. Too much vitamin A can damage the fetus.)

'"Morning sickness" is a myth.' (It bloody isn't.)

'You should try to hide your "bump".' (Oh for God's sake!)

AFTER THE BABY ARRIVES

'Breastfeeding/bottlefeeding is bad for your baby.' (It's your choice.)

'There's no need to use a baby restraint in the car for every trip, particularly short ones.' (This is potentially lethal, and can lead to terrible injuries.)

'Put the baby to sleep on its tummy.' (This is a sudden infant death syndrome – SIDS – risk.)

'Throwing the baby into the air is perfectly okay.' (No, this can be as damaging to the brain and eyes as shaking a baby.)

'Put honey on a dummy.' (It rots teeth and can create a 'sweet' dependency.)

'Always leave a baby to cry/never leave a baby to cry even for 30 seconds.' (Both of these are extreme.)

'That child is being "bad".' (This targets the child, not the behaviour.)

'Of course I can drop around without ringing to check if it's convenient – I'm a relative.' (Aaaargghhhh!)

'Give small children lots of lollies and sugared soft drinks as a treat or a reward. And milk or juice in their night-time bottles is fine.' (All these are a major cause of children having to have first teeth removed under anaesthetic because they've got holes.)

'Insist on a sleep routine/refuse to follow a sleep routine.' (Whatever works for you is fine.)

'Hitting, smacking and threats are good disciplinary measures.' (These teach the child to hit or threaten other children and creatures smaller than they are.)

'You need talcum powder when changing a nappy.' (No, and its fine particles can be bad for lungs, especially in premmie bubs.)

'It'll be okay if I smoke outside.' (If you can smell smoke on someone, don't let them hold the baby. Be firm.)

Grandparents might say, 'But we did this with you and you turned out fine.' Rather than replying, 'Well, that was bloody lucky then, wasn't it?', try saying, in the case of safety issues, 'You did the right thing then, but they've done all this new research and the right thing to do now is…'. When all else fails, just say, 'I really need it to be done this way.' In the case of safety issues, if a friend or relative is likely to ignore your wishes, it's safer for you to be there whenever they have access to the baby or your children.

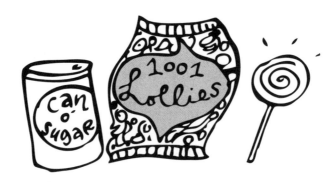

confusing advice

Advice from experts and pregnancy websites and books is often conflicting, which can be confusing. You only need to experience the midwife-shift changeovers at a hospital when you're learning how to breastfeed to find out just how varied professional opinion can be. It can be tricky to filter it, and – as always – you need to assess the individual you're dealing with, whether it be a physiotherapist conducting an antenatal class, a breastfeeding consultant or a paediatrician after the baby's born.

Choose to talk to the more cheerful, relaxed, experienced midwives at the hospital. And find women who you relate to who have had children, especially recently. Ask them anything you need to know, and they'll tell you their experiences. But bear in mind you're just researching – your experiences will not be exactly the same, and you may get pointed in different directions. New mums will have a few hints about settling babies or the best nappies, that kind of useful stuff. Mums whose kids are older may have forgotten the details.

Average approximate fetus length this week from head to bum

1

2

3

4

5

6

7

8

9

10

11

12

13

14

15

16

17

18

19

20

21

22

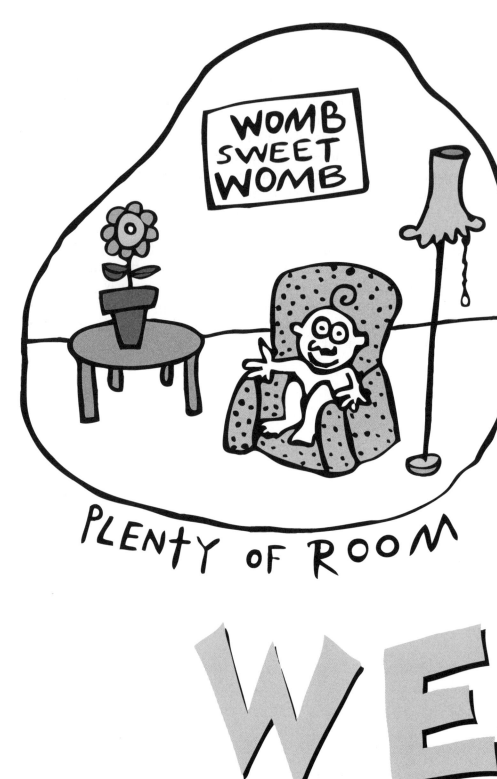

WOMB SWEET WOMB

PLENTY OF ROOM

WE

what's going on
Your waistline is missing, presumed obliterated. You may have backache, skin pigment changes, and a tendency to vague … somethingorother. The fetus still has plenty of room to move around in the amniotic sac, but it's a tighter fit than, say, a pear in a bucket of water – that's why, if you haven't already, you will feel movements any time from now on.

Its muscles have developed enough for the fetus to be doing loop-the-loops, and it can get itself tangled and untangled in the umbilical cord. The fetus is putting on brown-coloured fat deposits, which produce heat to keep it warm.

Weight: about 260 grams.

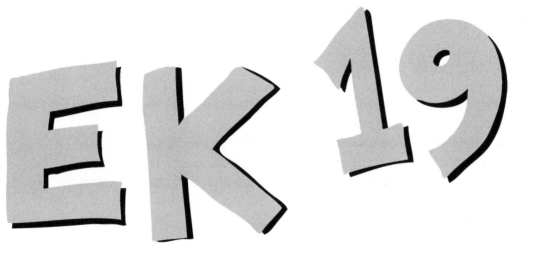
EK 19

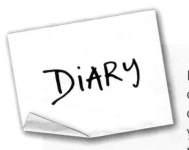

I have been reading Sheila Kitzinger. She abandons comparing the fetus size to fruit for a moment to solemnly declare 'You may notice that you are putting on weight on your buttocks'. Actually I've been noticing that for the last nineteen weeks, sunshine. If they get any bigger, people will start to think I'm shoplifting a futon.

Jane, who'll probably be a godmother without the God bit, and Geoff come to this week's ultrasound. I'm a bit nervy. In my heart I feel that everything is fine but my head is saying, well, things do go wrong. My left ankle just doesn't know what to think. Actually it probably has nothing to do with my head – instead it's got a microchip implanted by Aunt Julie to flash signals at me regularly throughout life: 'TERRIBLE things can happen'.

It all turns out all right. Going by the pictures on the screen the fetus is eighteen weeks four days, but ultrasounds are only 'guesstimates'. Jane is pretty gobsmacked. I think she was expecting it to be a fairly static side view. Instead, the camera goes in from all angles – top of head, soles of feet – and measures the length of the thighbone and the arm bone, and thankfully everything's all right and connected to the other right bits.

The fetus's face still looks pretty spooky, sort of like a skeleton face with black shapes where the eyes should be. The shot of the spine makes our little darling look like the remains of a flounder on a dinner plate. It's hard not to think it's really waving or having a chat or playing peekaboo when really all it's doing is instinctively having a rowdy time, practising grabbing, sucking and Morris dancing. The sonographer takes quite some time and is very thorough, checking the four valves of the heart, measuring a whole lot of circumferences and lengths and widths. She speaks very quietly to her assistant, who types it all into a computer. She says it's all good.

Suddenly sleeping properly and floating through the days. If I didn't know better, I'd say I was on drugs.

Another thing I have started noticing: people who warn you against unsolicited advice already have their own. 'Don't listen to any busybodies', they say. 'What you'll need to do is…'

The finance experts in magazines and on the radio all suggest that when you stop using contraception you should start saving for all the stuff you're going to need, especially because one person is probably going to drop an income for a while. Accordingly, we are spending money like there's no tomorrow.

I have £82 left in the bank. We've got bars on the windows, we've got built-in wardrobes coming, we've got trees going into the garden. We've got new maternity clothes. For some reason I'm in a demented frenzy and keep wanting to buy towels even though we've got enough. Must be some innate memory of all those films where the baby's come early and some gnarled old trusty shouts, 'Boil some towels and splice the mainsail!'. Or perhaps I'm thinking of pirate movies. 'I've boiled the water and trained the parrot, dear. Everything's going to be fine.'

If it wasn't for the phone, I'd never have any social life. All my childless friends are flat out at work (so am I) and the ones with kids are worse. I never go out at night any more, and when I do I leave parties at about 10 p.m. stone-cold sober, wishing people wouldn't smoke. Miss Francine was right. My life is over...

info

placenta praevia (low-lying placenta)

This is one of the things your ultrasound anomaly scan will look for. Placenta praevia means the placenta is attached to the lower part of the uterine wall, instead of the upper part, partially or completely blocking the way out. In the late stages of pregnancy, as the uterus stretches and the cervix ripens (becomes thinner and softer, ready to 'dilate' – open wide – enough for the baby to pass through during birth), a placenta attached to the lower uterus can become detached, causing painless bleeding.

The risk of having placenta praevia is increased if you have uterine scarring from previous pregnancies or surgery, you're older, you smoke, or there's more than one baby in there. If the bleeding is severe, you may need to have an emergency caesarean, but sometimes your obstetrician will adopt a 'wait and see' approach after mild bleeding, especially if the obstetrician wants the baby to develop a bit more before it comes out.

pregnancy clothes hints

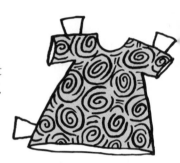

ⓖ Let's not forget that both Pamela Anderson and
the Queen have been pregnant. Women's tastes don't
become all the same just because they're up the duff.
There are a berzillion maternity clothes shops now,
many of them online, with everything from bizarre
stripper outfits to princessy pink stuff with bows.
And many high-street chains now have maternity
sections too.

ⓖ Length does matter when it comes to 'maternity wear'. If you weren't the
type to wear a miniskirt before you were pregnant, why would you wear one
during pregnancy? If you want a fairly normal dress that ends in the vicinity
of your knee, rather than a micro-mini the size of a beer towel (or a frock so
voluminous you could use it as a duvet cover), try something stretchy like
cotton jersey.

ⓖ Always remember: this is a TEMPORARY wardrobe. Don't spend a
fortune unless you're a diamond heiress, in which case stop reading this
book and go invade Corsica or something.

ⓖ Borrow everything you can from a previously pregnant friend, but
only things you know you'll wear. Don't clutter up your
drawers with stuff that doesn't fit or you wouldn't wear.
Write down who has lent you what – with the label and
description recorded – so you can give it all back. (Some
friends will just say you can pass it on.)

ⓖ Don't borrow anything really flash if the person you're
borrowing from wants it back. You never know what could
happen to it, and it might be a financial hardship to replace it, even if you
could still buy that style, which is unlikely.

ⓖ Check out the racks in the following sections: sports, dance and other
stretchy stuff, men's, and full-figured women's clothes. Bear in mind that in
the last month or two of pregnancy just 'big' may not do it. You'll probably
need at least a couple of items that have the properly designed stomach bits
you only get in maternity clothes.

⑥ Don't worry if your maternity wardrobe is all black, or all navy, or all incredibly boring in some way or other. At least everything will match. You'll be so sick of the sight of everything by the time you give birth, anyway, that it doesn't matter.

⑥ The maternity fashion police will tell you not to wear men's shirts or tight trousers or flat shoes because they are unflattering. May I just say that from about the thirty-second week of the pregnancy, you might as well be wearing an armoured tank: *nothing* is flattering.

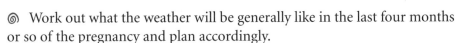

⑥ To cut down on searching every morning, look through your wardrobe ONCE, now. Put all the possible maternity clothes up one end of the wardrobe and clear a drawer for the non-hanging possible clothes and maternity undies and bras. As each item of normal clothing outlives its usefulness, put it in the normal-person part of the wardrobe or chest of drawers.

⑥ Work out what the weather will be generally like in the last four months or so of the pregnancy and plan accordingly.

winter

See if any of your friends have a swing-coat (also known as an A-line or knee-length overcoat) that you can borrow to get you through. If you're going to need to wear huge socks for the cold, you're probably going to have to buy a pair of gigantic shoes for the duration. A basic winter maternity wardrobe might include:

1 frock for best
1 skirt
2 pairs trousers
maternity jeans
4 pairs tights (you can wear them below the bump)
gigantic jumper or cardie
T-shirts
2 maternity-sized bras – maybe one pale and one black
gigantic cotton underpants
low-heeled, generous-sized shoes
a warm coat with plenty of room for a bump

summer

Please, just forget that polyester was ever invented. Go for cotton, or microfibre or a rayon if it's the cool, floaty kind. Corner a bloke and confiscate all his T-shirts and shirts. A basic summer maternity wardrobe could include:

1 frock for best
something floaty and pretty (remember any print should be little, as a large print will look like upholstery fabric and make you look more sofa-like)
1–2 everyday frocks or skirts
comfy maternity trousers or jeans
T-shirts
men's shirts
a light coat with room for a bump
shawl, wrap or giant jumper or cardie for cold evenings
(use a horse blanket if necessary)
2 maternity-sized bras – maybe one pale and one black
gigantic cotton underpants
flip-flops or sandals

undies

⑥ The most important word on undies is cotton.

⑥ If you wear a bikini style you can probably continue to wear your pre-pregnancy undies with the waistband sitting under your bump; or if you find up-to-the-waist styles more comfortable, you can probably just buy bigger sizes of your favourite brand. You'll have to see how you go – you might end up nipping down to M&S for some comfier larger ones, or even a packet of maternity ones. Undies department ladies are always excellent for this sort of thing and will have you sorted in no time.

⑥ Women who have bad backs, are overweight or are carrying twins may be told by their doctor to wear a maternity girdle to give some extra support late in the pregnancy. Using tight 'shape wear' is not a good idea during pregnancy – don't try to hide or squish your tum.

⑥ Real tights usually just don't fit at all as you progress in size. But why doesn't anyone make matt-black opaque maternity tights that don't fall down so you don't get that sagging gusset thing happening? Until they do, you could take a tip from Superman and wear your underpants OVER your tights to keep them up.

shoes

Yes, your feet are getting bigger – firstly, they're probably puffed up with extra fluid (and if you go on a plane they puff up like blowfish), and secondly, they're probably broader because of all that extra weight you're carrying. The ligaments in your feet are softer and stretchier than usual, so your feet will 'spread' and well-fitting, comfortable shoes are essential.

⊚ Your feet may end up one size bigger permanently. You may want to wait and see before buying lots of hideously expensive new shoes.

⊚ If you wear socks, buy thin ones or 'stocking' socks.

⊚ Buy a new, larger, all-purpose, flat-heeled pair of shoes to 'live in' for the duration – many very pregnant women wear trainers. Or pop a couple of canoes on your feet.

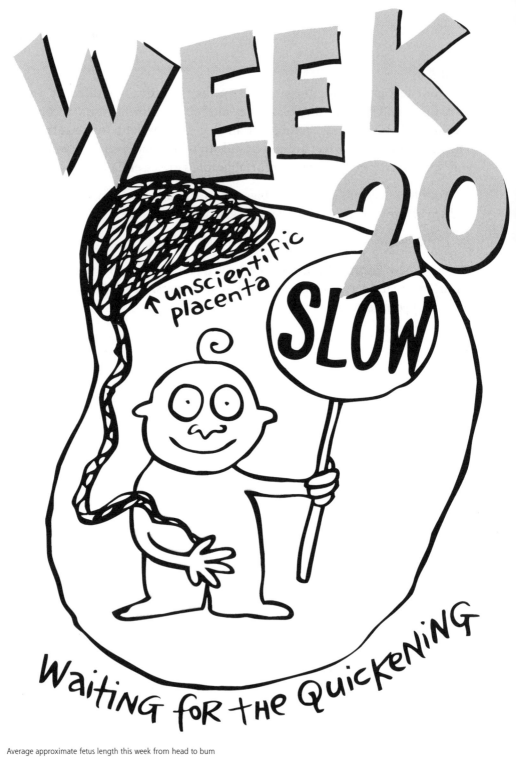

Average approximate fetus length this week from head to bum

cm   1   2   3   4   5   6   7   8   9   10   11   12   13

what's going on

Probably by now you will have felt the baby move, but maybe not. It's usual to laugh or cry the first time. Doing both at once is perfectly fine. It might still be too early for anyone else to be able to feel the movements from the outside. For a while it's your little secret bond.

The fetus puts on more muscle and tests it out by moving around. A girl fetus already has 6 or 7 million eggs in her ovaries. The skin's sebaceous glands (needed, of course, to make spots later) become active and make the oily stuff called vernix caseosa that covers the skin. It's the fetus's do-it-yourself wetsuit, made – disgustingly enough – of fatty material and dead skin cells. (If that doesn't make you feel sick, how's this: doctors say the coating looks like cheese.) Vernix caseosa waterproofs the skin against the amniotic fluid, and protects the fetus from scrapes when it bangs into the wall of the uterus. Weight: about 320 grams.

16   17   18   19   20   21   22   23   24   25   26   27   28   29   30

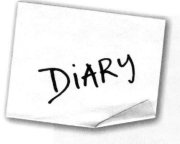
DIARY

I still haven't bloody well felt the baby move and I'm sick of all the books and websites I've read saying I should have. I think it's because there's so much fat between me and Cellsie. It makes me really anxious. I feel very cheated about it not kicking and really cross with them for making me feel like a freak because I haven't felt the 'quickening'.

Beck says 'You have felt the baby move, but you just don't know you have. You probably thought you were going to fart or something.' How romantic.

We go out to dinner and I think it won't do any harm to have a glass of French champagne. I have half a glass and it tastes like windscreen cleaner. (Well, like I think windscreen cleaner would taste. I'm not a connoisseur.) I sleep for eleven hours and only go to the toilet four or five times. Remarkable.

Feeling suddenly bigger, probably because it all seems like it's out the front there now. I really feel like I'm carrying weight – when I try to run, this hilarious galumphing tummy precedes me like a big beer belly. Geoff says soothing, private things like 'You are *not* a fat old baggage. You are the Tummy Princess.'

Suddenly feel connected to other mothers a bit – certainly more than I ever have before. Not all mothers. Well, obviously. Not Pamela Anderson or the Queen or anything.

Back, legs and neck all painful. Get hysterical. Ring the chiropractor at home. Make an appointment for the next afternoon, so of course I have another reasonable sleep (again only four or five wees during the night!) and by the next morning most of the symptoms are gone.

I am getting more and more worried because I haven't felt the baby move. Decide to phone Dr Sharma.

'Listen, Doc,' I say, 'all the books say by week 20 you should have felt the baby move, and it's week 20 and mine's gone out for coffee or enjoys a lot of kipping.'

Dr Sharma's opinion on the matter, basically, is bugger the books (except that Dr Sharma probably never says bugger), I'll feel it soon enough.

I realise that I don't know whether you keep feeling the baby once you've felt it for the first time or if you have to wait another week. Dr Sharma says once you feel it you feel it every day.

Quite often in the street I suddenly find myself rubbing my stomach in the unselfconscious way men scratch their scrotum or stick their hand up between their buttocks to arrest some pants making a bold upward bid for freedom. And I don't care who sees me. My stomach sticks way out in front and people ask 'When are you due?', and I say 'August', and they look at me as if I've got a bullock up my frock. Their next question is usually 'Is it twins?'.

I saw Peter X in the street today. Nothing like the wildly startled look of an old boyfriend who's about to say 'Hi, you look huge' and then has to restrain himself from fainting as he realises you're pregnant and he doesn't know what to say. His eyes rolled around in his head like the eyeballs of a mad dog – lots of white. Poor thing. I suspect that just for a split second he thought it might have had something to do with him – until he came to his senses and realised that six years' gestation is probably pushing it.

Yesterday I paid for all my literal slackness in not doing my pelvic-floor exercises. I sneezed and wet myself. Not a huge gush, but enough to make a tiny splash on the floor. Luckily I was standing on the wooden floor at home.

When I sneezed Geoff said 'You look absolutely mortified.'

'Well, I just wee-ed', I explained helpfully.

I am also having a recurring dream that I'm having an affair with a freelance sausage maker. I wonder if freelance sausage makers mind if you wet yourself.

My old friend Luke and his wife, Fatimah, call to offer a pram. Excellent. Uncle Mike insists on buying the cot even though he will no doubt complain for six weeks about how much it cost and express the view that the baby should be sleeping in a hammock in the open air dressed in a robe knitted from chamomile or something.

Susanne's getting on in her pregnancy now. She just rang to say she was in the shoe shop and a woman told her she had good posture. Suze, completely vague and stuffed full of pregnancy info, meant to tell the shop assistant that's because when she walks she 'leads with her sternum', the breastbone. Unfortunately what she actually said was she 'leads with her perineum', which is the area between the vagina and the anus. No wonder the shop assistant looked startled.

Susanne's not putting on enough weight to keep her doctor happy and I've got plenty extra. We're considering a transference.

info

weight gain

Weight gain is an important part of a healthy pregnancy. The right weight gain for you is different from the right one for somebody else (you know, depending on your height, weight and body frame when you became pregnant, and whether you give a stuff about it). The ranges nominated for a one-baby pregnancy vary from 12 kilograms to 16 kilograms and more. Many slender women put on 20–30 kilos during pregnancy and then lose them again afterwards.

About a third of the weight gain is baby, placenta and amniotic fluid; the rest is new bits of you – increased blood volume, breast growth, fluid and fat. The body needs to build up stores of fat during pregnancy, which is then used in breastfeeding. The weight you gain will probably be somewhere in the vicinity of:

> baby, placenta, amniotic fluid: 4.5 kilograms
> increased size of uterus: 1 kilo
> increased breast size: 0.5–1 kilo
> increased blood: 1 kilo
> retained fluid: 3 kilos
> increased fat and protein stores: 3 kilos

Most of the weight gain is between the fourth and seventh months of pregnancy.

At the birth you can lose up to 12 kilos at once, and in the days following the excess fluid will also be lost through sweat and urine.

Under normal circumstances you don't need to weigh yourself or be weighed by the doctor or midwife (see 'Eating and Supplements' in Week 2).

IF YOU'RE ITCHING ALL OVER

Report this to your doctor straight away. It could mean your liver enzymes are not working properly, which will need to be monitored with blood tests. It can be safer to have your baby delivered earlier than expected.

Your obstetrician or midwife will be on the alert for any unusual, wild or rapid increase in weight during the last ten weeks of pregnancy, which can be a sign of pre-eclampsia (see the info in Week 28). Some other conditions associated with considerable weight gain in pregnancy are gestational diabetes, high blood pressure, varicose veins, haemorrhoids and uncontrollable Magnum addictions. Shut. Up.

See 'Being Active' in Week 15 as well as 'Eating and Supplements' in Week 2.

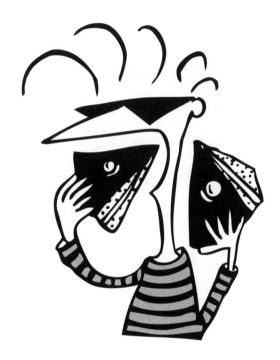

WEEK 21

what's going on You could start to get heartburn and indigestion. Get used to people judging your size – 'You're not very big for dates' and 'My giddy aunt, that's enormous!' – sometimes on the same day.

The fetal eyelids are still fused closed (until week 27). The brain has been developing very quickly, but its surface is still very smooth, not like the textbook pictures of walnut-looking adult brains that we're used to.

Weight: about 390 grams.

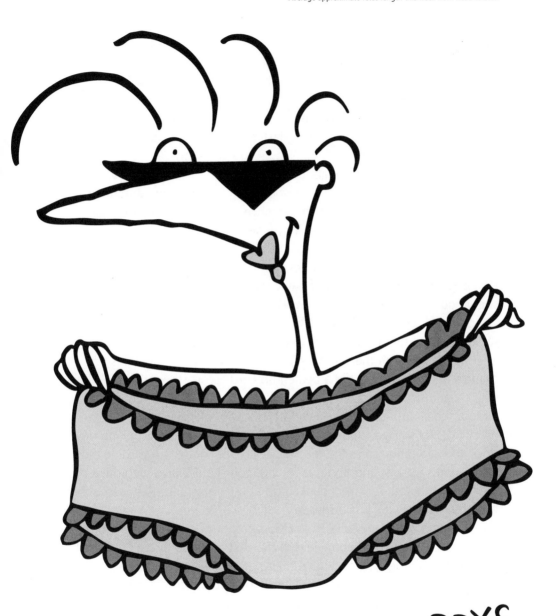

You could catch stingrays in my underpants

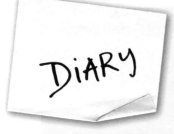
DiARY

I have new moles and skin tags everywhere. It's like my skin is hyperactive and throwing out extra bits wherever it can. Basically I'm getting extra tags and moles in every area I already have them, plus a whole new bunch of tags under each breast.

My hair also appears to be attempting an Afro at every available opportunity. It seems to be growing faster and getting thicker, but perhaps this is an optical illusion.

My tummy's sticking out about where the rest of the world used to be, so when I squeeze through to get out of the lift at work and automatically calculate I've got a 10-centimetre clearance I actually rub myself against someone, who starts to look very frightened at the idea of being groped by a pregnant woman.

Young men look me up and down in the street, and when they realise I'm pregnant there's this look of panic that crosses their face and they quickly swerve out of my way. It makes me want to rush over and get them in a vice-like grip and scream: 'The baby's coming! You'll have to do something!' I reckon most of them would faint dead away or just run.

I was standing in the street the other day waiting for the lights to change, and just as they did a beaten-up Ford Escort stopped and a bloke with dreadlocks and a cowboy hat stuck most of his body out the window and started shouting, and then the driver was honking his horn and wolf-whistling, so I started rubbing my big tummy up and down, pulling up my frock and vamping across the road – because of course it was some blokes from Geoff's work falling about laughing. You should have seen the looks on the faces of the other drivers banked up at the lights: like, this used to be a bad area but now it's just *disgusting*.

Shopping with Aunt Julie. Thank God no horror stories, although she does tell me encouragingly at some length that ALL first babies cry CONSTANTLY and wriggle all the time and drive their parents mad, and the parents *never* get any sleep, and this is the inevitable fault of the parents, who are necessarily inexperienced and tense so make the baby tense. Quite serene, this shopping caper.

See a small child in a clothes shop and say '*Hellooo*' in exactly the same tone Aunt Julie uses. Reel back in horror and hope I won't automatically start trying to feed small children grey mince on rice and boiled chops four nights a week. A few minutes later say 'Peekaboo' to another strange child just as if I am channelling Aunt Julie, who is at that moment looking at a pink floral suit and saying 'This is lovely, dear, unless it's a boy.' (She is very worried about cross-dressing babies.) The child seems to take it rather well and in the jaunty manner it was intended.

Shopping for baby clothes is actually just like being size 16 in a shop for grown-up women where all the sizes are 8 and 10. Everything's teeny tiny. Except there are slightly more snap fasteners at crotch level than usual. When shopping for myself I can still go into a shop and say, 'Yes, I'll have one of those in size ginormous, thank you.' If they have them. At this stage you could catch stingrays in my underpants.

Anyway, back to baby gear. Some kids' clothes are £30 a throw, even £60 a throw, for something that they must grow out of in a nanosecond. I'm thinking I might just coat my child in Vaseline to keep it warm. There are T-shirts and romper suit things you can buy with 'Baby' written on the front – you know, in case you think you've given birth to a ferret, or you get confused and start dressing your bedside lamp. 'No, that's right, tea cosy on the teapot, T-shirt on the BABY.'

And there are these hair bands with flowers on that go around a baby's head, and basically they're used on a baldy baby to indicate that it's a girl. Oh, say it loud and say it proud: 'The kid's bald.'

People keep asking me if it's going to be a boy or a girl and I say 'Yes, I believe so. So I've been led to understand. But we're not fussy. We're just hoping for a life form of some description.' They say 'Well, you should find out so you know what kind of clothes to buy for the baby.' I'm like: is it going to matter? Is somebody going to accuse a four-month-old child of cross-dressing?

And sometimes people ask 'What are you hoping for?' 'A giraffe. They're up running around the paddock an hour or so after birth and starting to feed themselves.'

Baby clothes sizes take some getting used to. They start with 'Tiny Baby' or 'Early Baby', for premmies. Next comes 'Newborn', but the clothes are still teeny-tiny; when I say that looks too small the sales assistant shows me a doll that's size 0–3 months and fair dos, it could play full-back for the Harlequins. There's no way something that big is going to come out of me without some kind of major rearrangement of the laws of physics. So 'Newborn' it is – about the size of one of those gowns that starlets wear to the Oscars, in fact. Don't get too much labelled 'Newborn' as your bub could grow out of that size pretty quickly. See how you go and you can always lay in some more. It's the sort of thing relatives will love doing.

I'm feeling much better, but still sleeping up to ten hours a night easily. The whole food thing is weird. I still eat when I'm hungry but nearly hurl at the sight or smell of any slight sliminess, like green leafy things more than a few minutes out of the ground. I can't go to the supermarket with Geoff any more because I go whey-faced the minute I smell the delicatessen section and have to go outside.

I watched a TV documentary on *Goon Show* hero Spike Milligan and was astonished to hear that after they divorced he refused to let his wife ever see their children: that's what the law allowed then because she had left him, even though he was a manic-depressive alcoholic. He later admitted he was an unfit father. His kids talked about how they used to write letters to fairies and leave them in the garden, and Spike would write back tiny, enchanting letters and they really believed there were fairies, well into their teens. It sounds lovely, a man trying to make his children's world so beautiful. But then his son sadly describes how completely ill-equipped this made him for the real world. Oh, who'd be a parent?

We're off to Geoff's work function. Geoff is given a nurseryman's achievement award (a very nice shovel), and his colleague Brenda makes a speech in front of the entire workforce of the nursery chain stores about how his extra work is really appreciated, especially as his 'wife' (apparently that's me) wouldn't appreciate him working on weekends with women in skimpy shorts (no, I really think lady gardeners should wear crinolines) but I had mounted the best strategy and got him pregnant.

I spend a good half an hour restraining myself from wrestling her to the floor and strangling her with a tablecloth.

About sixteen people handle my stomach without asking. Only one, Trina, asks whether she can. Her baby is a year old and she tries to flog me her cousin's pram. Crushed to hear we are already prammed up on a promise, she changes tack by looking at me critically.

'How are you going with your weight?' she asks, swaying in the wind on her go-go boots.

'Oh, stacking it on, thanks', I say cheerfully.

'Don't do what I did. I got up to 80 kilos.'

I break it to her gently. 'I'm already 80 kilos.'

'OH MY GOD! I've finally lost it all.'

'Breastfeeding?' I ask.

'No, it's harder than that', says Trina. 'As soon as

go-go boots

I stopped breastfeeding, I started starving myself and eating junk food. But I'll have to start eating properly again to set the baby a good example.' Fat chance.

At Lucretia's party that meat-faced old drunk Michael F comes up and tells me loudly I'm the last person he expected would ever get pregnant. I suggest he take a long look at himself.

'Babies love me', he says. 'I don't know why, but when they get a bit older they reject me.'

'Maybe it's because you smell like a bottle of mixed sherry and urine', I don't say. More bloody advice about how to get them to sleep from a man with four children by five different women, who thinks a hearty breakfast is a bottle of stout and a packet of Marlboros.

Today's newspaper says a new study shows that 'unborn babies' can hear at twenty weeks. I hope Cellsie didn't get a load of Brenda's speech. Mind you, I'm really not sure about the research methods in some of these surveys that provide quotable statistics. Ten pregnant women listened to one music tape in the twentieth week of pregnancy. Two to three weeks after birth the babies kicked less when those songs from the tape were played.

Well, this is just not enough information. Were the babies forced to listen to Garth Brooks, Celine Dion or Mating Calls of the Lesser Yak? Couldn't the lack of kicks have been incredulity?

info

at work

In a healthy pregnancy and a healthy workplace there is no reason why you shouldn't keep working for as long as you want to and your doctor and health and safety officer agree, especially because the money will come in handy. How close to your due date you work will depend on how you feel.

Most women value some time alone before they begin the horror! the horror! Oops. The extremely rewarding and divinely bondworthy, magnificent experience of childbirth and caring for a newborn baby. It's common to take maternity leave for at least the last four to six weeks of the pregnancy, and longer if you can afford it. You'll probably feel really tired and uncomfortable in the last few weeks. Resting well, exercising gently, eating right and thinking serene thoughts during the last weeks of the pregnancy certainly won't hurt.

From week 32 your heart, lungs and other vital organs are working really hard and getting more and more squished up by the growing uterus. The strain on your back, joints and muscles is increasingly intense, and you might be vaguing out a lot. Not to mention that by week 36 that baby head bouncing on your cervix can make you swear and jump around as if you've suddenly developed Tourette's syndrome: not a good look during a meeting.

If your job requires a lot of standing up, working in the last few weeks can get really difficult. Even a desk job can become hard. You might just want to lie on the couch and read magazines or watch DVDs.

Some doctors recommend that if your job has you on your feet more than four hours a day, you should stop work by week 24, and that if you need to stand half an hour of each working hour you ought to stop work by week 32.

Other work conditions that should be discussed with your doctor are exposure to possible teratogens – substances or environmental factors that could harm your baby (see the info in 'Protecting Your Pregnancy' in Week 4) – work that involves lots of lifting, carrying or bending, or shift work, which can upset sleep and eating patterns.

Being pregnant at work should probably be dealt with like any other personal issue: don't blab everything to everybody, especially gossipy people and ones who couldn't care less and drop off for a nap at the first sign of the word 'trimester'. This will also allow you to feel more professional for the time you are there and when you come back.

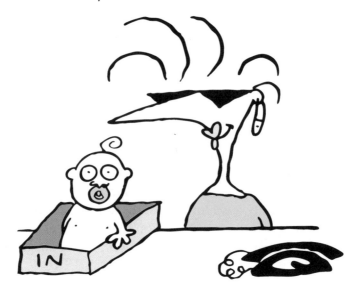

How managers view the whole deal of pregnancy and maternity leave can vary dramatically, regardless of what the law requires of them. Bosses in some large companies have done cost-benefit research and realised it's cheaper and smarter to give valued employees leave, then welcome them back with flexible working hours, than drive them out and start training new people (who may also get pregnant). Other bosses try to sack you as soon as they find out: this is illegal.

While you're busy being your same old reliable, efficient self, you might really be feeling very different, hiding how you feel and worrying that you might overlook something important. Here are some suggestions that might help.

⑥ Keep a stash of healthy snacks at work, which are useful for keeping your blood sugar up and nausea at bay during the first trimester, and for general nutrition the rest of the time.

⑥ Make yourself comfortable. Get horizontal when you can. Sit rather than stand. Have regular walks and stretches if you're bent over a desk for much of the day. Drink plenty of water. If you feel really tired, use your lunch hour to sleep in a spare office, organising to have someone wake you up at the end of the break. If you do this, don't forget to make time to eat.

⑥ Take it as easy as possible. See if you can work at home some days, or go home for a snooze when you can.

⑥ If work is stressful, try yoga or meditation classes and learn some good relaxation techniques.

⑥ Keep the best work diary you could imagine and religiously consult it every morning. Make lists. Invest in Post-it notes for reminders. Get colour-coded folders. Get staff pals or an assistant to remind you of things, including 'Go and have lunch'.

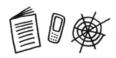

more info on **the workplace**

If you think you're being discriminated against, check your rights with your union, a lawyer or the government departments dealing with employment. Also see 'Work Entitlements' in the Getting Ready chapter.

what's going on

You may have back pain, cramps, varicose veins, vivid dreams, and feel strangely calm. You also put on the most weight in the second trimester. But of all the weight you put on, a relatively small proportion is the weight of the actual fetus. The rest is stuff you need, such as blood, amniotic fluid, larger bosoms, necessary fat stores and, um, cheesecake.

Downstairs there may well be some exhibition somersaulting going on. The inner ear has reached adult size. There are now eyebrows and head hair (unless you've got a baldy one). The lungs are starting to produce stuff called surfactant, a detergent-like substance that will help them to function properly by keeping them expanded after a breath. Weight: about 460 grams.

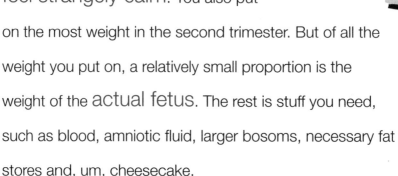

Average approximate fetus length this week from head to bum

| cm | 1 | 2 | 3 | 4 | 5 | 6 | 7 | 8 | 9 | 10 | 11 | 12 | 13 |

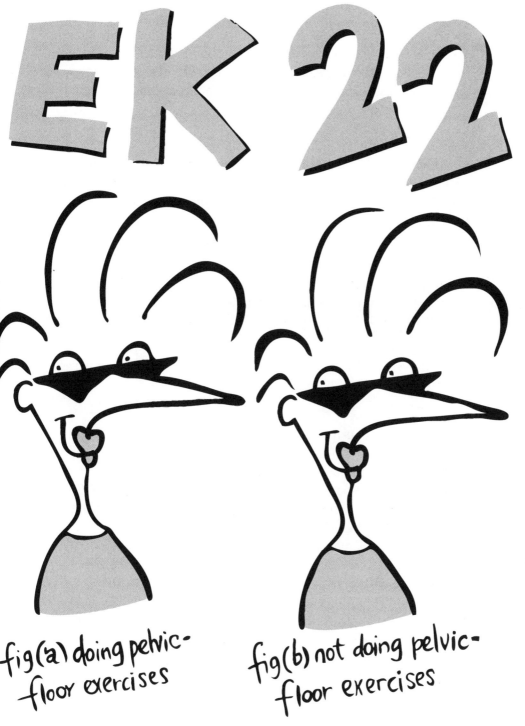

fig (a) doing pelvic-floor exercises

fig (b) not doing pelvic-floor exercises

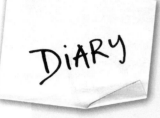
DiARY

My horoscope this week says: 'Dating is invested with potential. Those who are pair-bonded ought to beware sudden attractions to deeply inappropriate types'. In my case, I presume, this would mean … anybody else in the entire universe.

Geoff talks to all the men at work about weird things their wives do when pregnant. I don't have enough people to talk to about this stuff. Most of my friends who aren't childless have forgotten what it's like to be pregnant. Even a lot of my lesbian friends who want to have kids haven't got around to working out how yet. We are about to leave the baby-free zone.

I'm organising a nappy-wash service for Suze for when she gets out of hospital with the new baby. I send an email to all our friends.

> Hi All
>
> As you know, Susanne is about to have a baby any minute now. Possibly at this very moment. What you may not know is that newborn babies need their nappies changed up to sixty times a week. I'm getting her a gift account at Snappy Nappy – which will deliver clean nappies (and take away the other kind) each week, as soon as she gets home from hospital. Do you want to be in on this? Email or text me if you do and I'll organise the rest, including a card from all of us.
>
> Kaz xx

I am prostrate with exhaustion and self-admiration after such efficiency. Then I realise I've sent it to everyone in my email address book, including my boss, who doesn't know Susanne from a bar of soap.*

This not-feeling-the-baby-move business is getting embarrassing. Beck, with absolutely no tact in sight, tells me I'm 'a bit remedial'. She assures me again that I have felt the baby move but haven't realised it, and tells the story of a very large woman who came into A&E when Beck was a nurse.

The woman was complaining of terrible, sudden, intermittent abdominal pains. (You know what's coming, don't you? Well, she didn't.) The paramedics told the nursing staff the pains were coming at regular intervals and were probably labour contractions, although the woman kept saying she wasn't pregnant. Beck said to her 'But haven't you felt the baby move?'. 'It's just wind', the woman said, shortly before being joined by her offspring, whom she regarded with some astonishment.

* I eventually got a thank-you note from Suze confessing she switched to disposables after five weeks! Next time, she said, pay for a cleaner for a couple of weeks. Fair enough.

I've popped into Beck's clinic, after another visit to the chiropractor, to see if I'm in early labour or just constipated. What a glamorous job she has.

'I'm not giving you a laxative without feeling what's going on', she says. 'Otherwise you might be having a baby instead of a poo.'

Charming.

Speaking of wind, am nearly crippled by it in the babies' wear department of a gigantic department store this afternoon, and have to walk around bent in half and rubbing my stomach. People look rather concerned but I can hardly announce 'It's all right, move along, I think I just need to do an enormous FART.'

Once again some of the baby clothes have Paris couturier prices, and although I am careful I end up spending £85 on small hats, vests, cotton jumpsuity things and oh, all right, a couple of expensive cute things like a red denim jacket and matching leggings. Bought a few light blue items. Not because I think I'm having a boy but because that pale pink makes me feel queasy.

I think it's better if I stay out of babies' and children's wear departments. It will be cheaper, and I don't want to end up with a child resembling anything remotely like those demented-looking blond children with bowl haircuts you see in glossy kids' wear brochures, dressed in velvet frou-frou knickerbockers with matching bow ties, looking like their parents would have conniptions if they got dirty. I'm thinking of dressing Cellsie in a plastic mac from dawn till dusk and just hosing him or her down before bedtime.

Today I officially let myself go. I spent the entire day dressed in a hessian sack and moccasins, and I haven't washed my hair since Wednesday. I know the *Oprah* theme music by heart.

And I've been looking at the preggo websites again. One suggests that you could hint to your partner that you were pregnant by serving him a dinner comprised of veal, baby carrots, baby peas and baby spinach. And decorate the table with the white flowers called baby's breath. Geoff, at least, being a professional, could tell baby's breath from a bunch of cauliflower, but even he's unlikely to make the connection.

And the pregnancy magazines are full of aerobicised chicks in high heels. I haven't done any side-lying crunches and I don't swim the equivalent of the Channel every day. I have lifted no weights, cross-country skiing is a mystery to me, and I don't even know what an isometric abdominal is. I haven't done any pelvic-floor exercises. This means by Christmas I'll be incontinent, broke and 487 kilos. What I want to see is a few of these mags with women who were more than size 10 to start with and who've just had two nights of insomnia and half a Black Forest gateau; and instead of male models, I want to see proper blokes looking unshaven, and shell-shocked after seeing their first ballistic baby poo.

I've 'popped' again: another growth surge in the tummy region. I popped at four, five and, um, 5.425 months. It makes me go around singing the blues song by Howlin' Wolf, 'Three Hundred Pounds of (Heavenly) Joy'.

info

skin

A whole lot of stuff happens to your skin when you're pregnant. Everything is working overtime, generally resulting in more oil, sweat and pigment (colouring) being produced. More blood is flowing closer to your skin, making it warmer; and increased oil gland secretions, giving skin a shinier appearance, add to the pregnancy 'glow'. Retained fluid can give the skin a fuller, smoother appearance than usual. Necessary fat stores mean more 'cellulite' on buttocks and thighs for the duration.

It depends on the individual: although many women find their skin looks better than ever during pregnancy, some may be prone to oily skin or spots on their face, chest and back, because of rampant hormones, while others may find themselves with dry, scaly skin. Oestrogen slows down oil production, but progesterone promotes it – and they are both very active during pregnancy. Most skin changes, including some skin tags, are temporary, but some are permanent: you may end up with darker nipples forever, and a few more moles; stretch marks will stay too, but fade to be hardly noticeable unless you run around in the nuddy under fluorescent lights.

pigmentation changes
Pigmentation changes, also known as melanin or colour changes, are caused by increased production of melanocyte-stimulating hormone (MSH), which acts on the cells that affect the colour of your skin. These changes are usually more obvious on dark skin. The theory is that darker nipples make it easier for breastfeeding babies to find them. If you have fair skin and red hair the changes will probably be slight.

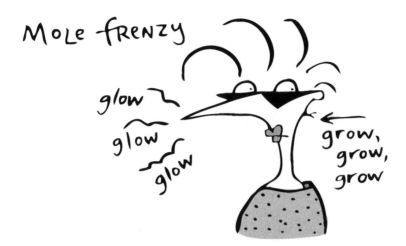

The area around and inside your navel can become darker. So can existing freckles and moles – but any changes to moles should be checked by your doctor. The skin under the eyes and arms, between the thighs and of the genitals may also be noticeably darker during pregnancy. Some pregnancy experts say the vagina turns purple. But who's game to look? It doesn't matter what colour it is. (Tell a lie. Lime green would be a worry.) Oh, let's just take their word for it.

linea nigra

The dark line called the linea nigra, which divides your tummy into halves along the site of the stretching rectus muscle (from your navel down to your pubic hair), often appears by week 14, though sometimes not until weeks later. (The line is actually there before pregnancy – imaginatively and inaccurately called the linea alba, the Latin for 'white line' – though it's not particularly noticeable on any skin colour.)

irregular patches

Irregular patches of slightly different-coloured skin might turn up on your face; these are called chloasma or, by doctors who like the movies, 'Zorro', the 'mask of pregnancy'. The patches are dark in women with light skin and light in women with dark skin.

Folic acid deficiency is linked to too much colour change in the skin. Exposure to the sun will intensify changes such as the face patches. A hat and a 15+ sunscreen cream will protect you.

stretch marks

Stretch marks, which look like thin pink, red or purplish lines on pale skin, and paler brown lines on dark skin, can happen on breasts, tummy, thighs and bottom. Relaxin, the hormone that makes ligaments relax during pregnancy, also has an effect on collagen, making it stretchier. But if weight gain is rapid (and sometimes you can't do anything about this because that's just the way it is, rather than the result of eating too many Magnums), the collagen expands too much and breaks, creating marks.

After pregnancy, stretch marks gradually fade to silvery lines in the skin, usually barely noticeable. How many you get and how quickly they fade will largely be determined by the skin and body type you inherited. Some skins have more stretchiness (more collagen and elastin) than others.

Gradual weight gain may help to minimise stretch marks, and a good diet that includes plenty of protein and vitamin C will help keep skin in a generally healthy condition. Many people swear by vitamin E cream, but there's no scientific research that proves it helps, and many women who use vitamin E cream still get stretch marks.

skin tags

Skin tags are little extra bits of skin that often develop in places where there is some friction, such as the bra line under your breasts, or under your arms. They are caused by small areas of skin getting overactive. Sometimes they disappear a few months after birth, sometimes you've got them forever (but dermatologists can remove them). Guess you'll just have to wait and see what happens to yours.

visible veins

Some people develop spider veins: threadlike, wiggly red lines, usually on the cheeks. They are small broken blood vessels caused by rapid dilation and constriction of the vessels when circulation increases during pregnancy.

Blue lines under the skin, on the breasts and on the tummy, just show some of the extra blood you're carrying. They will go away after the baby arrives.

Bulging varicose veins in the legs can be painful. Your doctor can tell you how to avoid them (usually: put your feet up when you can and wear special 'support' tights). They may eventually disappear or in severe cases have to be surgically removed.

rashes and spots

Heat rashes can be caused by the combination of increased circulation, body temperature, sweating and skin friction in pregnancy. Rashes might cause itchiness. It may help to dress in cotton clothes that allow good ventilation and to wash using a non-soap alternative or special oil (ask your pharmacist).

Red spots sometimes appear on the face, arms, torso, palms and soles of the feet. These too are caused by increased blood flow through dilated vessels, and go away after pregnancy.

Skin problems such as psoriasis and eczema are unpredictable during pregnancy. They may get worse or get better, disappear for the duration or appear for the first time. See a dermatologist (your GP can refer you), and tell them you're pregnant.

Some medications for acne, psoriasis and other skin problems can be dangerous for the developing fetus. Discuss any treatments, whether in tablet or ointment form, with your doctor or dermatologist.

Don't use any creams containing steriods on your face (whether you're pregnant or not): these come under various brand names and include ingredients such as hydrocortisol. They can cause a persistent facial rash called perioral dermatitis. (More never-ending glamour!)

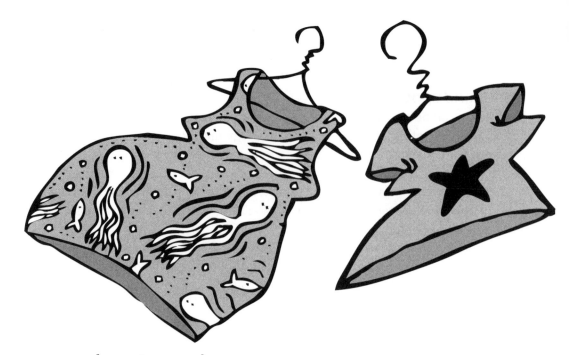

what's going on
Your bladder is getting squished, so you may need to wee more often. You might feel practice labour contractions from now on, called Braxton Hicks (or they may not start for weeks, or you might not ever experience them).

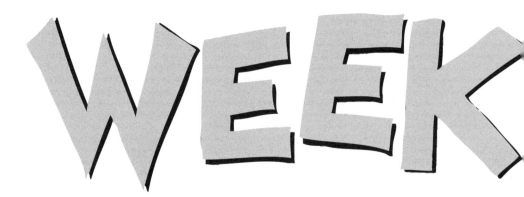

Average approximate fetus length this week from head to bum

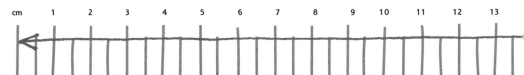

cm   1   2   3   4   5   6   7   8   9   10   11   12   13

The fetus is growing like crazy, and the brain is maturing. Some researchers believe the fetus has started to think. Others, to be safer, say we can't really tell when this happens, and it may be much later. (And even then, it's probably just stuff like 'Gee, I like to suck things' and 'La, la, la, whatever' or 'It's a bit wet in here, innit?'.) The skin is growing very quickly, but there's not much fat yet developed for plumping up underneath it, so it looks a bit pruney. Weight: about 580 grams.

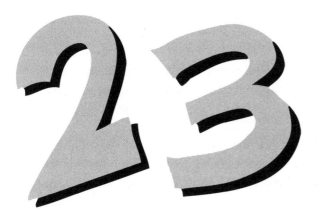

23

16   17   18   19   20   21   22   23   24   25   26   27   28   29   30

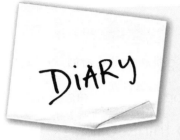
DiARY

Just ate entire block of chocolate. Feel sick. This won't stop me from having lunch, mind you. By this stage I find I am in need of some even more simply enormous underpants. They are the kind of thing you could wave if you were surrendering. Later I might recycle a pair as a duvet cover. I find it is infinitely more soothing not to think about the size of my bum.

The only time I can get a sense of weightlessness is in the bath. I'd rather be swimming, even if I did resemble the opening sequence of *Free Willy*, the whale movie. But I've let my healthclub membership lapse, and the public pools are infested with some hideous staphylococcus, germy thing that's front-page news. The reports include a hideous diagram of minute quantities of 'faecal matter' floating around public pools and spreading the bug. Not for me, thanks.

Susanne's baby has arrived. She's a very beautiful girl with gigantic feet and no name, but never mind that: Suze did the whole labour as Warrior Woman without painkillers! She had a trainee midwife who made her push too early – apparently the midwife thought the distension of the vaginal wall caused by the pushing was the baby's head! Suze's fanny, by this stage, was looking like it had been thoroughly bashed up. Poor Suze was very happy to see the obstetrician, who marched in, terribly calm, put a suction cup on the baby's head and pulled it outta there. He had to give her an episiotomy, so she has heaps of stitches.

Suze said she was in shock afterwards and thought she'd rather die than ever do that again, but a few days later she'd kind of forgotten. She has stories of over-bustly nurses coming in at all hours and patting the baby around as if she were a football, which unsettled her. So she told them all to bugger off and only let in the nicer nurses. She had the 'baby blues' day on day four when the real breast milk came into her breasts, but she reckons it wasn't too bad – she just let herself cry all day without feeling weird about it. She looks terribly glamorous and serene in her silky nightie, and the baby seems to be an old hand at the breast.

Suze's maternity ensemble reminds me I don't have anything suitable to wear in hospital. I head off to Oxford Street to get myself a nightie and dressing-gown because a T-shirt, hiking socks and an old overcoat obviously will not do. I also try to buy a back-supporting maternity-girdle-type thing. But when I mention the girdle, the saleslady asks sternly through cat's-bum lips 'Has your doctor told you to get one? They're not recommended these days. Have you told your doctor?'

'I don't want one to hide my stomach, I want it to support my back.'

'I see', she snapped. 'We haven't got any.'

What a ninny.

Boy, do I have this Nesting Thing really bad. All afternoon I daydream about moving the furniture. Why can't I live in a minimalist house like the ones in *Elle Decoration* magazine? Pout for a while. I collect more boxes to put things in and cut out magazine articles that introduce a new verb, 'de-cluttering'.

Thank God I am removed from the house for a few days by the necessity to travel up and down the country promoting the new fashion range. Realistic sizes are flavour of the month, but you watch – by summer every other fashion house will be back to toddler-sized persons jigging about in grown-ups' clothes. I have to do an interview at Classic FM, where it's so posh that as I'm eating a muffin out of a paper bag while I'm waiting to go in, somebody comes and gives me a plate so I won't 'have to be a savage'.

I'm supposed to say in the interview why I've chosen these bits of classical music – and I don't even know what they are. I got them all off this relaxing CD that my beautician plays while I'm having a facial. So the interviewer's going 'And why is this passage by Debussy a favourite of yours?', and I just take a punt and say 'Look, it's got a lot of piano, and if you're in the bath you can go underwater to wash off the shampoo, come back up and not feel like you've missed anything.'

And then the interviewer says: 'And you're pregnant. We had another pregnant lady in a while ago – or maybe she was breastfeeding, I can't remember.'

I say 'Well, did you see her bare bosoms? If you saw her bare bosoms, she probably had passed the pregnancy stage.'

Being in a huge city like London is really no fun in this condition. I flew back from Manchester to Heathrow and the queue for a taxi was 200 long and full of business people who look at you as if you're an alien and never offer to help with your luggage.

Meanwhile a local shopping centre has banned public breastfeeding in the food court because it's 'just exhibitionism'. Hear, hear. I am sick of these mothers pushing their prams around the streets in string bikinis, removing their nipple tassels and just flaunting themselves generally. I mean, it's too much. There are many people who don't know what a breast looks like, and when confronted with one in the street, for a split second before a bub wraps its gob round the pointy bit, people could lose their reason!

And everybody knows that when a woman is breastfeeding, it is impossible not to be reminded of such classic films as *Debbie Does Dulwich*, *Swedish Knockers Akimbo* and of course any *Carry On* film starring Barbara Windsor. In fact, breastfeeding is such a salacious and provocative act, I'm surprised it isn't banned altogether.

Obviously a lot of nursing mothers will pretend that they just want to feed their child to stop it from shrieking – but I think we all really know that it's just an excuse to behave like a strumpet and give all the blokes in the vicinity a bit of a saucy come-on. Apparently when you're getting 20 minutes of sleep a day and you spend your life cleaning up somebody else's poo and you haven't had time to wash your hair for three weeks, all you really want to do is have sex with strange men in public places. Can't help yourself.

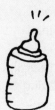

All the newspapers have gone wild with letters, including one from a member of the Breast Police who has managed to insult *everyone* by saying she finds mothers who *bottlefeed* their baby in public to be offensive because everyone must breastfeed. She's alienated all those mums who would love to breastfeed but can't. I hope her nipples rotate at night like propellers and keep her awake.

info

travelling

The best time for holiday travel is the middle trimester – you're probably not queasy, there's not much chance of labour starting, your energy levels are up, you're not too huge to get comfortable and you're less likely to be mistaken for a large wildebeest in the dark.

Think twice about going somewhere you're unaccustomed to that's hot, humid or otherwise a frenzied-mosquito festival. Pregnancy has already raised your body temperature. In addition, high-altitude destinations (over 2000 metres) are not recommended because of the lack of oxygen for you and your baby.

Plan a holiday that allows for good diet, rest and relaxation, and always check in with your midwife or obstetrician before making any bookings. This is no time to press on with that adventure trek across the Mongolian plains on the back of a goat just because you planned it two years ago.

And if you are lucky enough to live in a developed country, this is probably not the time to visit a developing one. Ask yourself 'Would I feel safe if my baby arrived early in this country?' You might have to be there for up to two or three months.

You might not be able to have the vaccinations you'll need for a developing country, and you'll be exposing yourself and the baby to diseases and the sort of medical care they make scary films about. If you insist on heading for regions where gastro bugs are common, pack diarrhoea medication recommended by your doctor or obstetrician for use during pregnancy, and drink lots of reliably bottled water to ensure you don't dehydrate.

Don't go anywhere where you'd need to take malaria prevention drugs. They're not safe in pregnancy – and neither is malaria.

If you travel overseas, get high-level travel insurance that includes medical costs. The most 'developed' country in the world, the US, has a freakishly expensive health system. If you have an annual policy you may find it has become invalid: be sure to check. Ask your obstetrician about how to find a doctor at your destination who literally speaks your language. Carry a brief medical history, including your blood group and allergies, and your obstetrician's phone numbers. Many people carry their full maternity notes. If you have a problem, call your doctor at home in the UK, even if you're in Burkina Faso. Worry about the phone bill when you get home.

by car
You can drive all through pregnancy as long as you don't rule yourself out for severe vagueness. (Driving yourself to the hospital in labour, however, is not on.)

⑥ Take snacks, drinks and a back support cushion if driving for long distances (and likewise on train trips). The only snacks you can buy in most places have the nutritional content of a battered Mars Bar and three times the calories.

⑥ Put the seatbelt's lap strap underneath your belly and the sash between belly and breast.

⑥ You can sit on a folded towel for the last couple of weeks of pregnancy in case your waters break when you're driving, so the amniotic fluid doesn't ruin the upholstery.

⑥ Stop, stretch and have rest breaks, and don't hold back if you need to wee: make sure you stop regularly and go to the toilet.

by plane

Most airlines refuse bookings from pregnant passengers during the last four to five weeks of the pregnancy in case you give birth prematurely on the flight. Restrictions and medical certificate requirements vary from airline to airline. Don't think you can fox them by just turning up, either – they may make an arbitrary decision not to let you fly if you can't prove your due date.

It's not safe to fly in an unpressurised aircraft when pregnant because of the lack of oxygen. Large planes all have pressurised cabins but smaller planes may not, and you need to find out about this from your travel agent. Oxygen levels can fluctuate even in pressurised aeroplane cabins, so if you are feeling lightheaded ask the flight attendant for some oxygen.

⑥ Check with your doctor to assess your risk of deep vein thrombosis (DVT) developing during air travel.

⑥ When booking flights, say you are pregnant and ask for an aisle seat (for access to the toilets and leg stretching) near the front of the plane (you can get on last, get off first and have better air quality).

⑥ Ask about food options, such as vegetarian or low-fat meals, that might be yummier and better for you.

⑥ If taking a short holiday or trip, try to limit yourself to hand luggage to save having to wait on arrival.

⑥ Wear comfortable shoes and thin socks because your feet will swell even more than they do on a long flight when you're not pregnant, and put on support tights if you have varicose veins. Puffiness may last for a day or so afterwards (see the info on swelling and fluid retention in Week 28).

⑥ On long flights avoid dehydration by drinking plenty of fluid – water, diluted fruit juice or milk – but not alcohol, tea or coffee. Bring your own healthy snacks.

⑥ Take plenty of walk and stretch breaks. Elevate, flex and rotate your feet while you are sitting, to help your circulation.

staying away

⑥ In your handbag, carry a few essentials such as tissues (you never know when your nose will run or stuff up or you'll need toilet paper), ear plugs and an eye mask.

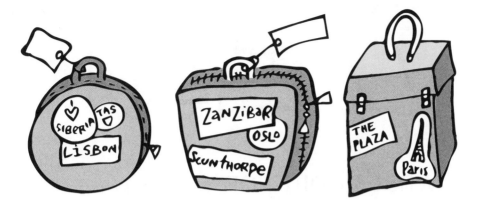

⊚ Pack versatile, lightweight clothes.

⊚ Don't even think about high heels.

⊚ Lighten your load as much as possible. Some marketing geniuses now make small cosmetic travelling kits for this very purpose. Cute but expensive – you can make up your own in tiny plastic bottles.

You are very obviously pregnant by now so if you'd like to avoid people asking you lots of questions on your train, bus or plane trip, read some erotic fiction with lurid book covers. You'd be surprised how much people leave you alone.

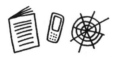

more info on **travel**

fco.gov.uk
>The website of the Foreign and Commonwealth Office. Click on 'Travelling and living overseas' for advice on which countries are safe to visit, travel health info and other tips.

The Rough Guide to Travel Health by Dr Nick Jones, Rough Guides, UK, 2004
>This is a useful pocket guide with lots of advice on travel during pregnancy (including the low-down on vaccinations and malarial prophylactics), plus country-by-country tips for trips. It has handy sections, too, on travel with … BABIES!

WEEK

what's going on
You may be feeling constipated. Changes in blood flow can mean your blood pressure drops and you may feel faint. This can happen when you lie flat on your back because the weight of the uterus can compress the big fat vein (the inferior vena cava) that carries blood from your lower parts back to your heart. If you do feel weird, stop lying on your back and you'll feel better again.

Many babies born at this stage have survived with the help of hospital intensive care, but this is by no means guaranteed. The biggest problem is that the lungs aren't really finished, so if the fetus came out early it would need help to breathe. The fetus still looks thin compared to the roly-poly Anne Geddes calendar-style baby, but is starting to get plumper. Weight: about 630 grams.

cm
1
2
3
4
5
6
7
8
9
10
11
12
13
14
15
16
17
18
19
20
21
22

Average approximate fetus length this week from head to bum

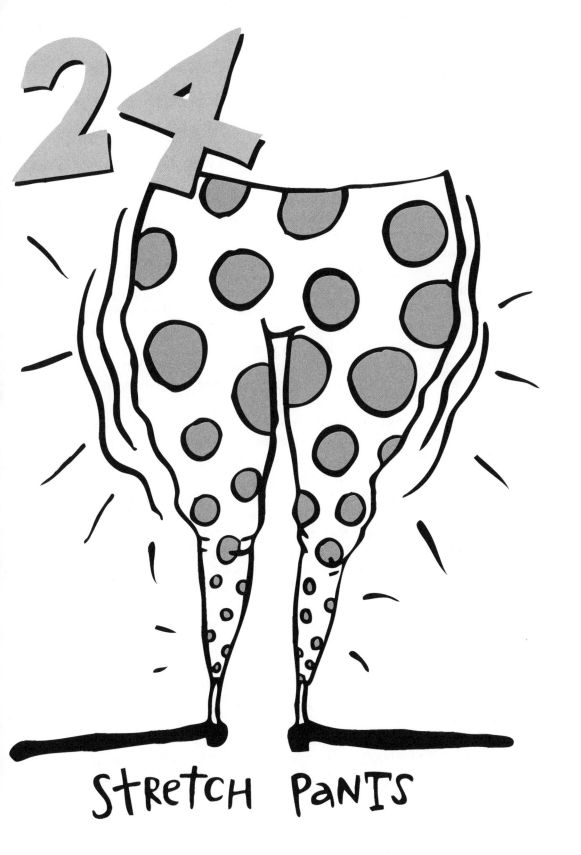

24

STRETCH PANTS

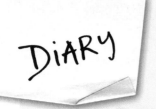
DiARY

Katie rings to say she's just been to an agricultural show, where there was a 'maternity ward' – a bustling pavilion full of twenty ewes, any one of which was 'lambing' (that is, giving birth) at any one time while a woman on a microphone made an incessant commentary and people stood around waving show bags and, depending on who they were, looking stunned (young men), completely horrified (young women), sympathetic (older women), stoical (older men), and antsy from eating their weight in candy floss (children).

So of course last night I dreamt that it is me and a whole lot of other pregnant women in the pavilion. I am wearing baby-doll jarmies and everyone else is in Laura-Ashley-style dressing-gowns. The commentator is sitting on a velour throne and saying 'Look at that woman. She can't give birth because she's wearing the wrong pyjamas.' I am mortified about the pyjama situation, but just then the woman in the next stall gives birth to a small lamb and confides to me over the fence that she'll 'make the best of it'.

I wish my hair wouldn't be quite so eccentric. One day it looks like a full-on Big Hair extravaganza, and the next it lies down like a couple of bad billiards players in a city pub.

I'm thinking more about the baby. The great festival of nesting continues. Rachel says every time she rings me up there is another tradesperson in the house. This time it's the carpenter, Crazy Axel (he doesn't call himself Crazy Axel, but he should). Crazy Axel makes my long-awaited built-in wardrobes in large pieces that he unloads off a trailer onto the pavement and then realises none of them will fit through the door, and he has to saw them in half.

Installation brings a whole new sense of horror, with great big bits gouged out of the wall, and Crazy Axel's frank admission that he hasn't thought about how to install the heavy top pieces. At one point I offer a crane, but luckily some Swedish circus performers who are staying next door come in and climb up the wall and help guide the pieces into place. If the bottom ever falls out of the flying-trapeze market, these gals should be able to get a job at IKEA.

Crazy Axel distinguishes himself by running into the gate in his car, leaving the job for hours at a time and walking back into the house without knocking. Finally he says he can't finish the job because it's all too upsetting, and drives away. Leaving his mobile phone in the wardrobe. Which rings in the middle of the night.

I'm still really sensitive to smells. I try to go to the supermarket again, but one foot into the deli section and I nearly faint and throw up at the same time. Luckily I don't try Fish – my head might have rotated.

Why do I bother to make those few social calls to remind myself I still have friends? I distinguish myself by leaving parties when most other people are arriving. It's impossible to keep up my previous, non-pregnant pace – but hard to slow down to a real pregnant pace. This leaves just the uncomfortable feeling of being boring and guilty at the same time.

My brain is suet pudding and I can't remember anything. I have stuck Post-it notes around my computer screen so many times it looks like a ruffle.

I'm sitting on the sofa watching *Playschool* (practice) when I feel a sort of a feeling that could be some lunch rearranging itself, only it's too low down, and might be a fart but isn't, and come to think of it, I've felt it before. There's a bear in there!

It's Cellsie! I feel intensely pleased with the world, and can't help patting my tummy in reply.

People are still trying to get us to find out if it's a girl or a boy. An article in the local paper asks 'Does discovering your unborn baby's sex spoil the surprise or does it allow for sensible planning?'. It says three-quarters of English women want to know the sex – but I'm sure it has to do with thinking of the baby more as a person, so you'll take any info you can get. If the doctor could tell whether or not the kid was going to have a natural talent at footy, you'd probably want to know that too – partly because there are so many unknowns and undercurrent worries that any hard and fast information can seem comforting. Apparently, people are more likely to find out the sex of babies when they have already had a child or children. I suppose that's the one thing they are not pre-warned about.

I squeeze into some old stretch pants and wear them down the street. And I do mean stretch pants. They are so thin that the tight grey pantery shows my bum crack (a fact helpfully imparted by Geoff when we arrive at the Tube station) and threatens to simply twang off my body at any moment. A rather narrow squeak for me, if I can use the words 'me' and 'narrow' in the same sentence.

info

antenatal classes

where?

Ask your midwife or GP for their recommendation regarding antenatal classes, and book as early as possible to make sure you get a place on the course you want. The provision of classes varies widely around the country. They may be run by your hospital, by your local midwife or health visitors, or by your own GP or health centre. The NCT (National Childbirth Trust) also runs classes, usually in the evening and at the home of whoever is running the course. Classes run by the NHS are usually provided free of charge except for refreshments. NCT classes can be well over a hundred pounds for you and a birth partner; but discounts are available for those on low incomes.

why?

The aim is to prepare you and your partner or birth support person psychologically and practically for labour and delivery. Well, as prepared as you can be if you've never done it before. And these classes are full of first-time parents. (Already-parents are probably at home having a lie-down.)

what?

Also known as parentcraft classes, childbirth education classes and the horror video club, antenatal classes typically comprise a series of weekly sessions of an hour or so in the third trimester of pregnancy. Ask about the style of the class before you book in. You may have found that pregnancy and childbirth websites and books often talk about the various schools of childbirth theory, such as Sheila Kitzinger's psychosexual approach to childbirth (birth as an earthy, sexual, visceral woman–baby thing) or Janet Balaskas's active-birth model. In practice, antenatal classes tend to provide a combo of the most helpful elements from various schools of thought as they relate to the experience and philosophy of the hospital maternity department or individual teacher.

man watching birth video

THE NCT

Set up fifty years ago, the NCT is a charitable organisation that offers educational advice and support for parents during pregnancy and birth, and on through the toddler years. The NCT has campaigned successfully to ensure that fathers have the right to attend their baby's birth and that babies are not separated from their mothers straight after birth. They continue to push for more women-centred postnatal care and a positive breastfeeding culture.

The NCT offers a wealth of well-researched information, maternity sales (equipment, books, bras, etc), and, most crucially, a network of antenatal courses – which offer you not only knowledge about pregnancy and babycare but also a local support group with other women and couples in the same boat. This may not sound like what you want right now but when a baby arrives along with your new life it may be just what you need.

The structure of NCT classes depends on your local branch (there are hundreds of branches across the UK – see 'More Info on Childbirth' coming up for contact details). The classes can be quite informal, and the content can be completely changed by what you and the other prospective parents are interested in finding out about. Most classes start towards the end of the second trimester (Week 26 or 27) and continue with weekly sessions for the next eight weeks. By the end of the classes, you will have a new gang of potential friends who will become part of your life, or a really good idea about the sort of parents you want to run away from – or a bit of both!

Some childbirth classes are run as a series of lectures; others may have an open structure, allowing for discussion. Some offer hands-on sessions for practising breathing and massage techniques; others may encourage the sharing of feelings about pregnancy and childbirth, or involve lying around on lumpy, brown corduroy beanbags discussing your innermost feelings with total strangers.

Other antenatal classes focus specifically on fitness or yoga during pregnancy and after delivery.

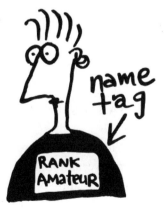

These may be found through hospital antenatal clinics, or local sports, recreation or yoga centres (see also the Active Birth Centre in 'More Info' coming up).

Ideally the person running the class will impartially present the pros and cons on issues such as hospital vs home birth and pain relief, without saying things like 'Anyone who has an epidural is a big girlie wussbag' or 'Anyone who doesn't have an epidural is a mad feral hippie'.

If the teacher seems to be going in a direction you don't like, try another teacher. Good classes should ensure you develop realistic expectations about what labour will be like, providing a balance between childbirth as a joyful, amazing event and the things that might go wrong or go against your picture of the ideal birth. Ask lots of questions (reading the relevant chapters in this book may also help to answer them). Classes are there to give you the information *you* want.

Typical classes will provide information on how to recognise the onset of labour; when to go to the hospital or birth centre, or call in the home birth troops; pain relief; and body positions that might help during labour. They almost always show videos of childbirth, provide a tour of a birth centre or labour ward, and include advice on antenatal and postnatal exercise, caesarean section, induced labour, the partner's or birth support person's role, breastfeeding, unsettled babies, how to reduce the risk of sudden infant death syndrome, and how to recognise postnatal depression.

who?

You can go to birth classes on your own (and some classes are run especially for single women), but it makes sense to go with your partner or birth support person. This makes it less likely that they'll be asking questions during the real thing such as 'What happens now?' and 'Can I have some of those drugs?' Check whether partners are welcome before you book your course: on some courses, partners are only invited to one or two sessions.

BABIES BORN EARLY

With specialist care, some, but not all, babies born as early as 24 weeks can survive, although they face ongoing medical problems. (There's detailed info on premature birth and premmie babies in Weeks 29 and 30.)

Blokes, you can learn a lot at such gatherings and may also find yourselves a part of the invaluable support networks that come about through classes. In other words, you can make parenting friends and meet helpful babysitters you can 'swap kids' with. Life is about to change big time, and allies can be a great part of that.

how much?

Two hours is plenty on labour. No need to go for weeks and weeks. Labour is one day of your life – parenting is forever. So pick a childbirth class that also includes stuff on breastfeeding, looking after a baby and other info for L-plate parents.

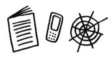

more info on **childbirth**

nctpregnancyandbabycare.com
From the main page, choose 'In your area' then 'Course finder' to check out which NCT classes are handy to your work or home.
Enquiries line: 0300 3300 770

activebirthcentre.com
Click 'Classes and training' then (at the bottom of the page) 'Active birth teachers UK and international' to search for teachers of pregnancy yoga.

Read one of the books about how to care for a baby listed in Week 43. It will give you an inkling of what you're in for.

WEEK 25

what's going on The fetus is about due to start putting pressure on your ribs and also on your digestive system. You could get pains down the sides of your tummy from now on as the uterus stretches. The fetus looks pretty much like a baby at birth. It will definitely have developed its own sleeping patterns: usually awake when you're asleep and vice versa as your movements soothe it to sleep. (This is why babies can be rocked to sleep once they come out.) The fetus may be startled by loud music and start bashing you up when it hears a certain tune. Or maybe that's just dancing. This is a good time to play it music, talk to it and see if you get a reaction. Weight: about 700 grams.

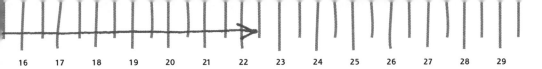

| 16 | 17 | 18 | 19 | 20 | 21 | 22 | 23 | 24 | 25 | 26 | 27 | 28 | 29 |

Average approximate fetus length this week from head to bum

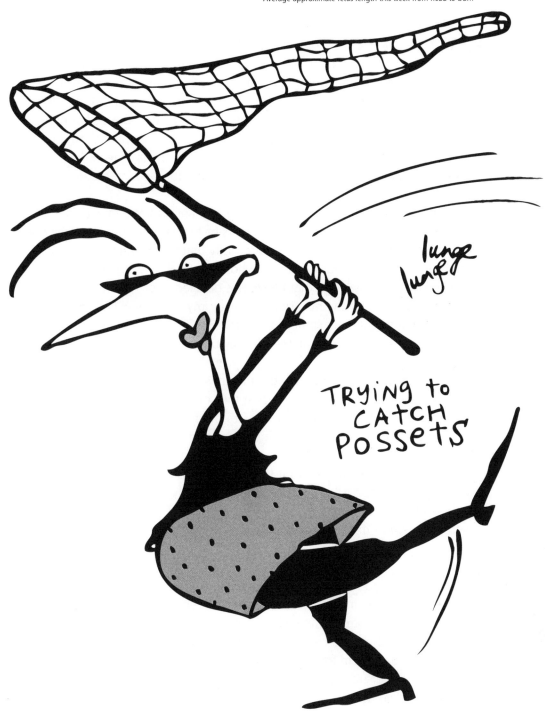

TRYING to CATCH POSSETS

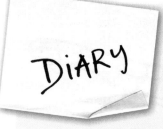
DiARY

I keep forgetting where I am in the middle of sentences: it reminds me of all those times recovering from endometriosis operations, when the general anaesthetic seemed to temporarily wipe out most of my vocabulary.

I have covered the house with a confetti of Post-it notes, and I keep paper and pencil AND a tape recorder next to the bed at night. So far I have written down really helpful stuff like 'Remember the thing', and mumbled thoroughly unintelligible words into the tape recorder, then dropped it and stood on it on the way to the loo for the nine-hundredth time.

Geoff inquires whether, now that I'm pregnant, I intend to eat his head. Turns out he has been watching a wonders-of-nature programme on the telly about black widow spiders. I point out loftily that the praying mantis eats the head – the black widow eats the whole lot. Strangely, he doesn't look soothed by the knowledge that I have this detailed information.

A weirdy man on the bus tries to look up my skirt. I feel like saying 'Careful. You might meet someone coming the other way!' I've heard about men who are affected in an unseemly way by pregnancy, and here is the proof.

It takes some effort to think about what will happen after the baby arrives as I can't seem to stretch my mind past the concept of childbirth, but it must be done. Oh my God. It's not just that I'm pregnant; there's actually going to be another person along any minute, and they haven't even got their own room.

Actually I don't really mind if the baby spends the first few weeks sleeping in a cardboard box, but it would probably upset Aunt Julie. We have completely run out of money, but these are some of the things the books and websites seem to think we should be purchasing:

✳ a gigantic industrial-strength washing machine

✳ a fridge with a freezer big enough to store frozen casseroles for the weeks after the birth. The fridge-freezer we have is a legacy of the old shared-house days. The freezer compartment is a lot more used to ever-emptying bottles of vodka and tubs of ice-cream with a spoon frozen into them. Right now it has only enough room for four sausages, a frozen pizza and eight ice lollies. Unless it has over-frosted again, and the door has frozen shut. We just *can't* have a baby, we haven't got the right fridge

☀ a Moses basket. This is the one thing Susanne also says I will need: a nice basket with sheet lining, and a stand and handles so you can cart it around from room to room. I quite like the idea of having a baby in a basket and it seems you can use it instead of a cot for the first few months

☀ 'muslin squares for catching possets'. Oh for God's sake. I don't intend to go hunting. If possets are required, I'll just buy them at the supermarket. (Later it turns out that this means a 'piece of cloth to put over your shoulder that the baby can vomit onto'. Why don't they just say so?)

☀ 56,000 nappies

☀ a 'nursery', a word which previously had connotations only of seedlings – will need to strip boyfriend of personal space, manhood and shed-like environment by taking over his private room to achieve this

☀ a 'bonnet'. I presume they mean hat. Or is it compulsory to get something with bobbles on it?

☀ a nursery floor covering, as in 'The floor covering of the nursery should be linoleum or cork tiles'. Ours is carpet. Maybe we could just throw a tarpaulin down for the first couple of years

☀ a dimmer switch, 'installed for night feeds'. Have a dimmer switch installed?! How much money do these books assume you have? What, now I have to sleep with an electrician? Give me a break. Might as well say 'Install a surround sound system with wall-sized video screen to simulate the sound and light show of the womb'. We'll make do with an old lamp, thank you. Or I could park the cot near a window that lets in street light. Or gaffer tape a bicycle lamp to my head

☀ a small sink with running water – some pregnancy books actually suggest you install one in the corner of the room. Oh and perhaps a turret might be nice.

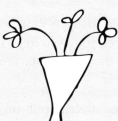

info

baby clothes and nappies

The exact quantity of clothing you'll need will depend on things such as whether you have a very vomity baby, how often you will be washing, and whether you use cloth or disposable nappies (cloth nappies tend to create more clothes washing because their 'containment' is not as efficient as that of disposables).

It's not a bad idea to get your baby's clothes before you get too big to go charging around shops and bargain outlets. Here's what you'll need.

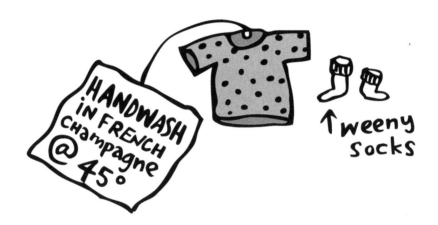

HANDWASH iN FRENCH CHampagne @ 45°

↑weeny socks

clothes
Basic newborn-baby wardrobe

⑥ 6 vests (aka bodysuits) with wide or envelope necks (usually short-sleeved with poppers at the crotch but no legs)

⑥ 6–8 front- or crotch-opening babygros (aka stretchsuits, sleepsuits or grow-suits) with or without feet; you need to go up a size in babygros with 'feet' as soon as they fit snugly or they will start to hurt your baby's feet and stop legs stretching out properly

⑥ 2–3 pairs of cotton socks, or stretchy, pull-on, machine-washable bootees – forget ribbons, forget handknits except for show, and you won't need socks

at all if the weather is very hot, or if you plan to use babygros with feet all
the time

⑥ 8 swaddling blankets: these are easily washed flannelette squares used for
wrapping a baby up – wrapping is the key to helping a new baby settle and
sleep (see the 'Wrap Party' box in Week 40). They can also be tucked around
the baby in a cot or pram, and laid on a floor or table as a nappy-change
surface

⑥ 10 muslin squares, which are easily washed and dried and become
indispensable – used as over-the-shoulder protection after feeds or general
mopping-up cloths, placed on the changing mat to make it more comfy for
baby, and put in the Moses basket to collect dribbles from the mouth (so
cutting down on the need for endless laundering of crib sheets)

⑥ bibs – you don't need these straight away, and the number will depend
on whether your baby vomits or dribbles a lot. To be honest, all babies
dribble a lot. Get big towelling bibs without ribbon ties (Velcro's good);
plastic-backed ones are stiff and no good for wiping faces. You'll need about
eight bibs once the baby starts eating solid foods (and maybe a shovel and
nine bath towels). For breastfeeding, people usually just have a cloth nappy
or a muslin square handy to mop up possets (little vomits)

⑥ forget mittens, and hats that can slip over faces, and anything with
strings, tassels, cords or long ties

⑥ a few weeks or months later – one or two quilted-cotton or flannelette
baby sleeping bags with sleeves but no hood, dangly lace, ribbon or
drawstrings. These washable, zip-up bags are both very cosy and safe (see
'Baby's Bed' in Week 26) and come in a variety of togs (warmth ratings)
suitable for different times of the year.

Summer baby   The baby may need grow-suits with short sleeves and legs,
or may be more comfy in just a vest and nappy as long as the insects are kept
away.
     A summer baby won't need as many swaddling blankets as listed, but a
couple won't go astray for cool nights. Substitute a few soft, absorbent muslin
or gauze squares for wrapping (you can make these yourself or get them from
baby shops).

Winter baby The baby will need three to four outer items: cardigans or jackets are easiest to change. If you use jumpers, make sure they have two buttons at the neck or are very stretchy. Fabrics such as velour, thick cotton jersey or thermal materials are more practical than woollen knits, which are harder to wash and dry and can be itchy.

Hints from mothers

⊚ Buy natural fabrics.

⊚ All clothes you get should be able to be soaked, machine washed, and tumble dried if you need a dryer.

⊚ Good vests have really generous neck and arm holes so that you can get them on your baby quickly and easily.

⊚ Babygros are so much easier to change if they have press-studs that run from the neck to the crotch and right down the inside of both legs. DO NOT BUY A SINGLE THING THAT BUTTONS DOWN THE BACK OR LACKS CROTCH FASTENERS.

⊚ If you buy those headbands with a bow on them for a girl baby your child will look like a demented Easter egg in a nappy.

⊚ A small baby doesn't need shoes except for show. Warm, snug socks are fine – they're not going hiking any time soon.

⊚ A tiny baby hates being dressed and undressed. To help make changes quicker and less traumatic, choose soft, stretchy cotton or cotton-blend clothes and envelope necks that are easy to get over the head.

⊚ Go to bargain places, but be careful to check why the stock is cheap. Small marks that will wash out are fine, but clothes likely to spontaneously combust or fall apart in the first wash are not.

⊚ Borrow as much as you can. If it has to be returned, keep a list! Don't ask people repeatedly to lend you baby clothes – they will offer if they want to. Sometimes they are keeping their baby clothes in case they decide to have another one, and it's all too psychologically confronting to give away their supplies.

⊚ Buy or borrow the minimum number of tiny-sized clothes: they don't get worn for very long and some big babies can skip the newborn size and go straight into 0–3 month size.

⑥ Babies grow out of things so quickly you could well match up with someone with a slightly bigger baby and someone with a slightly smaller baby to become part of a clothes chain.

⑥ Cheaper chain stores can have very good babies' and children's wear departments: sometimes the best clothes are the cheapest because they're not fiddly and made for show. At this early stage they won't need to last unless you're passing them down the line to other children. Don't overbuy, even though the clothes are so cute: your baby will grow quickly.

nappies

A newborn baby needs about sixty nappy changes a week on average. Later, you use fewer nappies, but more goes into them. (That was delicately put, wasn't it?)

Cloth   Depending on your washing plans, you need about 36 nappies. Cotton cloth nappies (like tea towels) are usually for very tiny babies, who graduate to more absorbent towelling ones. There are various nappy companies offering all sorts of modern designs and systems, including Velcro fastenings, fitted pant-nappies, bright colours, quick-drying fabrics, inner liners and plastic over-pants.

Washing your own nappies could be easier in the summer when there's (hopefully) plenty of sunshine and warm breezes for line drying. In wet weather, and especially in the winter, you may need a stable of clothes horses or an electric dryer to ensure a steady supply of dry nappies. Generally, the idea is to put any solid poo into the toilet (especially as babies and their poo gets bigger) and wash the nappy to re-use it. People usually have a nappy bin in the laundry, with its lid kept tightly on – because of the smell, but also because if it's filled with water to soak the nappies it's a drowning risk for toddlers and other kids. Nappy-wash services are also available, which take away their plastic bin full of dirty nappies and swap it for a new one and a stack of clean, sterilised nappies. Usually they visit once a week – at a price, of course.

Most of the people who choose re-usable nappies do so because they're cheaper in the long run, and because of concerns about the undeniable problem of landfill waste caused by disposables. But it's important to also factor in your own circumstances and the amount of water and chemical soaps you use: which is worse for the environment, cloth or disposable nappies, is often a dead-heat in environmental studies. Some local councils provide incentives for using cloth nappies.

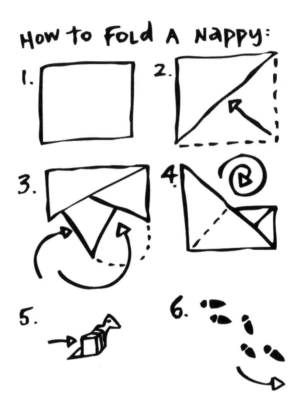

Disposables The worst nappy choice is cheap disposables, which are hopeless. If you can, buy a more expensive, big-name brand in newborn-baby size, which, despite the cost, will be good value for money because they are much more efficient.

Even if you plan to use only disposables, buy ten to twelve cloth nappies: perfect for over-the-shoulder protection after feeds and for general mopping up. You'll also be confronted with an occasional bottom so comprehensively pooey that cottonwool balls will get you nowhere. When this happens, dip a clean cloth nappy in warm water, squeeze out the excess and go in valiantly. Always use a cloth nappy to cover the change mat, which otherwise can be a bit too plasticky and cold (or sweaty) to put a baby on.

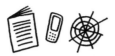

more info on baby clothes and nappies

Many of the pregnancy websites reviewed in Week 1 have ads for, and forums that recommend, baby clothes outlets. Buyers beware! For second-hand clothes, also try charity shops, jumble sales and reliable online stores.

nctpregnancyandbabycare.com

On the home page, select 'nearly new sales' and enter your postcode for listings of sales in your area. As well as baby clothes, they'll include equipment and toys.

goreal.org.uk

Tips for reducing the environmental impact of cloth nappies, and help finding places to buy cloth nappies and nappy-wash services in your area. It does describe home washing as a breeze, though … which isn't true for everyone.

which.net

The website of *Which?*, the independent consumers' association, has stats on nappies and their effect on the environment (search 'nappies').

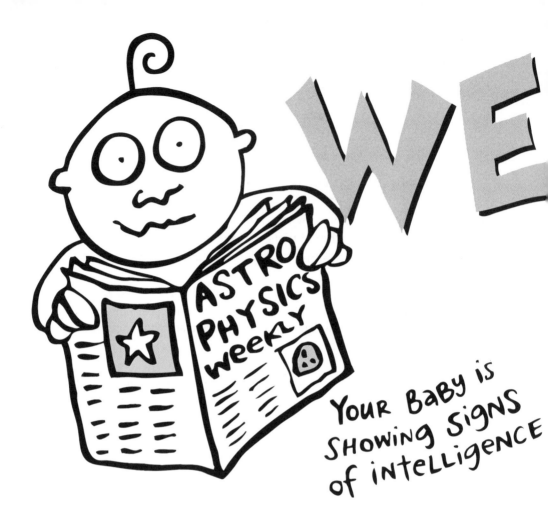

WE

YOUR BABY is
SHOWING SiGNS
of iNTeLLiGENCE

what's going on Get lots of rest and
exercise. (You should also get gifts consisting of large
gems, but this is unlikely.) If you haven't worked it out
already, stop wearing shoes with really high heels, and
don't do any climbing or hurling yourself about: remember
your centre of gravity has changed and you need to
protect your tummy. You will be steadily gaining weight.

Average approximate fetus length this week from head to bum

| cm | 1 | 2 | 3 | 4 | 5 | 6 | 7 | 8 | 9 | 10 | 11 | 12 | 13 |

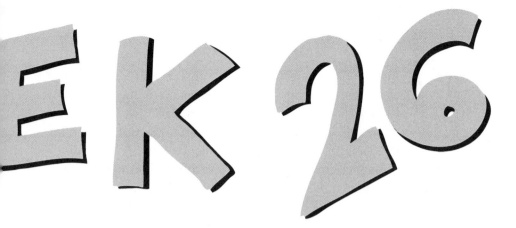

EK 26

This coming month the fetus will really spend time putting on more fat and muscle. Each week its chances of survival outside the uterus increase as it makes more surfactant for the lungs. According to one pregnancy expert, this week in the uterus your baby 'is showing signs of sensitivity, awareness and intelligence'. So if you put a little calculator in there your fetus could probably estimate the Gross National Product of Botswana. It can detect light even through its still-closed eyelids, smell (sadly for the fetus the only thing on offer is the amniotic fluid, which smells like a swamp), hear, and possibly play the slide guitar. The baby will recognise other voices from now on: friends, Daddy, aunties and Dusty Springfield singing 'Son of a Preacher Man'. Weight: about 820 grams.

16   17   18   19   20   21   22   23   24   25   26   27   28   29   30

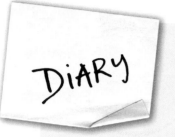
DiARY

Are the leg cramps causing insomnia, or can I feel the leg cramps because I'm awake in the middle of the night? What a fascinating philosophical question. Beck says there are two things that might be causing sore calves: blood pooling in the veins, or lack of calcium or magnesium – in my case probably a lack of magnesium as I am taking enough calcium to turn into a tusk. For the itchy, runny nose and sneezing she suggests a special garlic-and-horseradish dose.

'What about this gigantic tummy?'

'That will settle down in a few weeks.'

My tummy is now not just a big ball out the front, but a bulge all around the sides, the supporting tissue wrapping quite tightly, like wide bandages under the skin. Not quite like love handles – too curvy to really get a grip on.

Did I mention shocking heartburn and indigestion?

Pregnancy is just an absurd strain on the body, and we don't expect that any more. We expect there to be a pill or an exercise or a mantra or a caring discussion that will alleviate 'discomfort' – and 'pain'. Nope. It's just a pure and simple pain in the arse (and the rest) for a few months. I'm sorry, but I'm not finding this a sublimely spiritual experience. It's a deeply PHYSICAL experience.

The feeling of a baby moving must be different for everybody. Some books say it feels like wind, or feathers, or gentle patting. Sometimes I think it feels like someone's twanging a ligament as they might test out a harp string; sometimes it's like a bit of inside bongo work – all these feelings still all very low down in my tummy. Although the bump seems to start under the bozoom, the top of the uterus is actually just at navel level. All the stuff above is displaced bits making way for the uterus.

This morning's paper reports that a computerised baby doll is being used to help teenagers realise how much work a baby is. The baby doll is taken home from school over a weekend, and is programmed to cry constantly or several times, day and night. A special sound indicates how often the nappy must be changed, and the student must decide how often the baby needs to be fed. One student who had the baby doll for the weekend said 'It really put me off having kids.' You should try pregnancy, love.

What an incredibly raunchy life it is: so far this week I've had half a glass of red wine, nine orange ice lollies and a Magnum, some calcium tablets, and I'm about to get my daffodils in. AND WHAT'S MORE I am becoming a stately pregnant lady and am now so considerably fattened up that THE

THING has happened. THE THING where your thighs rub together up the top. If I wore corduroy trousers while I was walking, I'd sound like a sword fight.

Time to pay a visit to the midwife. I spend bloody ages in the waiting room looking at pictures of thin people in magazines, then am hustled into the room by a matronly, old-school-style midwife, who while clearly competent and replete with all her marbles doesn't have the bedside manner of Dr Sharma, and indeed doesn't even help me to sit up after examining me. She tells me with a disapproving look that I have put on 14 kilos since the start of my pregnancy.

'Most people', she says, 'have put on 8 to 10 by this stage.' Why she didn't just call me Mrs Blimpy I don't know.

Afterwards I go to visit Beck to say 'Help me, I'm Mrs Blimpy.'

She says 'Bollocks!' (I do love a medical adviser who says bollocks.) 'Some people put on 20 kilos when they're pregnant.'

However, we agree that if I can nourish the baby and not get fatter myself, this will be a lot easier to carry around. So I must keep taking the special pregnancy multi-vitamin-supplement thingy. I must stop eating Magnums. And stop toasted muesli for breakfast. I must have porridge with some apple or half a banana in it.

'Can I have sultanas in it?' I whine piteously.

'You can have four', she says.

I strike her.

Then I go out to dinner and have lemon tart with ice cream. Oh well, fuck it.

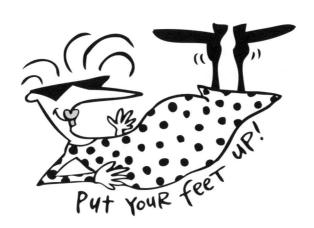

PuT YouR feeT uP!

info

baby equipment

You're about to enter the world of safety warnings – try to keep in mind that most babies are robust little critters, but they still need to be protected. All the baby-wrangling gear listed below needs to be safe and should conform to the relevant British, European or international standards (see capt.org.uk in 'More Info' coming up). Always check the label. Don't assume that if you can buy it then it must be safe or will comply with safety regulations or laws.

As with buying baby clothes, do the shopping now while you still feel energetic, especially if you're going to do a lot of it on foot. The major items can be bought from department stores and specialist baby shops (some of which will hire gear). Smaller stuff can be bought at supermarkets or chemists. You can get second-hand baby equipment through trading papers, second-hand shops, NCT sales, friends and notices on mother-and-baby health-centre pinboards. If you get stuff second-hand, replace any worn straps and all of the Velcro.

baby restraint for the car

Baby restraints are compulsory for transporting a baby in a car. A baby restraint is a specially designed seat secured to the car via a seat belt or (preferably) via 'ISOFIX' anchor points (these are internationally standardised attachment points which must be fitted to an older car – new ones have them). You're legally required to buy a restraint that complies with the United Nations standard, ECE Regulation 44-03. UK consumer group *Which?* rates some as better than others. Before buying, you will need to check with the manufacturer that the seat you are considering is suitable for your car(s). Get installation of a restraint checked for safety by your local council's Road Safety team – many people have unsafe car seats due to dodgy installation. (See 'More Info' coming up for how to go about this.)

Don't buy a second-hand one unless it's in very good condition and you know its age and history. Ask your local council about hiring one if you don't want to buy or can't afford to buy a new one. (Replace any Velcro.)

Estate cars and some huge four-wheel drives will need an extension strap to reach the anchor point, and a cargo barrier to stop flying shopping or dogs injuring the baby if you have to slam on the brakes. A warning: don't leave a baby sleeping unattended in a baby restraint you may have brought in from the car. Their little head can slump forward and their airway can get blocked. Most babies will rouse themselves; a few won't be able to.

baby's bed

Whether you choose a carrycot, Moses basket, cradle (rocking crib) or cot for your baby's first weeks, it should conform to the relevant British or European safety standard. This is no time to skimp or save money: peace of mind means a safe baby and a better sleep for you. Whatever you choose will need a firm, well-fitting mattress, two mattress protectors made of waterproof-backed fabric, and at least three sheets. You can buy fitted baby sheets of towelling or flannelette (it's not necessary to buy the sheets made of fine linen with ittle wuvvly la la duckies embroidered on them, which cost a bomb and would be covered in green liquid poo as soon as look at them); or you can cut up adult bed sheets. The easiest way to make sure babies don't get tangled up is to use only a lower, tightly tucked or fitted sheet with nothing on top. Up to three or four months old, your bub can be wrapped securely in a muslin or a swaddling blanket; after that they should be put to bed in a safe sleeping-bag suit with arms but no hood (from babywear outlets) – see the 'Wrap Party' box in Week 40 for more on safe sleeping. A duvet can cut off the air supply and smother a baby. If you feel that your baby may need a bedcover as they get older, two or three cotton cellular blankets that can be firmly tucked in are safest. The cot should be made up at the bottom end, so there is no danger of the baby wriggling down under the blankets (new babies tend to wriggle in a direction away from their feet). Pillows, stuffed toys and cot bumpers are also dangerous. Tiny babies don't need any of these things.

Cradles, carrycots and Moses baskets are only for very young babies, so you need to ask yourself if you really need one since your baby will be going into a cot within a few months anyway. Before you choose a Moses basket, you need to consider whether you will want to leave your baby unattended in one.

It's not easy to find a basket with a firm, tight-fitting mattress. And if you have it on the floor a lot, will you hurt your back lifting it and the baby?

The rocking motion of a cradle is soothing; but the soothing motion can be replicated by gently patting your baby in a cot, or rolling the baby in a pram back and forth for an arm's length. Don't leave the baby to sleep unattended in the pram, though, as they can wiggle into danger – always keep them where you can see them, not wheeled into another room.

Many cot designs on the market are potentially dangerous. Babies can be trapped, be injured on sharp protrusions, or get stuck down between the mattress and the side of the cot. A mattress should be firm and fit snugly, with no more than a 2.5-centimetre gap between it and the cot on all sides. Other important factors include the spacing of bars, the security of a drop side, the efficiency of wheel brakes, what the cot is made of and painted with, and the position of the mattress relative to the height of the sides. Make sure you get the latest information on the British or European safety standard before you get a new or used cot.

prams and pushchairs

Technically, a pram is the huge, old-fashioned type, with gigantic wheels, that a Mary-Poppins-style nanny would push around with the sixty-seventh Earl of Whatever inside. The name for the newer, lighter designs that can be converted into a pushchair (aka stroller or buggy), with the baby facing away, is pramette, but no one except shop assistants ever calls them that. They're all prams to us.

Again, lots of prams on the market are not considered safe. As well as safety, you'll need to consider cost, durability and adaptability.

Start off with a pram that faces you so that when you're walking the baby can see you. Babies learn to talk and relate to you – and other people – by you talking and relating to them. If a baby can't see you they will assume you're not there (baby brains aren't developed enough to understand you're behind them, out of sight, pushing the pram). And if you're always talking on the mobile to somebody the baby can't see, they won't understand that you're not talking to them or why. You don't need to talk to a baby 24/7, but try to make really long calls or lots of calls when the baby's asleep. (You also need to have a baby in sight at all times – see the box 'Pram Safety' in Week 27.) Later, when they can sit up and are more interested in life around them, a buggy lets toddlers look at the world going by.

Make sure there are no open parts on the side of the pram through which the wind can blow, and that it has a rain cover and, if you're feeling optimistic, a sunshade. If you don't go jogging or hiking you probably don't need a flash-looking three-wheeler. Is the pram light and easy to fold if you are going to put it in the car or on a bus a lot? (Don't take the manufacturer's or sales assistant's word for it – fold it up and down yourself a few times in the shop.) Is the pram comfortable for you and your partner to push? Is the handle height right, or adjustable? Can you walk freely or do your feet bump into the undercarriage? Do you want it to convert to a pushchair later? Make sure a pushchair has a five-point harness for the baby, good brakes and a shelf or basket underneath large enough to hold your baby-changing bag or shopping.

changing table

You will be changing gerzillions of nappies, so it makes sense to do it as comfortably as possible. If you can't afford a changing table, improvise by buying a plastic-covered, hard foam changing mat, with built-up sides, and putting it on a hip- or waist-height table or dresser. Even if you have a changing table, one of these is useful to throw in the car when you're travelling or out. If you can afford a flash changing table, go for a solid timber one with lockable wheels – don't buy the flimsy wire ones. Timber ones usually have a few shelves underneath, which are very handy for nappies, a change of baby clothes and baby wipes. Everything you need to change a nappy must be placed within arm's length beforehand because you can't take your hand off a baby on a changing table.

bath venue

Early on it is so much easier to wash a baby in a clean kitchen sink or bathroom basin (being careful of fixed taps that could bump a baby's head) than to lug a heavy, full plastic bath around. But if you do need a separate bath, consider buying a plastic laundry bowl, which can be recycled for non-baby uses later.

You'll also need two or three soft bath towels. These are great for wrapping a baby in after a bath, but for drying sensitive newborn-baby creases and crannies you can also use a muslin square, clean flannel nappy or swaddling blanket. You can buy towels with a hood to keep baby's head warm.

For toiletries, buy a baby bath liquid or soap alternative, or an unscented bath oil; blunt-ended nail scissors; a nappy-change lotion; cottonwool balls or nappy wipes (but wipes are more expensive) or wash cloths and a water container; and a barrier cream such as zinc and castor oil or some other nappy-rash cream. Ask around to find out what products people recommend, then buy small sizes to test on your baby. Don't use talc or any other powder because it can phoof into the baby's lungs and cause damage as it's released into the air.

feeding gear

You'll need nursing bras and nursing bra pads if you breastfeed. The pads, which soak up any leaking milk before it hits your clothes, can be bought as paper-based disposables or fabric washables. Have some disposables at least in your handbag for emergencies.

Hilarious but brilliant new-generation thin, bendy, clear plastic nipple shields, worn while the baby is breastfeeding, can help prevent and heal cracks. Always get the 'large' ones, however small your nipples are. Some folk warn that the shields can confuse the baby about what a nipple should feel like and interfere with attaching, others say the new-generation shields are not a problem because they're so much thinner and bendier. For some mums, this can make the difference between being able to continue breastfeeding and not. Definitely worth trying before giving up.

A breast pump is handy for expressing milk if you're ready for a night off, your breasts are painfully full, or you need to go to work. Electric ones are better than hand pumps for expressing often; say, for going to work. You can buy or hire them online or from pharmacies and lactation consultants. For expressed breastmilk feeds, you'll also need one or two bottles and teats, a sterilising unit (or you can just boil things) and bottle- and teat-cleaning brushes. You can freeze portions of breast milk in special plastic bags available in pharmacies.

For bottlefeeding, you'll need six to eight bottles and teats, bottle- and teat-cleaning brushes, formula, perhaps a measuring jug (although bottles should have measurements on them), a sterilising unit and an insulated bottle-carrier. To avoid bacteria, bottles should always be kept very cold and then warmed just before use.

bottom re-upholstering accoutrements

Two nappy buckets with a lid are essential if you're washing your own nappies. But everyone needs one because any clothes and bedding that come into contact with poo will need to go in a bucket of water and sterilising (not just 'whitening' or 'brightening') soaking powder before being machine-washed.

light for night-time feeding

Either a dimmer setting for the main light in the baby's room or a small, low-wattage lamp, which provides just enough light for you to change and feed by, is useful. A bright light can create sleep problems, so if you need to keep a light on in the baby's room all night make it very dim and indirect. A dim light helps to say to a baby 'It's still night-time. Have a quiet feed, no chatting, do the business and back to sleep.'

even more stuff

You'll probably find the following items useful:

ⓖ a baby-changing bag – any big bag that has a shoulder-strap handle will do, but some are specially designed to fold out into a changing mat. (For details of what goes in it, check out the info in Week 43)

ⓖ a baby monitor – like a one-way walkie-talkie set, this is helpful if the baby's room is out of earshot

ⓖ a hands-free mobile phone kit or a speaker phone on the home phone

ⓖ a sheepskin (also called a lambswool) or two – some people like to have these under the cot sheet, or thrown on the floor or placed in the pram for the baby to lie on. They need to be washed regularly, otherwise they can harbour gerzillions of dust mites, but can be machine washed and tumble dried

ⓖ a baby carrier or sling – great for comforting a fretty or crying baby while getting on with whatever else you need to do. Wearing a carrier or sling is a good way to have walks or go shopping when the baby is little, though it can be hard on the back when the baby starts to stack on weight. A baby should only spend one or two hours in it at a time before having a stretch and a kick. Try it on before you buy it: look for well-padded shoulder straps, sturdy fabric, detachable dribble bibs, a head support and secure and easy-to-use clasps. Babies outgrow slings by five or six months

ⓖ a safe heater – compare the safety and environmental features of heaters on the market before you buy. You can also dry clothes in front of one when the weather's bad.

A few months further down the line you will need a highchair, and may also want to buy a mobile, a playpen, a fold-up buggy, a backpack, a travel cot, and a large aircraft carrier to put them all in.

Do not buy walkers, bouncers or swings. They can hold back development and be dangerous. All you need are a rug and the floor.

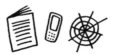

more info on **safe baby equipment**

which.co.uk

Which?, the UK's largest consumers' association, has tested many baby and children's products, and reviews are available on their website. You'll need to become a subscriber to access the full range of reports, and to receive their magazine, *Which?*

capt.org.uk

The website of the Child Accident Prevention Trust charity. Click on 'Samples of our leaflets' then 'Keep your baby safe' for a booklet covering cots, prams, car seats and more: it lists the relevant British or European safety standards, and offers advice on choosing equipment, as well as pointers on safe sleeping, bathing and nappy-changing habits.

childcarseats.org.uk

The Royal Society for the Prevention of Accidents' child car seats website provides clear guidance on choosing, fitting and using child restraints. Also includes details of checkpoints around the country where you can get your installation checked – click on 'Search for local help and advice'.

Also see 'Safety' in Week 27.

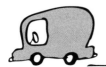

THE GREAT DUMMY DEBATE

You'll find many of the baby experts sternly frown on using a dummy, especially after the baby is three months old, but mother-and-baby sleep clinics often use them. Dummies aren't supposed to be used automatically as soon as a baby cries. But if a baby is fed, clean and burped and yet has got into a hideous, sobbing, can't-remember-why-I'm-crying-but-I'm-hysterical-now-and-can't-stop-yelling state, a dummy is heavenly. Take no notice of what the books say; the authors aren't there to hold the baby when you're going nuts. Wait and see if your baby is like this before buying a dummy.

But if you do decide to use one, here's the huge drawback nobody tells you about: the baby may become 'addicted' to it, and if so there'll be a period when the dummy will actually make the baby cry more because when a dummy falls out the only way a young baby can get it back in is to cry for you to come and put it in – several times a night. These weeks can be just not worth it. And experts say that once your baby is six to eight weeks old you need to chuck dummies out or you'll be creating a dependence and maybe speech delay, crooked teeth and mouth development problems.

You don't have to get a whizzbang, way-expensive dummy. Buy a cheap but safe one from a chemist or supermarket: make sure you get the right size and one that meets the British Standard. Let the baby suck it into their mouth so you know their tongue is in the right place.

what's going on

Hurrah, you're in the third trimester. Hire a brass band: bah de bah, bah de bah. If people don't stand up for you on public transport, say 'Excuse me, I'm pregnant. Could I sit down?' About twelve people will rise from their seats as if given 140 volts up the fundament. Your moles may be getting bigger and you may have small skin tags, especially under the arms and breasts. You need a lot more fluids from now until the birth. You can forget about moving gracefully. People will not be saying, 'Aren't you Audrey Hepburn?' You need to put your feet up when you can: at work, if possible on another chair – better still, make the boss massage your feet.

The fetus has grown so much it is running out of room, and it takes a little longer to manoeuvre about and turn upside down and sideways. Babies born now have a very good chance of surviving (they're called 'viable' in doctorspeak). The fetus has been practising breathing here and there, but from now on its breathing will become more rhythmic and constant. Folds and grooves appear on the surface of the brain, which is developing very quickly.

| 16 | 17 | 18 | 19 | 20 | 21 | 22 | 23 | 24 | 25 | 26 | 27 | 28 | 29 |

Average approximate fetus length this week from head to bum

(Of course if the fetus is born early, all this developing will continue outside the uterus, usually in an incubator with ventilators and other monitors attached.) Weight: about 950 grams.

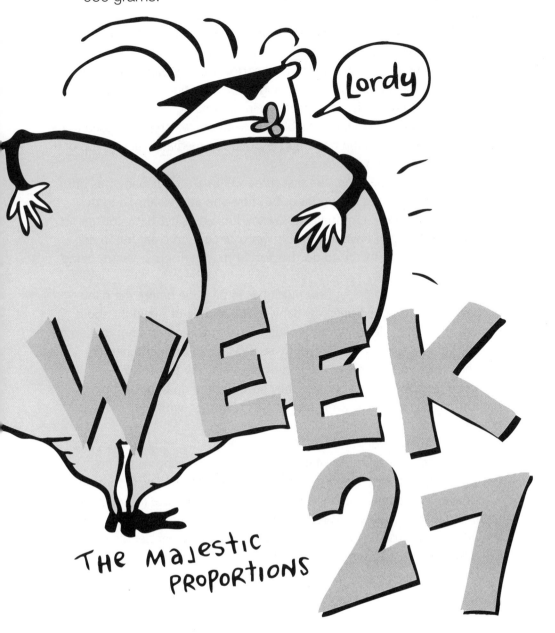

THE MAJESTIC PROPORTIONS

WEEK 27

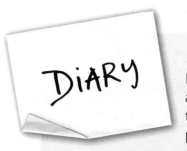
DIARY

It's true, you can spend an entire week in a dressing gown, although I accessorise it differently at work. I find when teamed with battery-operated earrings and a beehive people tend not to notice the dressing gown. I have developed approximately sixteen billion skin tags and my moles are all getting bigger. I am looking like a currant bun, so instead of calling Cellsie Cellsie we have started to call it Chelsea (a relative of the currant bun, how intensely hilarious).

Maybe I'm practising not getting much sleep because I wake up for an hour or so every night and lie there with vaguely aching legs, listening to the blood swishing in my ears or my heartbeat in the silence. It is very disconcerting. My blood sounds like languid wobble-board music and I don't really want to be reminded of Rolf Harris in the wee hours.

I have purchased a giant inflatable ball to sit on, which is supposed to be good for strengthening the back muscles. Geoff immediately lies on top of it and rolls head-first into a bookcase.

Jo rings to say she spent the first three weeks after her baby was born looking at him and feeling nothing, but now she adores him, and do I want some babygros? Liz emails to say she looked at her baby for the first time and said 'Now I have to put this weird screaming creature on my breast? What would I want to do that for?' I'm grateful people are being so honest.

I'm getting scared about how much has to be done before the baby is born. After two hours' sleepless panic in the middle of the night about coping with it all, I decide to drop another day at work: if I'm not fooling myself, I'm not going to fool anybody else. (Maybe I can get that on a letterhead.) Besides which, at the end of every day my feet smell like the world is ending – and because they have swelled up to aubergine proportions all I can wear is my pair of Hush Puppies, with the elasticky bit cut.

It's becoming harder and harder to manoeuvre the body around, and I am sad to say that grunting while changing position is by no means unknown. I find it very difficult to believe that Geoff would want to have sex with me, and he admits that he doesn't want to ask because (a) I seem so tired, and (b) my body seems rather preoccupied, but he does want to have sex with me because he loves me. This is the sort of answer people should win a three-piece suite for on quiz shows.

We try having sex but it is really quite an absurd proposition. It is impossible to avoid the conclusion that there are three of us involved. Well, there are. I wish I could unstrap Chelsea for a couple of hours.

I can now see cellulite on my thighs without having to pinch the skin together. Geoff says 'It's for a reason', and 'It's temporary', and 'It doesn't matter' (give the man another sofa, please), but if THIS is what size I am at six months pregnant, I am terrified to think of me at nine months. Especially the little matter of getting it OUT.

To add to the glamour of my relationship, apparently I am snoring like a demented tractor every night.

info

safety

The only way to childproof a house is to never let a kid in it. But you can try to make it safer.

The older the baby gets, the more dangerous the house gets. Baby websites and books such as *The Rough Guide to Babies and Toddlers* will tell you what tricks your baby is likely to be up to next (yes, that was a plug). Remember that there's a wide age range for milestones: your baby could be an early roller; your toddler could be an early climber.

As said in 'Baby Equipment' in Week 26, every baby-relevant item needs to be safe: cots, prams, car restraints, baby chairs, toys, changing tables, clothes, dummies – the lot. Remember, when you are preparing the house for small persons, that the most common causes of death and injury in little kids include car and pedestrian accidents – often in their own driveway – drowning, suffocation, falling, burns, poisoning and electrical accidents.

Blokes and other support staff: make yourself useful! Crawl around your house at baby and toddler level, thinking like an inquisitive kiddie, and identify risk areas.

Here's what needs to be organised:

⑥ a hot-water service set to 50° Celsius (which takes longer to burn the skin than the usual, hotter setting)

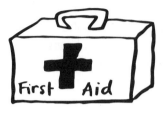 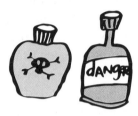

◎ a tamper-proof cabinet for any garden poisons and chemicals, and a first-aid kit placed higher than a child on a chair or the kitchen work-top could reach

◎ cupboards in which the following have been moved to a higher position household poisons such as cleaning agents and detergents; medicines; alcohol; batteries; pesticides; mothballs and camphor; soaps and shampoos; cigarettes; matches and lighters; cosmetics and perfumes; essential oils; foods that could cause choking, such as peanuts and marshmallows; plastic bags (and go through wardrobes to get rid of dry-cleaning bags); glasses and other breakables; objects with sharp bits Babies and toddlers can be both gymnastic and inquisitive. You can also get baby-proof catches to 'lock' cupboards

◎ an extinguisher for the kitchen, and check that your smoke alarms are working

◎ electrical circuit breakers and plug-socket covers

◎ electrical cords placed off the floor and out of reach – curled cords on kettles and irons are good

◎ topple-proof TV sets and computer screens

◎ fireguards for heaters and open fires

◎ hairdryers kept away from water

◎ stair and doorway barriers

◎ a fence or cover for any pool or pond in your garden.

Don't forget: never assume when you buy something that it complies with British or European safety standards. A lot of stuff doesn't.

other people

Never hesitate to ask people to smoke outside the house, stop drinking hot tea or coffee while nursing your baby, support the head properly when holding the bub, and not bounce the baby up and down if it's young or has just had a feed. They'll probably be glad of the instruction: many non-baby-wrangling friends want some guidance.

Rogue grandparents or older friends and relations may need a firmer hand. As mentioned in Week 18, many practices from their own parenting days, such as not using a baby safety restraint in a car, are unsafe. Their homes will also need to be checked if they babysit there, especially once your baby can roll, crawl and walk.

prevention

⊚ Always remove a bib before putting a baby to bed, and don't attach a dummy to a baby's clothes with a ribbon or string ('Baby Clothes and Nappies' in Week 25 has more info on safety with baby's clothing).

⊚ Don't leave a baby, even for a second, unsupervised on a changing table, a bed or any other raised surface. Here's the rule: when your eyes are off the baby your hand must be on them.

⊚ Don't leave a baby to feed unsupervised from a propped-up bottle.

⊚ *Never* leave a baby or young child in a bath if you go out of the room, no matter how briefly.

⊚ Always empty baths and toddlers' paddling pools after use, and keep a lid on nappy buckets at all times. Your baby might walk before 12 months and crawl way before that, and babies can drown in a tiny amount of water, so be aware of all water dangers.

⊚ Put cots, prams and baby chairs out of reach of any dangly curtain ties or blind cords and stoves, heaters, fires and plug sockets.

⊚ Turn all pan handles towards the back of the stove.

⊚ Never leave a small baby unattended with another small child, a dog or a cat. Never allow a child, a dog and food to be together. Most cats will give babies a wide berth anyway (but you can't assume this will always be the case). Some cats will get very cross about baby's crying or any high-pitched squeals and could lash out if close to the baby. (Cats will usually wriggle away from toddlers when they want to and must be allowed to do so – otherwise nasty scratches are likely.) Cats shouldn't be allowed on prams or on baby's bed and must be stopped from licking a baby.

⑥ When you are travelling or at someone else's place, you might need to bring safety stuff with you and be a bit more vigilant, particularly where there are other young children and dogs.

emergencies

Keep a contact list near the phone or add emergency numbers to your direct-dial system. The numbers should cover your GP and NHS Direct (England and Wales, 0845 4647) or NHS 24 (Scotland, 08454 242424). Babysitters should be told about it. You can do an infant and child first aid and resuscitation course with the Red Cross or the St John Ambulance Service, or get an instructor to come to your playgroup.

Add a digital thermometer and baby paracetamol to the family medicine cupboard and/or your baby-changing bag. Ask your GP when you can use the paracetamol.

PRAM SAFETY

Mobile phones can dangerously distract you from your baby's safety. A hands-free phone kit for walking is essential.

And if you do stop the pram to talk on the phone – or for any other reason – park it on flat ground with its brake on so that it can't roll into danger. Even so, don't take your eyes off the baby.

It's not safe to leave a baby sleeping in a pram – or a toddler sleeping in a buggy – unsupervised for even a few minutes.

Don't push a pram or buggy out in front of you onto the road first when crossing. This puts your child in danger.

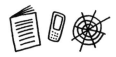

more info on **safety**

First Aid for Babies and Children Fast Dorling Kindersley, UK, 2006
Produced in association with the British Red Cross, this is a handy first port of call for everything from basic first aid through to life-saving procedures. Clear illustrations and colour-coded for when you're in a hurry.

childsafetyweek.org.uk
Created by the Child Accident Prevention Trust, this website has safety advice by age group, plus info on what to do about burns, scalds, poisons, fire and electrical hazards. From the home page, click on 'Parents' section'.

cm	1	2	3	4	5	6	7	8	9	10	11	12	13

Average approximate baby length this week from head to bum

what's going on For you, just more of the same, really.

Your baby may be hiccuping. It will usually decide to party while you are resting or asleep. Its eyes are partially opened – quite sensibly as who would want to open their eyes wide in a yukky swirl of amniotic fluid? The baby is now covered all over with vernix, so it looks a bit like one of those cross-channel swimmers smothered in gunk. Except babies have got more brains than to try to swim from Dover to Calais. They just hang out in the uterus growing their bodies so their heads don't look too big. Weight: just over 1 kilo.

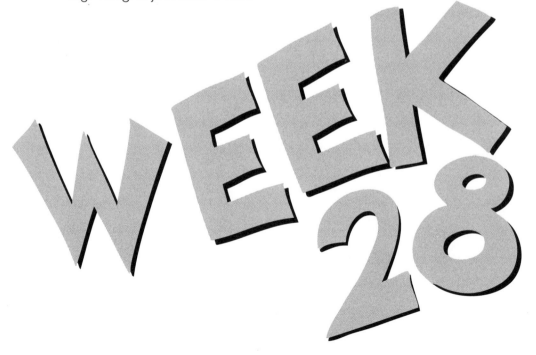

WEEK 28

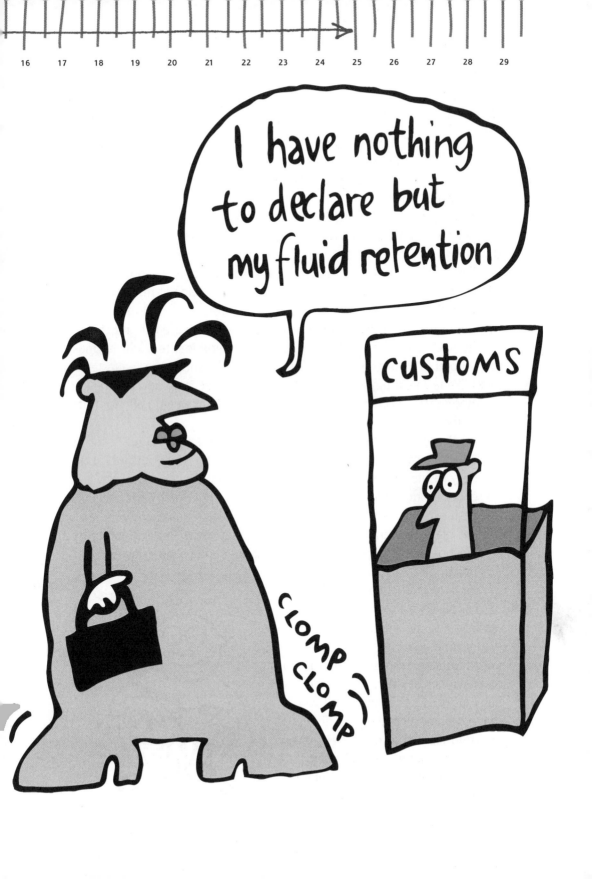

My feet hurt to walk, and my tummy's really starting to pull forward, so of course it's time to go travelling again. I've come to Fashion Week in Milan. The usual lot get all the publicity, and if anyone mentions Romeo Gigli to me again I shall have to have them killed. There's nothing wrong with a lacy wisp of froth and a scrinch of lace webbing between your headlights, but it's not like you can actually DO anything in it other than accept your best-supporting-actress-in-a-drama BAFTA. As one does. Yes I am bitter, and shut up.

Planes always make my feet swell up, but now it seems to work on the whole body. My fluid retention after I get off the plane at midday is clearly visible to the naked eye. Have gone quite bullfroggy around the face, and the indent marks on the ankles where the socks finish are like trenches. Luckily Beck had suggested I pack some dandelion-leaf tea, which I make at my hotel in a coffee plunger I buy in the lobby shop. The tea tastes and looks like lawn clippings. I get so desperate, I make it up and plunge mid-afternoon instead of waiting until morning, and am weeing all night. It works, though.

People now have their routine down pat: 'When are you due?', followed by 'Do you know if it's a boy or a girl?', followed by 'Is it your first?' I go to a very Fashion Weeky cocktail party (vodka icepoles instead of devils-on-horseback – but not for me) and meet the lead singer of Thrash Esky, who asks 'Is it exciting?' I think this a much better question and earbash him until his eyes glaze over and he staggers to the refreshment tent, supported by an elfin keyboard player from a visiting Canadian band called Prince Phillip's Undies.

Sometimes Chelsea kicks really hard and I get a shock. Quite often I am forced to move because the baby is stretching against me somewhere uncomfortable. It's fascinating that so many women say they love to feel their baby move, but they never tell you that sometimes it's really horribly uncomfortable and sometimes it even hurts. Last night in the bath things got really freaky when my rounded tummy momentarily went up into a

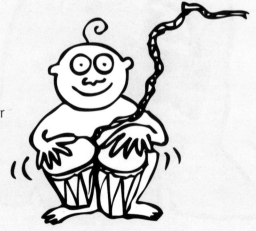

tent-like shape with a point. At any moment I thought Sigourney Weaver (out of *Aliens*) might appear in a vest.

I have a marvellously glamorous moment in a restaurant debriefing the boss about Fashion Week. As I squeeze between tables on the way to the toilet, I attempt to keep my bump off a nearby table and instead sweep my arse along the table behind me in a majestic arc, taking the two menus and a good bit of the tablecloth with me. Talk about dignity.

info

third trimester hassles

These three complaints can start earlier, but usually bug pregnant women the most in the last three months.

heartburn

What is it? Heartburn is that burning sensation you feel behind the breastbone, sometimes accompanied by the taste of small amounts of regurgitated food and stomach acid. It doesn't affect the baby.

Why does it happen? Because of the high levels of progesterone during pregnancy, which relaxes muscles, the muscular valve between the stomach and the oesophagus (the tube connecting stomach and mouth) relaxes, and so stomach acid flows up into the oesophagus and sometimes the mouth. It doesn't help that later in the pregnancy your uterus is encroaching on your tummy and squeezing it upwards.

What can you do?

⑥ Eat several small meals slowly, rather than wolfing down three main ones.

⑥ Avoid spicy, highly seasoned, fried or fatty foods, chocolate, coffee, alcohol, carbonated drinks, spearmint and peppermint, and anything with lots of chemical additives.

⑥ Wear loose clothing around your tummy.

⑥ Don't fold yourself up on the sofa because that squashes your tummy, and bend from the knees, not the waist, to pick things up.

⑥ If the heartburn is worse when you lie flat, try elevating your head by at least 15 centimetres with pillows, which will help to stop the yukky stuff flowing up into your mouth.

⑥ Avoid gaining too much weight – hate that one.

⑥ Don't smoke. (Duh.)

⑥ Try foods such as milk or yoghurt that help to neutralise the stomach acid.

⑥ Don't eat too late in the evening before bed.

⑥ If none of this helps, ask your doctor to recommend an antacid that is suitable for use during pregnancy. (Avoid preparations containing sodium or sodium bicarbonate.)

backache

Why does it happen?   Progesterone and relaxin relax the ligaments and joints of the spine and around the pelvis. This jollies everything along for childbirth, but makes it hard to have good posture, especially when the weight of the baby puts pressure on your lower back and weakened tummy muscles, and pulls the spine forward.

Lower back and leg pain can be caused by the pressure of the enlarging uterus on the sciatic nerve. The pain may pass as the baby's position changes. If it is very severe, you may have to go to bed for an extended period (not as much fun as it sounds).

What can you do to help prevent it?

⑥ Avoid standing and sitting for long periods of time. When you are standing, tilt your pelvis forward so that your bum tucks under, and keep your shoulders back; when sitting, get yourself well back into the seat, and put your legs up on another chair if possible.

⑥ Do some gentle stretching exercises recommended by your hospital obstetric physiotherapist or a yoga teacher experienced in pregnancy.

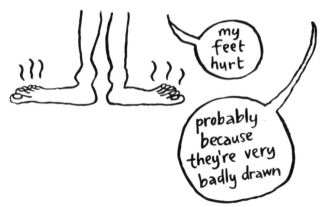

⑥ Avoid twisting movements.

⑥ Bend from the knees when lifting things.

⑥ Try not to put on too much extra weight.

⑥ Wear flat shoes, with good support – the flatter the better. This is no time for sparkly, aqua-go-green, platform thigh boots. Sadly.

What can you do for the pain?

⑥ Have a massage from a qualified masseur with pregnancy knowledge.

⑥ Relax in a warm bath or aim the shower spray at the painful area.

⑥ Apply a warm (not hot) hot-water bottle or heat pack.

⑥ If the pain is particularly bad, ask your doctor to prescribe an analgesic safe for use during pregnancy.

⑥ If the pain is severe, ask your doctor to refer you to a fully qualified, experienced physiotherapist, osteopath or chiropractor specialising in backache during pregnancy.

swelling and fluid retention

What is it?   Swelling, most noticeably of the fingers, legs, ankles and feet, also called oedema, occurs because the body retains more fluid during pregnancy. (Your face can also swell, due to the effects of natural oestrogen and cortisol, a steroid hormone, changing the distribution of fat in the body.)

Some fluid retention and swelling is perfectly normal and should cause no more than mild discomfort. However, if you feel that you are excessively puffy or if the oedema persists for more than 24 hours at a time, you should see your GP or midwife. This can be normal, but it may be an early sign of pre-eclampsia (see 'Pre-eclampsia' later in this chapter).

Why does it happen?   Hormonal changes can prompt the kidneys to hang on to salt, leading to fluid retention. There is much more fluid in your body to maintain the level of amniotic fluid, and increase the water level in your blood to help the kidneys to get rid of waste.

Hot weather, standing or sitting for long periods of time and high blood pressure are the most common causes of mild oedema. It also occurs more commonly later in the day, as fluid pools in the ankles and feet – that's gravity for you.

In the mornings you might see more puffiness in your eyelids and jawline. It is more likely if you're carrying a multiple pregnancy or excess weight.

What can you do?

⑥ Get horizontal as much as possible.

⑥ Lie down on your left side, or on your back supported by a cushion under your right side so that your back is tilted 10 degrees or more.

⑥ Wear comfortable shoes.

⑥ Avoid socks or stockings with elasticised tops.

⑥ If the oedema really bothers you, check out the range of support tights (available in pregnancy fittings with extra tummy room) and knee-high socks – and remember to put these on in the morning, when the swelling is less.

⑥ Don't add salt to any food.

⑥ Drink plenty of water to flush the body of waste products. Drinking extra water won't increase fluid retention – it may even reduce it.

⑥ If your fingers swell, remember to take off any rings before they become uncomfortably tight.

⑥ Exercise feet and ankles. Rotate in both directions, point and flex feet.

more tests

The following tests may be offered around week 28.

anaemia and antibodies

Around week 28 you should have another blood test. The blood sample will be checked for a low haemoglobin level indicating anaemia (not enough iron). You can take iron tablets for this. The sample will also be checked for a few other unusual things that could affect the baby.

gestational diabetes

This is a temporary form of diabetes: the body does not produce enough insulin to keep pace with the increased blood sugar caused by pregnancy. (Some pregnancy hormones act against insulin.) Some maternity units screen for this, at about week 28. The test involves drinking glucose, waiting an hour and then having a blood test. However, most maternity units will only carry out this test if a routine urine test shows glucose in the urine. You're more at risk if you're over 40 or weigh more than 100 kilos or so.

Gestational diabetes is usually managed by modifying what you eat – not many women need to take insulin. If it's diagnosed, you'll need to monitor your own blood sugar levels with a simple pricking device, and your doctor will monitor your fetus's progress. You may be induced (have your labour brought on a bit early), as going to full term can risk the baby's life.

↑ sky

← baby

↙ ↓ feet

pre-eclampsia

what is it?

Pre-eclampsia is high blood pressure that only ever happens in pregnancy. (It used to be called pre-eclamptic toxaemia – if your mum or nanna had it that's what it would have been called.) It can interfere with the placenta, stunting the baby's growth and depriving it of oxygen. It can cause the baby to come early, and damage the mother's kidneys, liver, nervous system and blood vessels.

Pre-eclampsia affects about 5 percent of pregnant women, usually in the second half of pregnancy. Occasionally the onset will coincide with labour and, rarely, it can occur after delivery.

The cause has still not been established, but you're more likely to get pre-eclampsia if you had high blood pressure before you were pregnant; have a family history of pre-eclampsia or high blood pressure; had or have kidney disease; have diabetes; have had or are having a multiple pregnancy; had pre-eclampsia in a previous pregnancy; are a teenager or an older mum; are carrying more weight than is considered healthy, or are in your first pregnancy.

Severe pre-eclampsia can escalate into eclampsia, which is a life-threatening condition for mother and fetus, but now extremely rare because of better medical monitoring. Eclampsia can cause convulsions, kidney failure and coma.

how do you know if you have it?

It's diagnosed from a combination of signs and symptoms, including a rise in blood pressure; swelling of the ankles, feet, hands and face; sudden weight gain due to fluid retention; visual disturbance (tell your doctor about any weird or blurred vision); and protein in your wee. Most women with pre-eclampsia don't show any obvious symptoms and are diagnosed after a high blood pressure result.

Early detection and treatment mean pre-eclampsia is better managed, although it can't be prevented. Your blood pressure is checked at each antenatal visit and you should tell your pregnancy carer about any puffiness or swelling. (Having only one of the pre-eclampsia symptoms, such as fluid retention, doesn't mean you have pre-eclampsia.)

Sometimes pre-eclampsia can get worse really quickly: symptoms (in addition to the ones mentioned) may include persistent headache, 'seeing' flashing lights, upper- or mid-abdominal pain, irritability, nausea and vomiting. Women being treated for pre-eclampsia should get emergency medical treatment at the onset of any of these symptoms.

treatment

There is no conclusive evidence, but many people believe that good levels of calcium in your diet can reduce the risk of pre-eclampsia. Treatment for very mild pre-eclampsia may include bed rest, changing what you eat, and careful monitoring of you and your baby. Tests include several blood and urine checks, monitoring of the fetal heart rate, and ultrasounds.

If the condition progresses or is advanced when diagnosed, you'll need to go to hospital. You may need medication to wrestle your blood pressure into submission, and your labour might be induced, or you might have a caesarean, depending on whether you respond to treatment and whether you and your baby are ready for birth.

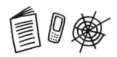

more info on **pre-eclampsia**

apec.org.uk
  Helpline: 020 8427 4217
  The site for UK charity Action on Pre-eclampsia has information about risk factors, symptoms and treatment. There's also a forum (click the speechmarks icon on the home page) – there's very little recent activity, but it's still a useful archive of others' experiences.

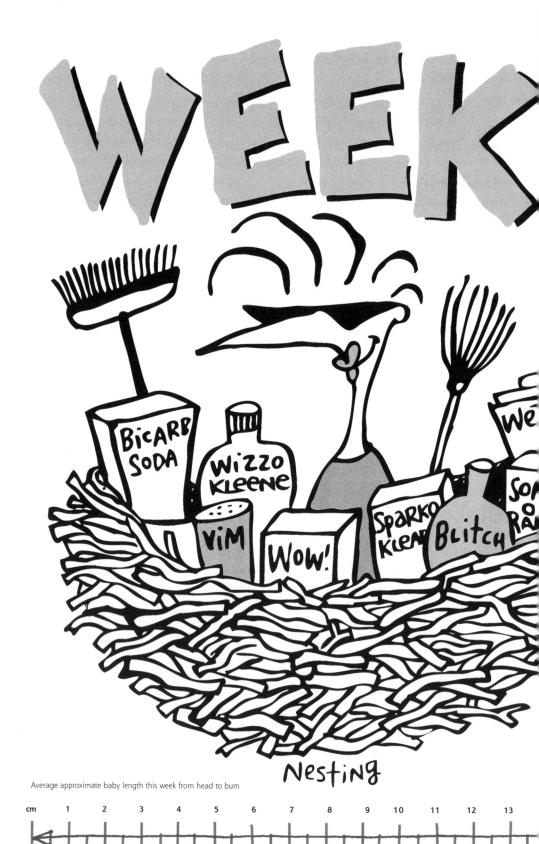

Nesting

Average approximate baby length this week from head to bum

cm 1 2 3 4 5 6 7 8 9 10 11 12 13

29

what's going on You may be hard pressed to find a comfy sleeping position. If you feel uncomfortable lying on your back, especially into late pregnancy, that's because the baby is pressing down on the main vein that pumps blood back to your heart. If it doesn't make you uncomfortable, sleeping on your back is fine. Most women who experience discomfort or faintness will automatically move position, even when they're asleep. (You shouldn't be examined by a dentist, or massaged, while flat on your back. Make sure there's a cushion under your right hip so you're slightly tilted to the left. Nothing makes a dentist flappier than a fainting pregnant woman.)

The baby is looking very babyesque at this point – plumper and rounder. The newborn-baby breathing rhythm is developing steadily; it's more regular, with fewer stops and starts. Weight: about 1.2 kilos.

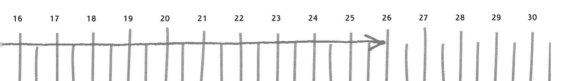

16   17   18   19   20   21   22   23   24   25   26   27   28   29   30

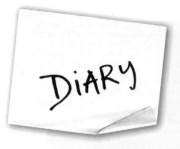

DiARY

I think I've got interior design nesting rather than cleaning nesting. (Typical. Even when I'm nesting I don't want to do the dishes, I'd rather arrange some vases fairly artfully in the hallway. Tremendously useful skill around the house.) I am putting things in boxes and getting mates to come to the house to help Geoff move furniture from room to room.

Maybe it's not just about making a nest, but about chucking out stuff from the past, stuff you don't need, and working out what you do want. That sounds a bit deep. Luckily I'm so scatterbrained my mind, having thought, immediately moves on … to … Not. Thinking. Or … wait. What?

Random thoughts

Glamour check: I have discovered that pregnancy makes you sweat more – it's as if Mrs Fluid has come to visit. If you're not retaining it, you're leaking it – or sometimes both at once. Not to mention all that extra blood in there. I tried a strong anti-perspirant, but it only blocked my pores and I felt like I was carrying a marble around in my armpit for a couple of days. I had to go without any and then went back to deodorant. I can remember at sixteen weeks when I skipped ahead in the books and thought 'God, look at 28 weeks.' It seemed so far away. But now I'm here, in a flash. Better take some photos while I'm looking pregnant.

Weeing a zillion times a night. Trying to remember to do pelvic-floor exercises. Too boring for words.

My walking shoes smell more and more disgusting. I am spraying them with a French perfume called Fracas.

Pop into the hospital for another blood test. Apparently it's to check whether I've developed anaemia.

Childbirth classes start this week. I don't want to go. For some reason it feels like having to go to Sunday School. I can't stand those things where the woman at the front of the classroom asks us all to share our feelings. I've already done the physio classes, dammit. If I wanted to share my feelings with strangers I'd hire a billboard. I don't want to bond with the group. They're not going to be there when I have the child, or when it grows up. I don't care what they think or what they do, really. Perhaps I should just wear a name tag saying 'Hi! I'm a Churlish Cow'.

Our first childbirth class goes like this: a young blonde midwife named Melissa wearing a cuddly blue cashmere cardie and black leggings gives us all a sticky-label name tag as we walk in the door. We have to interview another couple (everyone is in a couple! – what's the world coming to?), and then introduce them to the class. 'Garry and Diane are drug dealers. They conceived accidentally during a police raid. Diane intends to take at least a year off.' Unfortunately not quite that interesting.

We are divided into men's and women's groups. I put my middle name on the name tag out of perversity so Geoff has to keep squinting at my chest and saying things like 'Um ... Mildred here is going out to work and I'm staying home.' I feel it would be more entertaining if he could just admit he's forgotten the name of the mother of his child. Anyway, each group is asked to come up with a list of questions they would like the class to answer.

WOMEN

Can we eat during labour? (Yes, a bit in the early stages, but you'll probably throw it up. It's doubtful that you'll feel like eating, anyway.)

Tell us every single pain-relief option. (Certainly.)

What about if it's an emergency that this small hospital can't deal with? (We have facilities for a sick mother. A sick baby will be sent to a larger hospital by ambulance. We can look after the baby adequately until the ambulance arrives.)

Is there a modem link in the delivery suite, because I'd like my overseas relatives to see the birth live on my blog site? (That's a very weird question, but I'm way too polite to say so.)

Can I have 27 people in the room when I'm giving birth? (No. You're a fruitcake.)

Do men ever display the nesting instinct? (Frankly, no.)

MEN

How do we know when it starts? (We'll be covering this.)

What is the man's role during labour? (Do whatever she tells you and be quick about it.)

Do WE get any drugs? (Good one, Geoff.)

What if we faint? (Keep up your meals and drinks during labour and sit down if you think you might faint.)

What if the baby comes early and quickly? (Ring the ambulance and follow their instructions.)

What to bring and wear? (Ball gown.)

What to have ready at home? (Champagne.)

Melissa explains that the first lesson will be on signs that labour isn't far off (maybe hours or days). Signs include the 'show', which is the mucus plug coming out (she says that it might be the size of a 20p piece on your undies, and possibly bloody and mucusy); and the 'waters breaking' – actually when the membranes break and let out the amniotic fluid – usually in a rush, like a cup or a litre or two gushing out, but sometimes more like a slow leak (she says don't get it on the car upholstery because it rots it, so from 35 weeks I'll be sitting on a tarpaulin and four towels in the passenger seat of Geoff's precious van). I ask if it's true the waters smell of pickles. Melissa looks sideways and lets us know it's a sweet smell that's actually, ahem, like semen.

Other signs that labour may begin soon are: tummy 'dropping' as the baby's head engages with the pelvis, nesting and cleaning, more Braxton Hicks practice contractions, increased vaginal secretions, pelvic pressure and heaviness in the groin, and a decrease in fetal movements.

Then Melissa points to a chart and explains the following parts of a pregnant woman's anatomy: the vagina ('If you didn't know where that was, you wouldn't be here'), cervix (the bit between the vagina and the uterus), fetus and fundus (the top of the uterus). She explains that labour contractions begin in the fundus and the pain radiates down to period-cramp territory in the lower abdomen. Our bags should be packed by 35 weeks as 37 weeks is considered 'full term'.

Two hours of this and I'm ready for a whisky. Ready, willing, but not able.

info

premature labour

Even if you're feeling like pregnancy has gone on quite long enough, the idea that it's happening 'too early', or even a bit early, may be cause for huge anxiety. It's important to take comfort from the fact that neonatal facilities for premmie babies are now very advanced and getting better all the time. As already mentioned, many babies born as early as 24 weeks do survive with specialist care (the details on 'Premature Babies' are in Week 30).

why does it happen?

About half the time medical people don't know why premature labour happens, except it's not because you've done something wrong. Here are some possibilities:

⊚ the uterus gets 'too big' because there's more than one baby or too much amniotic fluid

⊚ the placenta detaches itself from the wall of the uterus and stops feeding the baby properly, so the body decides it's safer to bail out the baby (see 'Late Bleeding' coming up)

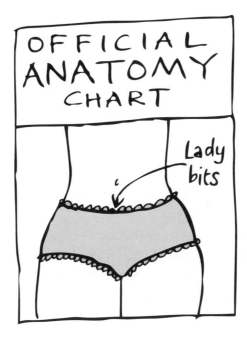

⊚ your 'waters' break early – a rupture in the amniotic sac lets the fluid out

⊚ you've developed pre-eclampsia high blood pressure (see 'Pre-eclampsia' in Week 28)

⊚ a medical condition or infection makes the body decide the baby would be better off out of it

⊚ you have a misbehaving cervix, which doesn't stay closed tightly enough

⊚ a diabetic pregnancy leads to the bub needing to come out before the due date, for optimum safety for the baby and you (see 'Gestational Diabetes' in Week 28)

⊚ the baby has died in the uterus (this is very rare).

what to look for

A premature birth has the same signs and symptoms of labour as a full-term one, but they happen earlier than expected: premature birth is defined as before 37 weeks. Symptoms may include cramp-like regular uterus contractions, possibly accompanied by diarrhoea or lower back pain or ache; the sensation of strong downward pressure on your pelvic floor; and your waters breaking. ('Labour' in Week 34 has more on all this.)

If you experience any (or all) of these symptoms, you need to immediately speak to your obstetrician or midwife: that doesn't mean leaving a message for them to get back to you the next day. Tell the person who answers the phone why you're calling, and say you need a medical person to speak to you now or to call you straight back. If the amniotic sac is ruptured (usually the cause of the waters breaking) you'll need to be examined by a doctor straight away – go to hospital immediately (ring on the way).

The good news is that having these symptoms early doesn't make birth inevitable. You may just need some bed rest or other treatment to hold on for a few more days or weeks. In some cases it's safer for the mum and baby if the bub comes out early; in other cases it's better if the baby is kept inside for as long as possible up to the due date.

GROUP B STREPTOCOCCUS (GBS)

This bacteria can be found in the vagina and although it will cause no problems for the mother, babies can become really sick if they travel to the outside world down a vagina with GBS in it. If your baby is considered at increased risk of developing a GBS infection – for instance because GBS has been detected from a vaginal swab or urine test taken for another reason, you have previously had a baby that developed a GBS infection, your waters break early or there are other signs of early labour – you'll be given antibiotics in an intravenous drip during labour.

late bleeding

Some light bleeding or spotting in the second and third trimesters is usually okay, but you need to have any bleeding checked out immediately by your obstetrician or midwife to be absolutely sure. Two uncommon conditions that cause bleeding late in pregnancy are placenta praevia (see Week 19) and placental abruption.

placental abruption or separation

Placental abruption (abruptio placentae) is when the placenta comes away from the uterine wall too early, and it usually hurts. The amount of bleeding and pain depends on how much of the placenta comes away. The cause is unknown, but it tends to be more common in women who have had two or more children, women with raised blood pressure, and smokers. Sometimes the problem resolves itself and the pregnancy continues as normal. Sometimes the birth must be induced; in serious, sudden cases a caesarean is necessary.

WEEK 30

confronted with the knitted uterus

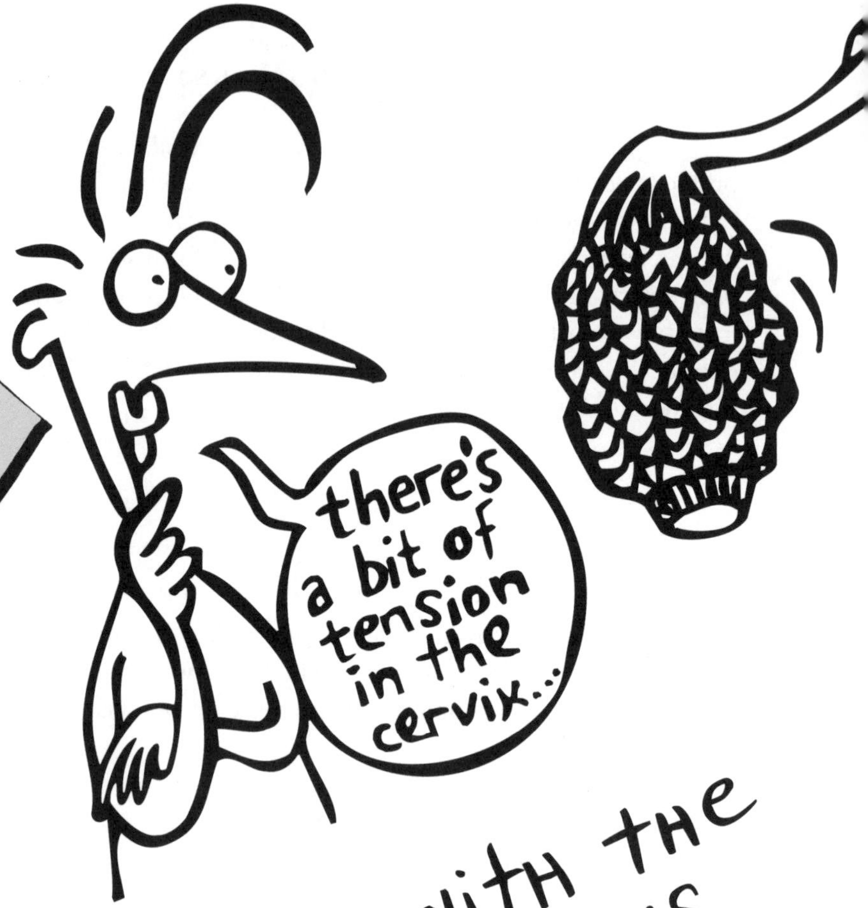

what's going on Your breasts are

STILL getting bigger. Will they ever stop? Yes. You might

be feeling Braxton Hicks practice contractions now,

although most people don't feel them until the last weeks.

Proper contractions last for about a minute each, come at

intervals of five minutes or less and go on for at least an

hour, and then after a while a baby comes out. So if that

happens, you're probably really in labour.

This week and the following three, the baby puts

on fat at a greater rate. The skin is still a bit wrinkled, so

there's room for the new fat underneath. The lanugo will

start to fall out, although a full head of hair may stay.

The eyes are fully open, but it can't be very interesting

just watching all that hair floating around. Baby hiccuping

starts to get more violent: you can feel the little jerks.

The baby may be jiggled around by the Braxton Hicks

contractions. Weight: about 1.4 kilos.

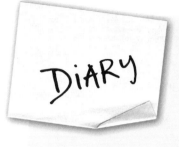

DIARY

Thank God I go to see Suze's baby, Gloria. It reminds me that there's a reward at the end of all this. Suze is full of advice about the changing-table arrangement, the best nappies and nipple creams, etc. I must start taking notes.

Also go to the clinic and see Jill the midwife. The receptionist takes my name and gives me a big smile, saying 'It must be soon.'

'Soon!' I shriek. 'It's ten weeks away. I can't even begin to tell you what I have to get done before it arrives!'

When Jill examines me, she smiles and says 'Your baby is big and healthy. She agrees I have put on a lot of weight, but says 'Worry about it after the baby is born. Just don't eat junk food.'

All the skinny girls at work put on more than 20 kilos during their pregnancy and lose it again afterwards. You can't go on a weight-loss diet during pregnancy. You (well, all right then, I) can stop eating a Magnum a day, though, which might help. I tell myself that it would be more dangerous for the baby if I don't put on enough weight during pregnancy than if I end up looking like a pivotal protagonist in *Moby Dick: The Mini-series*.

For a fashion designer, I've got bugger all to wear. But how selfish, I think. I'd better shop for the baby. (Besides which, shopping is no fun any more because after you've been walking for 15 minutes your feet feel like someone's been whacking them rhythmically with a baton for an hour.) I go to a posh shop and accidentally spend £150 on baby things like babygros and vests – honestly, I didn't buy anything flash at all. I become quite stupidly emotional over a tiny pair of socks for a newborn baby and start crying. Good God. Let's face it, I'm liable to burst into tears during a tampon ad.

Geoff is being a prince – well, a prince's servant – still doing all the dishes and cooking most nights. (He tends to cut things up into infinitesimally small pieces, but never look a gift dinner in the mixed metaphorical mouth, I say.)

Hired the removalists again to move more furniture around. Getting there. This weekend had better go and look for a changing table, and that cot Uncle Mike said he'd pay for. More shelves being delivered. Geoff just stands back and lets it all happen, and occasionally shakes his head and mutters like one of the witches in *Macbeth*. At least I think he said 'bubble'.

Second week of childbirth classes. And tonight our special project is: Normal Labour. Melissa is slightly less perky. Perhaps she's been delivering babies for 36 hours.

She gives us the old line about having faith in your body and the pain being part of a natural process. While I have always thought childbirth was actually a design fault, it is strangely comforting to know that millions of women have done it.

What Melissa says is that the average for a first-time labour is 12 or more hours. The time is counted from the start of getting regular painful contractions. (Statistically, second and subsequent babies slither out after about 7 hours.) I'm still not clear about this 12 or more hours. It's roughly made up of 10 to 12 hours of activity as the cervix dilates from 3 to 10 centimetres during the first stage, and then, say, 2 hours of pushing and shouting at people (second stage) before the baby comes out, as far as I can ascertain. After that there is a third stage of labour, when the placenta comes out, which nobody seems particularly interested in. If an injection of oxytocin is given, this takes between 5 and 10 minutes. If the placenta comes out naturally, it's usually under an hour.

Next Melissa produces from her handbag a very startling pink knitted uterus with a cream-coloured cuff on it, which represents the cervix. I don't know where she got the pattern. She says your waters can break at any time before or during the labour, even right at the very end. At first the contractions are like a period cramp and can last for 30–60 seconds and come every 5–20 minutes. By late in the first stage the contractions are very intense and 2–4 minutes apart.

The end of the first stage of labour is heralded by the 'transition', when the cervix completely dilates – wide enough for the baby's head to fit through. Ow. Ow ow OW. The contractions seem to come one after the other without a pause and last for up to 90 seconds. This is usually the time when women scream for an epidural and are often refused because it's too late.

'If you're abusive we know you're nearly there', says Melissa.

This sounds like a horrible stage when you can be shaky and vomit from the shock and stress, and you flake out for those tiny minutes between contractions.

At this point most of the men in the class move closer to their partners and take their hands. (You can tell they're thinking 'Oh you poor dear' and then 'Glad I don't have to do that bit.') They will not be so free with their fingers during the real thing: support people are advised that only two fingers be gripped by the labouring woman as any more fingers are easier to squish together, and even break. Support people are also advised to eat and drink and take rests.

After this stage, as far as I can see, a soft-toy baby comes out of a knitted uterus into a stuffed pelvis. Melissa advises us not to be too energetic in the early stages of labour before going to hospital as we'll need our strength later.

Apparently the very end of labour feels exactly like the urge to poo. Some women keep changing positions; some have their baby on all fours or a birth stool, or sitting up on the bed. Squatting is not something we do a lot of, so unless you're on one of those giant inflatable birth balls they have in some labour rooms it will probably be too much for your leg muscles.

This week was probably the perfect week to consider some of the mechanics of childbirth, as I am just changing from major denial (well yes, I know I'm pregnant, but I don't think I actually want to go through childbirth) to major denial (look, I know I'm pregnant, but I really don't want to think about how this baby everyone keeps saying is so HUGE is going to get out – I feel like I'm going to give birth to a small apartment block).

Melissa says we can massage the perineum (the area in front of your anus) for weeks before the birth, but there's no proof this is any use. Sounds like an excuse for being at yourself to me. (Dr Sharma's view is that it's a complete waste of time.)

A couple of attendees pipe up with their ideas. One woman says she has a 'vaginal balloon' she inflates in there to 'stretch things'. Someone else mumbles they've been using an economy-sized vibrator. Melissa says that unless these things are stretching your vagina to ten centimetres wide there's no point. Also, don't worry – when the vagina's supposed to stretch, it will. And go back.

'Often we ask the dad if he wants to cut the cord', Melissa says. For some reason every woman in the class packs up laughing. 'Once the head is through, that's the hard bit done – unless you've got a really big baby and then the shoulders can be difficult.' Oh dear.

Melissa then talks about the third stage of labour, which involves the expulsion of a large stuffed red stocking, with a veil around the edge that makes it look like a giant jellyfish, and a twisty grey dressing-gown cord hanging from it, which is the placenta and umbilical cord. At this point

Melissa admits that somewhere she has a knitted breast as well. I hate to think what her tea cosies look like.

Then we watch two videos. The first one is narrated by a serious bloke who says things like 'some of the joy and happiness brought about by this happy event' and 'this stained mucus plug' as if he were reading the nine o'clock news. This happy event and the stained mucus plug are both brought to us by somebody called Julie, who wears a yellow jumper until the second stage of labour, when she changes into a mauve silk negligee (bad move, really). At the hospital Julie wanders the corridors like Lady Macbeth and then ends up panting, which Melissa has said is not good so early in the labour. An obstetrician turns up in a hideous patterned jumper and holds one of Julie's legs while Scott, her husband, holds the other. Being in labour is probably the only time a woman wouldn't even notice this happening. Then the midwife squirts some cold detergent on Julie's private parts, which Melissa says is shocking behaviour as it gives Julie quite a fright. 'We like to give you a quick, warm wash', she says. The whole video is 15 minutes long, which I think is a little misleading.

The midwife holds the baby back so it doesn't come out in too much of a rush and tear Julie, and then the head comes out a very grey-blue and turns slowly before the rest slips out. By about this stage nearly every man in the room has gone into shock and half of them have tried to crawl into their partner's lap – forgetting that, with a seven-month-pregnant woman, lap space is at a premium.

We watch a second video, starring a rather more hippie couple. (Why is it that in every picture, drawing and video to do with pregnancy and childbirth the husband has frightening facial hair?) Anyway, this woman gives birth on all fours and then scoops the baby up as if she does it every day.

Neither woman needs stitches. As if.

Back at home poor old Geoff is squished into an area of the bed that's the size of an envelope. I waddle to the toilet about six times a night and have taken to having under-desk naps at work.

And the mood swings! Geoff never knows whether he's coming home to Medusa or Mrs Bunnikins.

One of the male models looks at me in the lift at work and blurts out 'What happens to all that stomach ... afterwards?'

'I'm giving it to the Salvation Army', I reply.

info

premature babies

Any baby born before 37 weeks is officially early or 'preterm'. If there is enough warning of a premature birth you'll be given a couple of steroid injections to improve your baby's lung development. Underdeveloped lungs is the most common serious health problem for premmie babies: some will need help with breathing when they first come out.

Some premmie babies are born by caesarean section because they may not be robust enough to make the journey or because they're trying to come bum – not head – first. Sometimes that decision will have to be made on the run as events overtake your previous expectations; sometimes there is time to discuss it and plan with your obstetrician.

Because a premmie baby can have health problems – perhaps as a result of their early arrival – they'll often need extra help to survive and thrive. As well as underdeveloped lungs, babies born before 32 weeks can have complications such as brain problems, bowel infections and even blindness. All premmie babies should have their eyes and ears tested before going home from hospital, or soon after.

Most premmie babies will steadily get stronger and grow up to be healthy kids and adults, but despite the very best efforts and skill of all the medical staff sometimes a baby is born way too early, or just isn't ready for life outside the womb, and they die. In these circumstances your doctor or hospital midwife will arrange for a counsellor to be available to help you. There's also useful information in the 'Grief and Loss' section of the Contacts and Resources chapter at the end of the book.

special care

All maternity hospitals have a special-care nursery where premmie babies are looked after; major maternity hospitals will have a neonatal intensive care unit especially equipped to help babies who have a health problem or are born before 32 weeks.

Babies born between 32 and 37 weeks usually need to stay in hospital until they would have been about 37 or 38 weeks inside. Babies born before week 32 usually need to stay in hospital a few weeks longer. They will probably do better if they're born in a major maternity hospital, with a neonatal intensive care unit. For babies born after 32 weeks this is usually not so important. If you have your baby at one of the smaller maternity hospitals, you and your bub may be transferred to the nearest hospital with a neonatal care unit.

When your baby is born they'll be given the Apgar test that all babies have to check their signs of health and energy (see 'Your Newborn Baby' in Week 37). This is usually repeated five minutes later to see if the baby is any perkier: premmie babies are usually rather sleepy because they're not quite ready to come out. They often need a little sucking tube to 'vacuum' their throat of fluid.

In the nursery they'll probably also be popped into an incubator, a special enclosed plastic cot with doors, which maintains a warm, even temperature, is safe from germs and allows the baby to have monitors taped to their body so that medical staff can check their vital signs at a glance. When they've grown to more than 1.8 kilos, they can usually be in an open hospital cot.

Seeing your baby all tiny and hooked up to machines can be very confronting and scary, but it really means they are as safe as the hospital can make them. Things that go beep can be stressful, but many functions are 'just in case' and show your baby is getting the best of care. The neonatal staff have heard and seen it all: ask them about anything that worries you.

Hygiene and germ control are very important in a neonatal unit because the babies are vulnerable to infection. Everybody washes their hands a lot. No visitors can come in if they have an illness, even a sniffle. This needs to be carefully explained to small brothers and sisters, who may not understand why they can't visit. Ask if they can visit if they wear a mask and wash their hands very thoroughly.

Most premature babies will develop jaundice after the birth, so they'll look a bit yellow. Some will need to lie with groovy eye shades on under a blue phototherapy lamp for a couple of days, which helps the liver to do its job properly and fixes the jaundice.

breathing help

Because of the steroid injections sometimes given to mums before the birth and given to babies when they come out, most premmie babies will be able to use their own lungs to breathe without help. Some may need extra oxygen in the incubator to keep their blood oxygen at safe levels. A few premmie babies will need the help of a tube in their nose or their windpipe. Babies on a breathing machine may be given surfactant down the tube: this artificial coating stands in for the natural lung-inflating stuff that babies usually finish developing during their last few weeks in the womb.

touching help

Ask if and when you and your partner can take your baby out for cuddles or stroke them through the gloves that connect the outside world to the inside of the incubator. The neonatal unit staff will be happy to help and to explain how to hold the baby and when it's okay to whisper or sing softly to the baby.

Premmie babies develop more quickly – and everyone feels better – if you can get some skin-to-skin contact, massage the baby and speak soothing words. So much the better if they can feel Mum's and Dad's heartbeat and their voice. Premmie babies tend to like gentle rocking, uterus-like movements.

If there is no comfortable chair you can use, make sure your obstetrician arranges for one to be brought to the unit. Mothers of premmie babies, especially those who've just had a caesarean, deserve and need to be comfortable with their babies. They shouldn't have to stand up or perch on stools, feeling they're in the way.

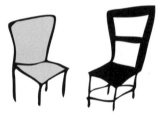

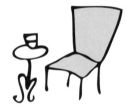

feeding help

If your baby is born before 36 weeks, they may not be good at sucking yet so they can't latch onto your breast. Instead they will be fed through a little tube; this is called nasogastric, or gavage, feeding. The milk can be either your expressed breast milk or a special formula, or both. Any breast milk you can produce – even a few drops – will help the baby's growth and immune system. This is something really positive you can do, even if you feel helpless.

common premmie characteristics
The following features are usually temporary.

⑥ Premmie babies weigh less and look tinier and skinnier than boombah full-term ones.

⑥ They're tired, and tire more easily. They like to stay curled up and asleep a lot. Remember, they're doing what they'd be doing if they were still inside. They're doing what they need to do to grow and develop.

⑥ They're not big on facial expressions, eye contact or reacting to being touched. They can be a bit irritable at arriving earlier than anybody thought.

⑥ They can be rather wrinkly and seem frail, with relatively large heads and hands.

⑥ Their skin can be pale and blood vessels can be seen beneath the skin (when they put on more fat this will change).

⑥ They're covered with a layer of fine downy hair, called lanugo.

⑥ Their party tricks such as breathing and feeding may need some work, and their cry will sound weak – some say almost kitten-like – until their lungs puff up and get stronger.

your feelings about having a premmie
You may feel:

⑥ guilt at not 'holding on longer' or being a 'good mum' who got to the 'right' week; this is common but not fair to you – treat yourself as you would a best friend going through the same thing

⑥ sadness and stress at the separation, caused by having to go home while your baby remains in hospital for a few days or weeks of special care

⑥ disconnected from the baby

⑥ frightened of touching the baby, of not feeling the 'right' things, and of taking the baby home and being alone without all the staff help of the hospital

⑥ incredibly tired, physically and emotionally, especially if you have had a caesarean or a traumatic birth.

Partners may have any of these emotions, plus a sense that they are irrelevant. They may feel frustrated that they can't solve the situation or fix the baby. In fact they have an incredibly important job: being there for the baby as much as possible and supporting you.

Partners are indispensable for getting expressed breast milk to the hospital when the mum has gone home before the baby but is exhausted and needs rest and recuperation. Partners can also be in charge of gate-keeping both at hospital and at home (letting people know if and when they can visit, according to the mum's wishes), and can take photos to show rellies who can't yet see the baby.

baby clothes

Neonatal staff will have a small supply of tiny clothes that fit a premmie baby. Dolls' clothes can also be useful (but are often not very tasteful!). Tiny babies prefer no-fuss, easy-to-get-off nighties and long T-shirts, with no long rows of buttons, ties or loopy or lacy bits that can entangle wee fingers, toes, ears or necks. Tiny caps can help keep them warm and win prizes for ultra-cuteness.

If rellies or friends are buying, knitting or crocheting clothes (it's a great way to make them feel useful), get them to choose closely stitched garments in soft silk or cotton fibre, not wool, which can irritate new skin, or non-breathing acrylic fibre, which can get itchy and hot. Feathery or shedding materials such as mohair shouldn't be used, as the bits could be inhaled.

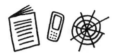

more info on premature babies

bliss.org.uk

Bliss is a national charity dedicated to supporting families of babies born 'too soon, too small or too sick'. From the main page of its website, click on 'Families and carers' then 'Information' for advice on what to expect. 'Having a baby in neonatal care' includes an online video showing what goes on inside a neonatal unit, with interviews with doctors and nurses. There is also a messageboard, and details of local support groups.
Helpline: 0500 618140

babycentre.co.uk

From the home page choose 'Baby' then 'Your Premature Baby'. Info on all aspects of caring for your premmie baby, including feeding and feelings.

preemie-l.org

A US-run website for parents of premmie babies (don't forget when web-surfing and searching that Americans spell premmies 'preemies'). This site has discussions, answers to common questions, fact sheets and links to other relevant sites.

The Premature Baby Book: Everything You Need to Know About Your Premature Baby from Birth to Age One by William Sears, MD, Robert Sears, MD, James Sears, MD, and Martha Sears, RN, Little, Brown, US, 2004

This is from an American family book business with a baby-centred attachment-parenting philosophy.

Preemies: The Essential Guide for Parents of Premature Babies by Dana Wechsler Linden, Emma Trenti Paroli and Mia Wechsler Doron, Pocket Books, US, 2000

Because this is an American book it uses the term preemies rather than premmies, but much of its info holds true for the UK.

what's going on Hello stretch marks here, there and possibly everywhere! What a splendid mauve, perhaps an attractive aubergine colour, or is it hot pink? Mind your posture, as your tummy will be putting you off balance.

The baby can blink or close its eyes when a bright light is shone onto your tummy. There's some brain action going on: receiving and sending lots of signals through the nervous system, maybe testing out the idea of thinking, possibly wondering how long it has to hang out in a hairy swamp. The baby's definite awake and sleeping times are still usually roughly the opposite of yours. Weight: about 1.6 kilos.

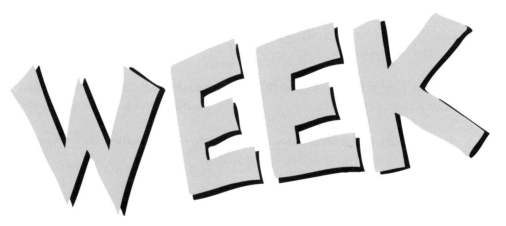

Average approximate baby length this week from head to bum

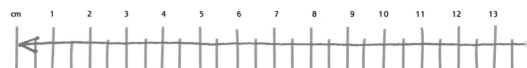

| cm | 1 | 2 | 3 | 4 | 5 | 6 | 7 | 8 | 9 | 10 | 11 | 12 | 13 |

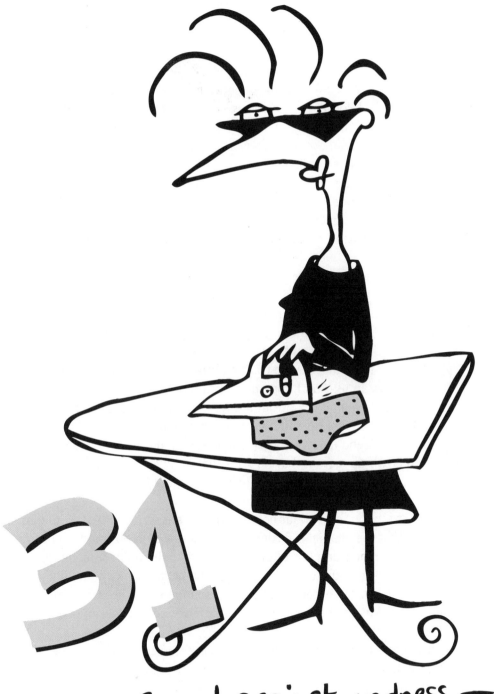

Guard against madness —
DON'T IRON YOUR UNDIES!

16 17 18 19 20 21 22 23 24 25 26 27 28 29 30

DIARY

I'm a little breathless because my lungs are all squished up. Unfortunately this does not make me sound like Marilyn Monroe singing 'Happy Birthday, Mr President'; it's more like an over-exerted warthog. Also I have a constant ache where the ligaments from the baby area extend down to the groin. Leg cramps keep waking me up at 4 a.m., and I can't get back to sleep.

Beck says it's probably not magnesium deficiency but a circulation problem and maybe I should walk shorter distances every day instead of two kilometres every second day. Maybe I get worse cramps during the nights when I don't walk.

During my walk today a huge truck pulled up at the park with rolls of wire in the back, and a big burly bloke in a reflective vest, denim shorts and steel-capped workboots got down from the cab, walked around to the passenger seat and collected a two-year-old girl with a Milly-Molly-Mandy haircut.

'Come on, darling', he said. And they went to feed the seagulls.

It made me think that having children brings out the best kindness and the worst temper in us. And I hope it will bring out the best in me, not the worst. Or at least when it brings out the worst there will be someone else to take up the slack while I go and bite some telegraph poles.

Geoff and I spend an afternoon looking at cots. It's amazing – some of them even LOOK dangerous, having gaps that a rhinoceros could practically climb out of. Not much more to buy now, but it would be nice if the washer-dryer fairy paid a visit.

Never speak too soon about household appliances. Just after I write that bit I notice that the enamel is flaking off the toaster onto our toast, so no doubt I've been ingesting bits of plutonium or aluminium or something.

Then this creepy guy turns up to service the heater, which I thought should have a new fan because the old one sounded a bit like Concorde landing. He opens up the front and says 'It's a wonder you're not dead.'

'Pardon?'

'This thing's been leaking carbon monoxide. You could have nodded off to sleep on the sofa and never woken up. I'm surprised you're still alive.'

Well.

Finally manage to hustle old Pollyanna With Spanner out the front door, burst into tears and call Geoff, only to get his voicemail. Damn, damn, damn, he is probably down the back of the garden centre explaining succulents to some dopey businessman who thinks hydroponics is a grunge band, so I call NHS Direct, who recommend I speak to the midwifery department at the hospital, where FINALLY, just before I think I'll go mad, a midwife explains that unless I have experienced the symptoms of carbon monoxide poisoning (severe nausea, severe headaches and severe lethargy and faintness) nothing will have crossed the placenta, and even if it has the likely result will have been a lack of oxygen getting to the baby, similar to what would happen if I smoked or walked around in the traffic all day, in which case the baby might be a little small.

'No', I assure her. 'The general consensus is that I am having a baby approximately the size of Danny DeVito.'

'Well,' she says, 'nothing to worry about then.'

Phew.

It is really very uncomfortable now. Beck has prescribed a grab-bag of different things (which she hates doing) to try to bring down my fluid retention. Vitamin C, dandelion-leaf tincture (at a very precisely calibrated dose as it won't work otherwise), a complicated specialist herbal mixture that tastes like a petroleum byproduct with bats' ears in it, and I'm sure if she thought it would help I would have to hang upside down every three hours as well. When I phone the surgery to check all this is okay with Dr Sharma, he just says he hopes it helps because he can't give me drugs.

Every now and then I forget I'm pregnant for a minute or two, and then the baby kicks or I have to move or something and remember. Geoff is being very sympathetic. I can't believe I have put on 17 kilos. From behind I look like two driver's-side airbags going off.

Go and buy some 100 percent cotton cot sheets – very hard to find. Another pregnant woman and I both put a hand on the last set. We look at each other.

She says graciously 'You take it, you're more pregnant than me.'

Sisterhood!

'Most people', says the shop assistant, 'don't buy 100 percent cotton because they have to iron the sheets.'

'Iron the sheets?!' I shriek. 'Are they mad?!'

Our third childbirth class: when to come to the hospital. Melissa says to come to hospital when your contractions are five minutes apart, the waters have broken or you're overwrought, but to ring first in case they've all stepped out for a daiquiri. No, to tell them what's been happening.

Here are the main points I shall have to memorise.

Early or 'practice' contractions are irregular, don't increase in intensity and usually go away if you lie down. They can happen weeks before your actual labour.

The waters breaking can be a tiny trickle or one to two litres of amniotic fluid coming out. Put on a pad. You're supposed to write down the time your waters break and note the quality and colour of the fluid. If there's an olivey greeny stain or blood in the waters, tell your midwife or hospital staff immediately, by phone, because it could mean the baby needs to come out quicker.

Don't ring everyone and tell them you're in labour or they'll all be round to the house or turning up at the hospital or getting times wrong and starting accidental rumours. Don't play hockey – conserve your energy for the labour.

Everyone is on the edge of their seat. This is what we came for – a bit of a chat about the real thing. Mind you, I thought there'd be a lot more beanbag action, and a lot more practice breathing. Apparently it's out of fashion. I am so glad Melissa is not the type to say 'Pinch your hand as hard as you can' each week to demonstrate the pain of labour. Because it's a bit like saying 'See that wee dinghy? It's kind of like an aircraft carrier'.

Melissa says not to worry if you poo during labour, and you probably won't because diarrhoea is often an early sign of labour so you'll have got rid of all the poo before you deliver. Anyway, now that I've done wee on my own floor because my pelvic-floor muscles are so hopeless, I suspect I can poo on the hospital floor, no worries.

Everyone is rather surprised by a few things. No wonder the baby comes out with its eyes closed – otherwise the first thing it would see is its mother's … ahem … arsehole. Also, after the baby comes out there's an enormous gush of fluid: the banked-up amniotic fluid – and usually up to 300 millilitres of blood.

At that point I thought things would be pretty much all over but I'd forgotten there's the third stage – the placenta comes out. (In order to demonstrate the placenta, Melissa drops the 'baby' on the carpet, which she promises not to do if she's assisting at any of our births.) And then the midwife or obstetrician will do a bit of classy embroidery on any tears or cuts. Melissa gives us the hospital's March stats: 252 deliveries, 124 intact perineums. Yikes.

Melissa tells us about three very different births in the last month.

'Oh my God', she begins (which is always a good sign in a story), 'we had a lady in the birth centre who demanded there be lavender all over the room when she gave birth. The obstetrician and midwife were having a complete lavender overdose, flopping around the room and trying to lie down in the beanbags, while the woman yelled her head off for three hours.

'Then on Thursday we had one of those rare quiet mums. She was just really focused and didn't say much, until eventually, in a tiny little voice, she said, "I think I'd quite like to start pushing now, if everyone thinks that would be all right." She didn't yell at all. I'd heard about women like that, but never seen one. It was amazing.

'And then yesterday a baby was being born right next door to this room, and the really mild-mannered mum just suddenly started yelling at me and the doctor. She was just shouting at us, "Scream at me to push the baby out, swear at me, swear at meee!!!" So the doctor was trying to help by yelling at the top of his voice "Push the fuckin' baby out!" just as a birthing class began in here. One of the dads got really scared and said to the birth class teacher, "Is it always like that?"'

info

your birth plan

what is it?

You write down all the things you want to happen during your labour. It's not a legal contract but rather a memo of understanding between you and your birth attendants: it can cover whether you want an epidural, right through to who's going to hold the baby first.

Your birth plan is also a starting point for discussion with your midwives or obstetrician about their usual procedure, the policies of the hospital or birth centre, and things such as playing the music of your choice during labour, family and friends being able to visit straight after the birth, and so on. You may not be able to have your own way on everything – this is the time to find out.

Discuss your birth plan with the midwives or obstetrician early, so that you're not still negotiating as the baby's coming out. The birth plan is usually incorporated into your antenatal notes. Tuck a copy away in your handbag. You need to realise, though, that labour rarely runs to order. Your midwives or obstetrician will probably encourage you to think of your birth plan as 'birth preferences', 'Plan A' or a 'wish list' and will ask you to keep an open mind about having a change.

Birth plans are good, to let everyone know how you'd like things to go, but the birth team is more important – you'll have to trust them to make the big decisions if anything unexpected happens.

what's in it?

You'll want your plan to be the best-case scenario for you. (You'll probably already have a vague idea about whether, for instance, you'd like the birth to be 'natural' or you'd be happy for it to be more 'medical' – see below.) But what if there are unexpected difficulties? For example, if you have a caesarean you will probably want to keep the baby with you, not have it whisked away immediately for weighing and measuring, as this time can be very important for bonding with your baby – you'll need your birth attendants to agree so it's good to have it in your birth plan.

Your plan may be a long and detailed list of what you want to happen at every stage of your labour, just a letter to your obstetrician or midwife saying what you want, or a point-form list of the stuff you think is most important. It might include:

⑥ who will be there

⑥ what you'd like to have around you to help you feel more comfortable and relaxed, such as music, massage oils and photos

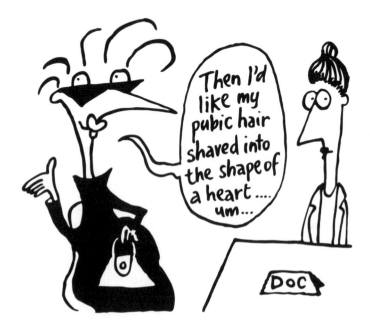

⊚ what clothes you would like to wear during the birth (hats and gloves are passé, and don't forget that anything that goes lower than your hips is likely to come off very second best in the stain department)

⊚ a reminder to yourself to trim your pubic hair if it's a bit unruly (a Brazilian is unnecessary – your baby doesn't need a landing strip!)

⊚ whether you want a tape recording, photos or a video of the birth, and who will be taking these

⊚ how, and how often, you would like to be monitored, if you have a say in this – some fetal monitors inhibit walking around

⊚ at what point you would like to be offered pain relief, and what your preferred pain-relief options are

⊚ what delivery position you'd prefer – squatting, sitting or on all fours perhaps

⊚ how you feel about an episiotomy – a cut made at the entrance to the vagina if your baby needs to come out in a hurry (it should never be just routinely done because most doctors agree it's better to tear, if possible, as healing is faster)

⊚ whether you would have a catheter to wee through if your obstetrician or midwives advised it

⊚ whether you want to touch your baby's head as it 'crowns' (peeps out for the first time)

⊚ who gets to lift the baby up first – maybe the baby's father, or you, or the obstetrician or midwife?

⊚ whether you want to be told the sex of your baby or find out for yourselves

⊚ who you would like to cut the umbilical cord

⊚ whether you want your baby placed on your chest for as long as you want immediately after birth. This skin-to-skin contact has many advantages for you and your baby and most hospitals have a 'baby-friendly' charter that includes this as a policy

⊚ whether you would accept drugs to speed up the normal delivery of the placenta.

'natural childbirth' vs medical intervention

'Natural childbirth' is agreed by most people to mean bringing your baby into the world without monitoring and medical intervention, including painkillers. The aim is to return decision-making and 'power' to the woman giving birth. Many birth activists advocate this philosophy, and they have plenty of websites.

shouldn't all women be able to give birth naturally?

Yes, and it would also be wonderful if childbirth didn't hurt and no women or children died. But I'm afraid Mother Nature couldn't give a rats about you personally. If several million women and babies die a year it's still within the natural scheme of things: Mother Nature only needs most, not all, people to survive birth in order to continue the species.

The truth is we're not all able to give birth naturally. Things go wrong for some of us. And a great many things can go right again with medical help. It's modern medicine, equipment and hygiene practices that save us from the high rate of baby and maternal injuries and deaths that still applies in many places around the world without proper hospital care.

the case against the 'medicalisation' of childbirth

The advocates of home birth and natural childbirth say that the medicalisation of birth has gone too far – that doctors and hospitals have created a culture of fear and dependence. They believe the very high rate of caesareans is scandalous and based on a blind belief in technology, the convenience of doctors and their fear of being sued.

They say that pregnancy and childbirth are not an illness; that women should use their intuition and instincts giving birth; and that routine monitoring and medical intervention can rob them of their right to a natural birth. They talk about women being empowered and in control of the birth, and being able to determine the outcome of their childbirth experience. They believe a midwife, doula or other birth attendant can ensure most women have a calm and natural birth.

the case for medically supervised childbirth

Midwives and doctors have seen hundreds, even thousands, of births, and all permutations from easy to scary and dangerous. They say that swift and skilful medical intervention does prevent brain or physical damage to the baby and save the mother's life, and they know because they've seen it over and over again.

Medical staff say that their training and experience mean they need to be the ones to monitor the progress of a birth and to be in control of decisions about urgent medical interventions such as blood transfusions, while a doula or other unqualified birth attendant may make a decision based on their ideology and wishes rather than on medical knowledge and necessity.

possible compromises

While almost everybody understands that labouring at home alone is dangerous, for a small but increasing minority of women a home birth supervised by properly equipped midwives strikes the right balance for them between natural childbirth and medical support. It may mean a more 'natural' childbirth than a hospital birth, but it needn't be entirely so: the midwives will be able to offer some pain relief and fetal monitoring, for example. And, most importantly, they will be on the look-out for developing complications and ready to transfer you to hospital if needed.

Another option is a birth centre. Many birth centres aim for a natural birth, but with medical help available if necessary (see 'Choosing Your Childbirth Place and Team' in Week 9). Of course, there are differences of opinion about whether birth centres are still too medical.

can we really choose?

It's important to understand and think about the issues. Make sure you're up to speed with the latest information. Some of the writing advocating natural childbirth is based on an overseas situation or on outdated info about the effects of drugs and procedures such as epidurals, which is not relevant to the new versions of these drugs and procedures. Check the facts with your obstetrician or midwife to make sure you're not getting old info.

It's good to know beforehand what you'd like to happen during labour (see 'Birth Plan' earlier) – so long as you know that many women change their choice about, say, painkillers during the actual birth. They may have thought they wouldn't want drugs and then found drugs helped them achieve the vaginal birth they wanted; or they may have assumed that they'd need drugs and then found themselves having a relatively easy and manageable birth.

But for some of us choice isn't possible, whatever our plans or philosophy. The vast majority of us who have a medical intervention such as a caesarean don't get to choose at all – events overtake us and the medical staff decide it's safer for mother or baby (see 'Caesarean Delivery' in Week 35 for more info). Only a very few women choose, and find an obstetrician who'll agree, to schedule an elective caesarean because they're 'too posh to push'.

trusting your childbirth team

Pretty much everybody accepts that a vaginal birth, if possible, is by far the best option for both mothers and babies, and wishes that childbirth was routinely natural, with babies arriving safely in their own time under the guidance of highly skilled midwives. Many of us would love to have a gentle birth at home, but many of us also reluctantly accept that 'just in case' means we trade off total control and a homey atmosphere for the safest possible outcome that medical skill and technology can give us.

Most obstetricians and medical staff say that they, too, are natural childbirth advocates, but only when it doesn't pose a risk to mother or baby. And natural childbirth advocates say they accept that caesareans are sometimes necessary. The disagreement is over whether monitoring is important; whether one medical intervention inevitably leads to another, more serious one; when during labour to declare a risk an 'unacceptable risk'; and how to decide when a caesarean or other intervention is wise or 'necessary'.

In some ways the debate is perhaps a difference of emphasis. Natural childbirth advocates focus on the journey and the process of birth; medical staff tend to focus on the outcome – a healthy baby and mother.

The reality for most women is this: if, in the middle of labour, an obstetrician or the midwives say you need a caesarean, or a forceps or vacuum delivery, you don't have much choice but to take their advice. They, after all, are down at the business end, with a great deal more experience. You need to trust them to make the right decisions for you and your baby.

In order to do this, women need to talk to each other about their childbirth experiences and the attitude and competence of the obstetrician or midwives who cared for them. Discussions with your midwives beforehand should reassure you that you are on the same philosophical page, and that they and the obstetrician on duty will make decisions based on your medical needs and your baby's health. If you are truly unhappy with the midwife that is caring for you, you can request a different midwife. This also applies to an obstetrician, but can be more difficult to arrange since the obstetrician who attends you in labour may be the only one on site.

more mum-centred medicine

Although many women may be intrigued by the idea of home birth, the truth is that the vast majority still choose to give birth in a hospital environment. And they should not be penalised for this choice: hospitals and birth centres should be a lot more mother-friendly than they often are, and provide top-notch care that, after the birth, makes the emotional health of mothers and bonding with babies the highest priority.

Hospitals and their staff would do women a big favour if they made sure that, essential medical processes aside, women had somewhere quiet to be after the birth. Women need to get back to a normal sort of room and cuddly atmosphere as soon as possible, rather than being parked on a trolley somewhere under floodlights while medical people do non-essential things such as measuring the length of the baby. Staff should be available to debrief with mums about difficult births or unexpected outcomes, as well as to help women feel comfortable and competent before they leave hospital.

In-hospital times are decreasing, partly because of the shortage of beds and the workload in maternity wards, and partly because women want to get out of the hospital atmosphere, especially when it isn't helping them learn how to breastfeed and care for their babies. Hospitals need to recognise that women shouldn't have to feel they're on a production line, or that they need to get out of the way because there's somebody else to take the bed.

Even though the birth is only one day, it's a day that is profoundly spiritually, mentally, emotionally and physically important to women and they deserve to have their wishes respected as much as possible. You never forget the birth.

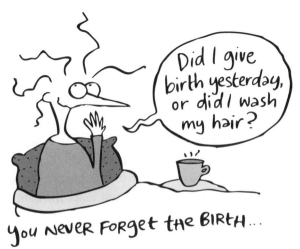

you NeVeR FoRget tHe BIRtH...

Politics and penny-pinching A big factor in all this is whether hospitals are properly staffed, with enough beds and maternity services. From now on if you're ever asked what influences your vote, please remember to say 'maternity health services'. And if you're booked in somewhere and you know it has a reputation for overcrowding, please call your local MP and put your case. The people who make the decisions about health services need to hear from us.

not having the childbirth you wanted

Some women who've been told that childbirth should be a spiritual experience and virtually pain-free, that they can transcend it by using 'calming techniques', meditation, hypnotherapy or hypno-birthing, or a breathing routine, or that it can be orgasmic or pleasurable, can be shocked when they find it hurts a lot more than they thought or they encounter an unexpected problem. Doctors and many midwives say the focus on natural childbirth has given some people unrealistic expectations, and this means that when things do not go the way they planned some new mums feel that they've failed or been cheated.

Needing pain relief or medical intervention is not a failure. (It doesn't help that sometimes medical staff unfortunately refer to a 'failure to progress' in labour: this is a medical term, not a description of the mother.) Self-blame or feelings of inadequacy are known to be high-risk factors in postnatal depression. Please don't regret it if you don't have a 'perfect birth', or feel that you weren't able to do it 'right' or that the birth didn't live up to your rosiest (maybe unrealistic) expectations. It's important to know that unexpected things can happen even if you're very healthy, eat well, do yoga and feel positive. What's that saying? 'Life is what happens to you when you're busy making other plans.'

If you do need a caesarean or other intervention, congratulate yourself on nurturing your baby up to the birth and keeping it alive and loved afterwards, and the fact that you and your team did a great job with the circumstances you had to work with. Acknowledge that, as usual, luck and random chance have more to do with your life than you'd like to think, and that some things are just out of your control. Women have enough ludicrous expectations thrown at them about being perfect without having to cop this weird idea that all of us can or must give birth without help. Mother Nature sometimes needs a big fat hand.

a difficult birth

Occasionally a birth can be very difficult and go on for many, many hours, or suddenly become life-threatening and need an emergency caesarean or other medical intervention. Even when a healthy baby is the result, a traumatic birth can leave you with physical complications and unresolved feelings of shock, guilt that you were responsible in some way, or anger about what happened. If this happens to you, it's important to be able to be upset, acknowledge your feelings, give yourself time to recuperate and heal, talk with professional medical staff and counsellors, mums' groups, friends, your midwife or health visitor, a phone counselling line – whoever seems helpful to you – and to move on. Also talk to your birth partner – it will likely have been traumatic for them too.

Make sure your medical team takes the time, when they can, to relive the birth with you and explain why decisions were taken. Sometimes clearing up misconceptions and getting a full explanation of why, for instance, you needed a particular intervention and how it ensured the best health outcome for you and your baby, can help immensely.

Take care of your emotional and physical self. You shouldn't have to suffer from fears or bad memories that overshadow your experience as a parent or make you afraid to have another baby. Whatever the reason, even if it's clear that bad things happened to you and shouldn't have, you will need to find a way to incorporate the experience into your life so you are not dominated by it. If you're always looking backwards with regret about that one day, rather than getting on with all the future days to come, find the psychological help you need.

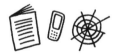

more info on 'natural childbirth' vs medical intervention

There are lots of natural childbirth websites. Get medical info from mainstream pregnancy or medical sites or your midwife or doctor.

Many of the pregnancy websites given in Week 1 have stories about natural births, caesareans and other variations (and also see 'More Info on Premature Babies' in Week 30).

homebirth.org.uk

The Home Birth Reference Site is a comprehensive website run by a home-birth advocate. Birth stories, pain-relief options, recommended books and DVDs, articles, and what to do if your GP opposes home birth.

newyorker.com

From the home page search 'The Score' by Atul Gawande to find a doctor's article about how medical intervention in birth became the norm, and an account of a caesarean.

pregnancy.com.au/natural_birth_can_go_wrong.htm

A personal story from an Australian woman 'desperate for a natural birth' who changed her mind after 35 hours of pushing.

pregnancy.about.com/od/birthstories/a/naturalbirth.htm

Some happy natural birth stories from the US.

Home Birth: A Practical Guide by Nicky Wesson, Pinter and Martin, UK, 2006

Home birth advocate Nicky Wesson, a herbalist and former NCT and NHS childbirth teacher, firmly states the case for the right to home birth, sets out her case for its safety, and advises women how to wade through the bureaucratic swamp and disapprovals where possible when fighting to get the sort of birth they want. She points out that if you're told you need to transfer to hospital while in labour it's best not to muck about. Contains stories by real women of their births, ranging from the gloriously exultant to the very sad, but all of them are honest and moving.

Birth Your Way: Choosing Birth At Home or In a Birth Centre by Sheila Kitzinger, Dorling Kindersley, UK, 2001

Home birth and breastfeeding guru Sheila Kitzinger's book is full-bottle on advocating non-hospital birth. She explains why and addresses lots of common worries or 'challenges' and possible queries from you or your birth partner. With lots of understanding about emotions and with practical (if astonishing) midwifery hints such as Sheila's get-the-placenta-out-by-blowing-over-a-bottle suggestion. Check any medical details and info on hospital and NHS policy, as this may be out of date.

Birth Stories for the Soul edited by Denis Walsh and Sheena Byrom, Quay Books, UK, 2009

Edited by midwives and billed as 'tales' of home and hospital, grief and hope, and incorporating the stories of dads, sibling and other relatives, this collection of stories from the UK, Australia, New Zealand, the US and Sweden is clearly built around a strong belief that the birth experience should be more 'humanised' as something that fosters family involvement and community feeling.

WEEK 32

what's going on

Your lungs are getting stronger, although because of all the pressure you may feel breathless if you overdo it. You may be starting to get a bit sick of the whole pregnancy thing. It's uncomfortable being this big, you're running out of outfits and as for sleeping well – ha!

The baby's lungs are stronger too, but not fully ready to go yet. The baby is filling out with fat, although it still looks a bit on the skinny side. It might be upside down in readiness for the lunge to the outside world. This is pretty much your complete baby item, covered in vernix. If the baby was born now it would open its eyes and take a peek at the world (except it can't focus on much at this age and will look endearingly cross-eyed). Weight: about 1.8 kilos.

cm   1   2   3   4   5   6   7   8   9   10   11   12   13

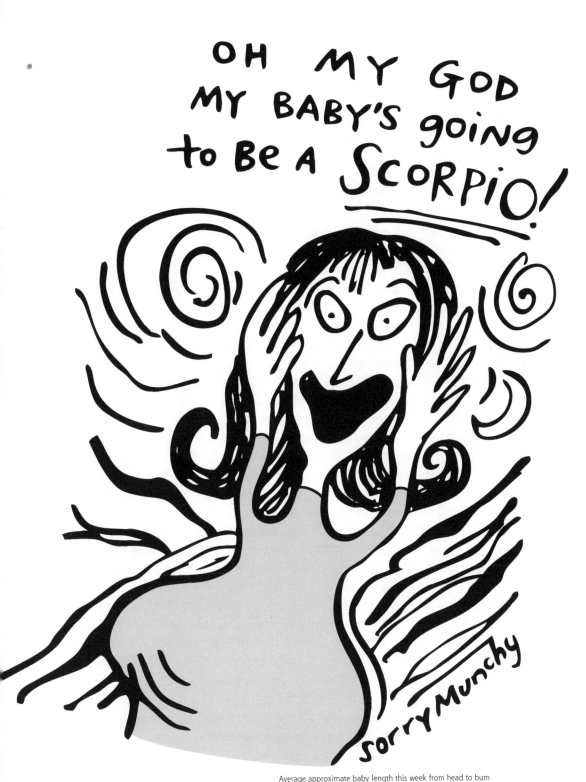

Average approximate baby length this week from head to bum

16   17   18   19   20   21   22   23   24   25   26   27   28   29   30

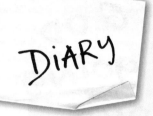
DiARY

I go for another check-up at the antenatal clinic. 'You look tired and bloated', says Claire, my midwife today. Charmed, I'm sure. She says the insomniac sore legs when lying down are probably due to the fluid retention. She listens to the baby's heartbeat, asks if the baby's moving (is it ever: Chelsea loves to rumba all night long), and measures the length of the uterus.

'The baby's doing beautifully – you're doing brilliantly well', she says.

It's very kind the way she does this sort of positive bit after she tells me I look like shit (in the nicest possible way).

There are no safe drugs for fluid retention during pregnancy, Claire explains.

'Why can't I take diuretics?' I whine.

'Two reasons. They reduce placental blood flow, and they can mask the symptoms of pre-eclampsia.'

Oh all right, smartypants.

She takes a couple of vials of blood to check if there's a high level of uric acid in the blood or my platelets are at all 'deranged' – both signs that I might be susceptible to pre-eclampsia. I quite like the idea of my platelets being deranged. I'm so responsible these days there should be some part of me acting like an idiot, but on second thoughts I can definitely do without pre-eclampsia. I have to come again next week because I'm retaining so much fluid Claire wants to keep an eye on it.

Week four of the childbirth class: Melissa's potted version of stuff that might happen that isn't your ideal plan. Forceps might be used if you're too tired to push any more, the baby seems to be staying put, you've been pushing for too long (one to two hours), or there are signs of fetal distress. Usually you'll get an epidural first. I can see why when Melissa holds up a pair of forceps. They look like very upmarket, Italian, oversized salad servers from one of those designer shops full of stuff that people don't really need but has 'Alessi' written all over it. There are three types: rotator forceps (also known as Kielland's forceps), lift-out forceps (aka Wrigley's forceps) and Neville Barnes forceps. I hope nobody ever says 'This is a job for Neville.' It never ceases to amaze me what men will name after themselves.

Then there's the rather sophisticated-sounding ventouse, a suction cup that they can stick on the baby's head and, well, pull it out. (It's a vacuum in the sense of the plumber's mate, not the type you do the carpet with.) Melissa sits there absent-mindedly playing with the soft-toy baby on her lap.

So far she's folded it in half and is waving one of its feet past its ear.

Emergency caesareans are performed if a large baby is stuck, the cervix just isn't getting any wider or the baby is really distressed, or for other reasons. Usually you'll get an epidural or a spinal block to numb the lower half of your body. After a caesarean you get morphine or pethidine – 'Hi baby! Mummy's reeeeally stoned!' Usually you're on a drip for up to 24 hours and have a catheter (tube) for weeing for up to 24 hours. The baby feeds as normal, and the dad, another helper or a staff member does the nappy changes and baths and stuff.

What about the bizarre-sounding 'induction' or 'inducement' (as in 'He offered me an illegal inducement, your worship, and I booked him for aggravated bribery')? An obstetrician may bring on ('induce') labour if you're more than one to two weeks overdue; if your little bub isn't growing well; or if you have pre-eclampsia. Melissa says she knows of a doctor who induced a baby because its mother didn't want a Scorpio, and a doctor who refused to induce a baby on the fourth of July for an American couple.

Then Melissa talks about stillbirth. Everyone in the room goes very quiet. She says she doesn't want to talk about it, but she has to because it does happen rarely that a baby is born dead, or is born with so many problems that it slips away from life a few days later. She says that in the case of a stillbirth, the baby often hasn't moved for a day or two before the labour. So always call your midwife if you haven't felt the baby move for 12 hours – although usually the baby's fine and just quiet, getting ready for labour.

If a baby is stillborn, the hospital organises to have photos taken and inked footprints on a card done, even if you don't want these mementoes at the time. (One bereaved mum called after three years to get hers.) Melissa's eyes fill with tears as she talks, and so do mine.

info

pain-relief options during labour

Way before you're due, the following people will give you advice on pain relief: your obstetrician, your midwife, your partner; plenty of people who haven't had a baby; plenty who have; and a large man called Trevor who you meet at a leather bar.

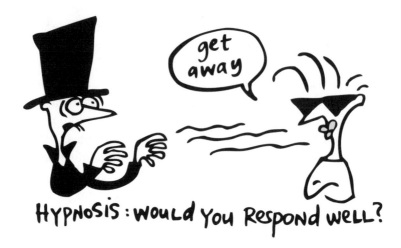

HYPNOSIS : WOULD YOU RESPOND WELL?

Everyone has a different perception of pain and how much they can put up with and for how long. Many women want to try childbirth without painkillers, but there's no shame or problem in changing your mind once you're in labour. There's only one absolute: painless birth is a myth. It's going to hurt. But with modern painkillers or other techniques, and your own decisions about these, you now have some control. Aren't you glad it isn't 1903?

The final decision rests with you. Beforehand you can choose the pain relief you'd like for an ideal delivery, but accept that you may have to have a back-up plan if, for example, the birth lasts longer or is more painful than you expected. That way you won't have to make any spur-of-the-moment decisions about pain relief during labour.

non-drug methods
The following non-drug methods of pain relief are often suggested (for each of these, faith in the method will help – if you're sceptical now, you may be a lot more so when you're yelling), but none of them stops the pain of labour:

⑥ moving around – keeping mobile can help take pressure off your back, as well as distracting you from the pain (some women find that standing or squatting is more comfortable)

⑥ acupuncture (mainly for people who use it regularly)

⑥ aromatherapy – this is *not* pain relief, it's just dickering with the atmosphere

⊚ massage – but once in labour almost all women say 'DON'T TOUCH ME' (except for hand squeezing)

⊚ hydrotherapy – a warm shower or bath will help to relax you; sitting in water can provide pain relief by supporting the abdominal wall and decreasing the pressure on muscles

⊚ localised heat – hot towels and wheat packs can help mask pain and reduce muscle cramps and spasms (there'll probably be a microwave nearby)

⊚ vocalisation – groaning, chanting or singing to 'release' pain, otherwise known as Just. Plain. Yelling. Yodelling is an option. And swearing.

⊚ transcutaneous electrical nerve stimulation (TENS) – with this, a machine delivers a very low electric current to your back, which offers slight pain relief

⊚ music – more dickering with the atmosphere (a lot of people make elaborate birth CDs or MP3 collections and end up throwing them across the labour room). Be warned: all birth teams are totally sick of bloody Enya.

the hard stuff

Epidural and spinal block   Many women request an epidural. First, a local anaesthetic is injected into your back. Next, a fine, hollow needle is inserted between two vertebrae in your lower back, then a catheter is inserted via the needle, and anaesthetic is injected into it. The catheter allows epidural drugs to be placed in the right spot in the back to block pain, and the continued administration of painkillers throughout labour and delivery if needed. The anaesthetic takes effect within a few minutes. The whole procedure usually takes less than half an hour and is always done by an experienced anaesthetist. 'Only an epidural or having the baby truly stops the pain', an experienced midwife says.

An epidural goes into the lower back tissue that surrounds the sac containing the spinal cord and spinal fluid, whereas a spinal block goes directly into the spinal fluid and so works more quickly (it is often used in a caesarean delivery when speed is important). Epidurals wear off after one or several hours depending on how much is used – they can be 'topped up' during a long labour. A spinal block is a one-off injection that lasts one to four hours. Modern epidurals are far more controlled and recovery times are getting speedier. You can have one early in labour (at a certain point it will no longer be an option as your baby will probably arrive before the anaesthetist).

Epidurals and spinal blocks are the only methods of pain relief currently available that take away all perception of pain yet allow you to stay conscious. That's why they are used for caesareans (see 'Caesarean Delivery' in Week 35).

Epidural anaesthetic is often used when women are in great pain, if the baby is in an awkward position (such as breech), if it's a multiple birth, or with a forceps or suction delivery. An epidural probably won't stop you from feeling pressure. Your doctor or midwife will tell you when to push. Some people choose to let the anaesthetic wear off a little towards the end so that they can feel the contractions again. Many epidurals can be controlled by you, the patient.

There is very little risk involved with having an epidural or a spinal block administered by an experienced anaesthetist. Occasionally an epidural only blocks pain in part of your abdomen, but the anaesthetist can often fix that. Less than one percent of women who have had an epidural report having a headache lasting up to a few days. Epidurals and spinals that block pain in labour without numbing the legs and bladder are now routine in most large maternity units. Having an epidural or spinal block in itself won't affect your baby.

Gas and air Gas and air, also known as inhalation analgesia, is nitrous oxide ('laughing gas') and oxygen under various brand names, inhaled during contractions through a mouth tube. It is generally accepted that it eases the perception of pain, but doesn't provide a complete block. Gas and air can be used safely throughout labour and appears to have very little effect on the baby, though it makes some people feel sick and light-headed. Because it can be used at any stage, it's an option in mid- to late labour if the window of opportunity for an epidural has passed.

Narcotics, including pethidine Heroin used to be given in childbirth; pethidine is now the most common narcotic still on offer but most birth teams want to avoid it. Narcotics, usually given as injections during the first stage of labour, dull the sensation of pain by stimulating opiate receptors in the brain and spinal cord.

An injection of pethidine takes about 20 minutes to work and it lasts 1–3 hours. Side effects can include vomiting, headache, blurred vision, mood changes, feeling well away with the fairies, and nausea. If given in large doses, it may make the baby sleepy and affect its breathing, so it is avoided once you are in advanced labour. If this does happen, the baby can be given a little oxygen or a drug called Narcan after the birth, to reverse the effects.

Local anaesthetic   The two most common forms of local anaesthesia given during labour are a pudendal nerve block, which involves an injection to numb the lower vagina and perineum before forceps or a vacuum instrument is used to pull the baby out; and perineal anaesthesia, injected into the perineum to reduce discomfort or, most commonly, to perform an episiotomy. Both types of anaesthetic take effect within a few minutes. Minimum doses are used so as not to affect the baby.

General anaesthetic   This is almost never used during labour, but is sometimes necessary in an emergency caesarean.

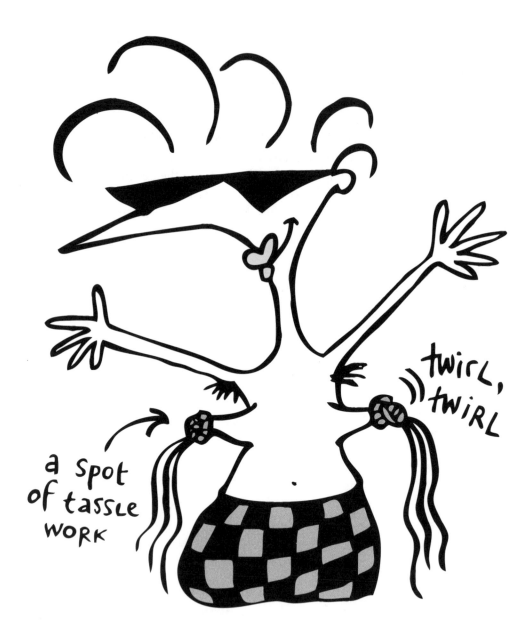

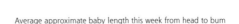

16 17 18 19 20 21 22 23 24 25 26 27 28 29

Average approximate baby length this week from head to bum

WEEK 33

what's going on You feel like there's not another thing that could be fitted inside you, not even a Mars Bar. Well, maybe a Mars Bar. Your navel is probably sticking out.

All the baby really needs is more surfactant to coat its lungs and some more fat. It has an excellent chance of survival if it comes out now, even though it would be early. As well as blinking, the baby is starting to learn to focus its eyes on close things like its own extremities and the umbilical cord. Weight: about 2 kilos.

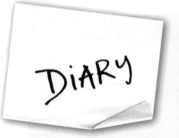
DiARy

I've been reading even more lists in books and hospital pamphlets about what to take to hospital: pillows, hot-water bottle and a birth ball; sanitary pads the size of the Isle of Wight; every beauty aid known to womankind, including 'setting equipment' (one book apparently thinks you'll be giving yourself a home perm) and a mascara for that touch-up during a difficult second stage of labour. PLUS: clothes for the baby, including bootees (get out), bonnet (oh shut up), undershirt, sleeper with legs (what?) and bunting with legs (stop it); cameras for still photos and videos (no thanks); change or a phone card to ring people up ('Hello, I'd like to order a bunting. No, I don't know what it is.'); your admission forms for hospital already filled in; books and magazines; your address book and notepaper to write thank-you letters for the flowers and presents (don't they know all you'll want to do is sleep?); and while you're about it, possibly some occasional furniture, a blunderbuss, and, oh, maybe a kayak.

I've checked the hospital's policy on giving out info about the birth: luckily they refuse to tell anyone anything. Having confirmed her presence with the switchboard, the parents of my friend Fatimah drove straight to the hospital when she was in labour and tried to force their way into the delivery room while she was yelling at them to go away. Most unseemly. And I won't be leaving a message on the answering machine saying we've gone to the hospital. In fact I'm going to leave a message saying 'I haven't gone to the hospital, I'm just not answering the phone. Do not call the hospital. Repeat, and this means you Aunt Julie, do not call the hospital. Leave a message.'

Another fluid-retention vigilance visit to the midwife to have blood pressure checked. The waiting room is an endless parade offering excellent people-watching opportunities. Today there is a couple who look straight out of the pages of Italian *Vogue*. Her: full, heavy make-up, hair done by the caring hands of a professional in the last five hours, Manolo Blahnik shoes, Armani suit, gold jewellery and diamonds the size of small mammals. Him: full-length suede overcoat, tailored suit, silk tie, designer specs, carefully cultivated two-day growth. Not a hair out of place, not a piece of lint. I can't imagine what they would do with a baby. Put it in a vase, maybe.

When it's my turn, I climb up on the bed thing, which is so narrow it always reminds me of being on a ship (especially when I was feeling sick). Jill's on duty today. She gets out her tape to measure the height of the uterus and feels my stomach and starts laughing.

'My, it's a whopper', she says.

Now, don't get me wrong. If I was on a fishing trip with somebody, or the boss was telling me about a pay rise, or an Italian sailor was taking off his strides in a sexual fantasy, the words 'My, it's a whopper' could be exceedingly welcome. When the phrase refers, however, to something that has to come out of your vagina, sometimes referred to amusingly as the birth canal in a pathetic attempt to make it sound bigger, like, say, the Panama Canal, well, it is a different kettle of episiotomies entirely.

Jill's approach to the big-baby question is basically to wait and see what happens during labour. She says that ultrasounds have proven notoriously unreliable in judging whether a baby's head will fit through the middle of its mum's elvis. I mean pelvis. I suppose I had better read a bit more about caesareans, just in case. I have a mental picture of a whole lot of people with miners' helmets on, carrying coils of rope, peering up my fanny and shouting 'Come out, you big bugger!'

Jill says I could get my GP to refer me to a skin specialist who can remove the moles and skin tags that have gone berserk, but she says all mole or tag removals should wait until at least three months after babies are born because they often disappear by themselves. (Not the babies, the moles.)

The fluid retention is really getting me down. Jill says I have to wait till after the birth, and then it will take days or weeks to 'wee it all out'. I'm from a generation that has been taught (wrongly as it happens) that you can be somehow in control of your body – even change its essential shape by diet and exercise, or surgery. The feeling of being totally OUT of control – along for the ride, part of a biology experiment – is kinda disconcerting. Now I'm told I have to get horizontal (sofa or bed? – spoilt for choice) to help rest the kidneys, whose job it is to flush this stuff out.

An uneasy feeling grows that David Attenborough is outside my house with a film crew, waiting to breathlessly narrate the next bit of my life. 'And now the Kaz has only six weeks to go', he whispers to the camera, as he crouches behind the hibiscus. 'Inside, she is groaning and puffing every time she lifts her enormous weight from the sofa. She is totally demented about getting the baby's room set up, and if her mate, Geoff, does not perform the act of cleaning his crap out of his office by the agreed deadline of 35 weeks, she will eat his head.'

Geoff, fully apprised of the whopperiness of our offspring, has taken to calling it Gigantor instead of Chelsea. I am running out of wry smiles.

My dreams are getting weirder and weirder. The night before last I dreamt that Geoff left me and took the furniture, and I forgot to ask him if he was interested in seeing the baby after it was born. Then last night I dreamt I had given birth and then one of the nurses (who were all dressed in pastel French maids' uniforms – a very sartorially satisfactory dream) said 'There was another cord hanging out so we followed it back in, and it was attached to another baby, which has been hiding behind the uterus the whole time. So now you've got two.'

Week 5 of childbirth classes: Melissa devotes the night to breastfeeding. I must admit I have kind of blanked out about breastfeeding. After Melissa wipes the floor with my illusions and severely bashes up my expectations, I fully realise that if I breastfeed I must accept that for several months I won't be able to (a) sleep, (b) work, (c) speak, (d) twirl tassels in opposite directions while they are attached to my nipples.

It's just that apparently you have to feed the little blighters at least every four hours in the early days, and apparently you're supposed to be awake while that happens. And get this. You can't schedule it. The *baby* decides when it's hungry and it could be ANY TIME. I'd also imagined I could pop out of a long office meeting and whack the baby on a gland for, say, seven minutes before handing it to a passer-by and rushing back in. But apparently babies can stay on for up to half an hour each side! And sometimes they want it and sometimes they don't! And it might not be the seven minutes you choose! And you can't just feed them when it suits you because it takes two to three hours to 'fill up' the breasts with milk again! Outrageous!

I can't imagine who designed this system. No wonder women in some other cultures aren't allowed to do any work or housework or even get out of bed for the first few weeks after childbirth.

And apparently, for the full benefits that everyone raves about (boosting the baby's immune system, annoying old fuddy-duddies who simply go gaga at the sight of a publicly bared bosom, etc), you need to breastfeed for a minimum of six months.

Melissa drops a few hints: go to the loo and wash your hands before you breastfeed, and have a set-up next to your chair with a glass of water, phone, etc on it.

There are an awful lot of instructions about breastfeeding, but at least everyone now admits it can be difficult. Plus Melissa is pretty sure that most of the midwives and lactation consultants (bet that looks good on a passport) at this hospital have their story straight, and we won't be plagued by seven different recommended methods while we're learning. Eventually ('they' say) you can whack a baby on your bosom upside down in the dark while riding a horse backwards side-saddle, but in the beginning it can be all rather laborious.

When your breasts get engorged – have too much milk – they get really big and hard and painful, and that's when you get some cabbage leaves out of the fridge and put one in each bra cup. Nobody really knows why it works, but I'd like to meet the person who worked it out.

The whole idea of expressing breast milk – pumping it out and putting it in bottles – which I'll have to do if I go back to work – seems damned weird. I can remember seeing rows and rows of dairy cows being milked and am starting to have visions of myself that are along the same lines.

I can't find my Fat Boots. In the vague frame of mind I'm in, they'll probably turn up in the toaster. I specialise in sentences that are in search of an endi...

info

what to organise before hospital

⑥ Go to an antenatal class, and do your reading. Labour and delivery are unpredictable, so you may as well at least have some vague idea of what you might be in for. (Midwives with years of experience are good to talk to.)

⑥ Write your birth plan (see the info in Week 31).

⑥ If you have another child or children, organise childcare for them now: this may need to be available at a moment's notice – even in the middle of the night – so it's a good idea to have a first choice and a back-up. Make sure the kids are well briefed on the plan so they are not freaked out when they find you gone.

⑥ Plan your transport to hospital; don't drive yourself. Avoid motorways if you can – they are hard to escape from when there's a traffic jam. And check out the car parking at the hospital – where you should park and how much it'll cost.

◎ If you haven't already, organise essential baby clothes and items, just in case (see 'Baby Clothes and Nappies' in Week 25 and 'Baby Equipment' in Week 26).

◎ Have a freezer stocked full of easy food, ready for the first few weeks at home. You could prepare soups, pasta sauces, quiches, pies, lasagnes or casseroles. Put it this way – you won't want to be plucking any chickens. When you go home your priorities will be (a) baby care, (b) sleep and (c) – there is no c.

◎ Have some light, nutritious early-labour food, such as homemade chicken or beef broth or puréed fruit, in the freezer.

◎ If you can afford it, arrange a house cleaner (friend, relative or agency) for the first few weeks at home, especially if you know you're having a caesarean.

◎ Make a sign for the door saying 'DO NOT KNOCK OR RING. New baby and mother asleep. GO AWAY QUIETLY', or use the one in my book *The Rough Guide to Babies and Toddlers*.

◎ Order a nappy-wash service, if you plan to use it – they generally only need a day's warning, but you may as well make a call putting them on notice while you have time. Or lay in a few packets of newborn-sized disposables.

◎ Fit the baby restraint in the car (see 'Baby Restraint for the Car' in Week 26), and practise buckling and unbuckling with a teddy bear. You'll need it to take the baby home.

◎ Find out what labour aids your hospital maternity section or birth centre can provide during labour and what you might need to bring in yourself – does it provide CD players, aromatherapy burners and birthing balls, for instance? Always double-check, when ringing to say you're coming in (see 'Labour' in Week 34), that whatever you need is still available just in case it's been booked by someone else. If you plan to use a TENS machine during your labour you need to book it now. Some hospitals provide them (sometimes for a small fee). Otherwise, some chemists rent them out for about £30 a month.

◎ If you are planning a home birth, check with your midwives what kit you need to provide and get it ready now. This might include plastic sheets to protect bed and carpet, mountains of old towels, and a bucket. You may want to pack a bag (see below) in case you need to transfer to hospital; if not, you'll still need most of the items listed, so it makes sense to put them all in one place so your midwife or birth partner can find them for you when needed.

to take to hospital

Your hospital or birth centre will give you a list in advance of what it recommends you bring in for yourself and the baby.

bag for labour

⑥ Labour aids might include: music CD or MP3 player; massage oil; massage roller (or rolling pin or tennis ball); a water sprayer and an aromatherapy refresher; lip cream; plenty of food and drink for your labour support person or people (you don't want to have to do without them while they go out hunter-gathering); warm socks with non-slip bottoms; glucose sweets or sugar-free lollipops; aromatherapy oils.

⑥ Take something to wear, such as a large T-shirt, giant-sized cotton shirt or cotton nightie. If you want to keep some semblance of being covered up during labour, go for a front-buttoning shirt (or back-to-front hospital gown) so you can have easy skin-to-skin contact and breastfeed your baby after delivery. Whatever you labour in is likely to get stuff all over it: whoever does your washing should soak blood stains in cold water and a stain remover before throwing it in the washing machine. You might also need a couple of pairs of dark undies and some pads to absorb leaking amniotic fluid while you're in labour.

⑥ Pack toiletries – soap, shampoo, conditioner, toothbrush and tooth-paste, moisturiser, hair elastics, hairbrush, hairdryer, shower cap – ear plugs, eye mask, and make-up if you want to joosh up a bit for visitors. You will probably also need a bath towel.

⑥ The support person's clothes should be comfortable, not too warm, and easy to wash. They should have a jacket or coat they can take on and off as they may flit into the colder outside world to make calls or get some fresh air. If your support person is likely to be, for instance, giving you pain-relief massage in the shower, they might also want to pack a swimming cossie or

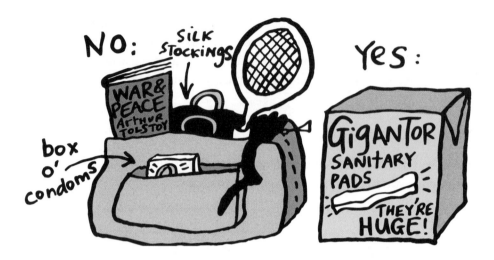

trunks, because hospitals do try to restrict the number of people running around in the nicky-noo-nar.

⑥ Apparently some people who are into 'creative visualisation' look at a photo of their dog. Of course they're obviously insane.

a bigger bag for the hospital stay

⑥ Take a few packs of super-soaker sanitary pads – these are sold as maternity pads. Do remember in your post-birth haze to put these on undies STICKY SIDE DOWN. Nobody needs a pad stuck to their episiotomy stitches or pubes.

⑥ Include a couple of front-opening nighties or PJs (for breastfeeding), a few pairs of black cotton undies (white ones will stain), a dressing gown and slippers. (Although you'll probably be home within 36 hours, and quite possibly a fair bit sooner, you may have to stay longer if you have a caesarean or any complications. It would be nice to have a clean nightie each morning and each night, and plenty of cotton undies – it's a leaky old time – so pack according to your helper's washing plans. Would the washing be done every couple of days, or not until you all get home?) You can wear regular day clothes in hospital, but the combination of a sore, tender and tired body, the high temperatures at which hospitals are generally kept and the number of times you'll need access to the business end makes cotton nighties a practical choice.

⑥ Take at least two very firm nursing bras for supporting tight, engorged breasts, and nursing pads to soak up the leaking breast milk when it 'comes in'.

⑥ Pack going-home clothes for you (maternity clothes because your tummy will still be big) and for the baby: include a cap/hat – mostly they're soft jersey (best not to have a pom-pom) – and a warm blanket if the weather's cold.

⑥ Take a newborn-baby-care book such as my *Rough Guide to Babies and Toddlers* or one of the others reviewed in Week 43 of this book, and a book of names if that debate is still dragging on.

⑥ If you have a toddler or young child, don't forget a wrapped present for them so they feel central to the action, and give them special status and lots of praise as new Big Brother or Sister. This is the beginning of a difficult time for them, and they will be nicer to the new baby if they think it's brought them a special present.

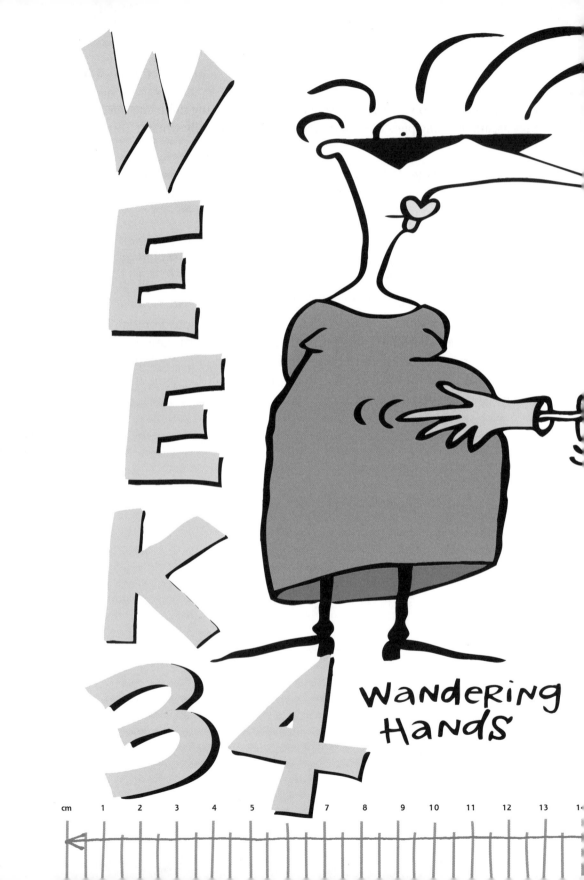

WEEK
34

Wandering
Hands

cm 1 2 3 4 5 6 7 8 9 10 11 12 13 14

what's going on From now on your baby will hog all available space and squash up anything silly enough to get in the way, like your lungs. If you do get breathless, sitting or standing up straight will help. So will taking it easy. If you're interested in going to childbirth classes but haven't organised this yet, you'd better make that phone call now. Lay in the 'layette' (baby's clothes).

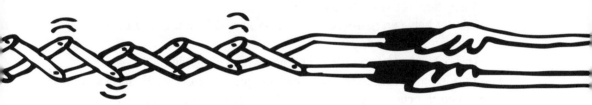

Your body is starting to put the final touches to the baby: it's the finishing-school stage. From now on your bub is pretty busy practising sucking, breathing, blinking, turning the head, grabbing things (such as its other hand) and stretching out the legs – but there's not quite enough room to actually do that. Hence the jarring kicks you may feel. The baby's skin is becoming smoother and less translucent – more like the final skin colour. Weight: about 2.3 kilos.

Average approximate baby length this week from head to bum

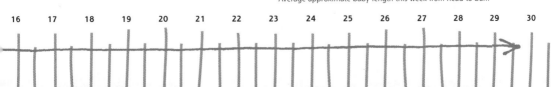

16 17 18 19 20 21 22 23 24 25 26 27 28 29 30

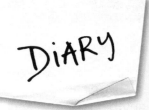

It's really hard to find comfy positions. If I lean back, I get heartburn. If I lean forward, I'm not resting, I'm listing. If I lie down, I can't get anything done. If I don't lie down, the fluid retention reaches epic proportions. If I lie down, my lower legs ache. If I walk around, I aggravate an ache in my groin. At the start of the day my face is all puffy. By the end of the day my ankles are all puffy. I'm starting to feel like one of those ballpoint pens with the liquid in the side: if you turn it upside down all the liquid falls down and the girl's bikini top comes off. Now I can't even adequately describe a novelty souvenir writing implement.

Make the mistake of trying to buy a frock in a flash boutique with three mirrors in the changing room. When I realise quite what I look like from behind, I have to sit down on it for a minute, in shock. And my arms look like the sort of arms that gigantic ladies get a few years after their wood-chopping days are over. Good grief.

I skitter between nausea and indigestion and faintness and wondering if that weird feeling is hunger.

This baby is a kicker. I try to imagine what else it will be like when it comes out. Still trying to get past the thoughts of labour itself, and wondering how on earth I can get all my work finished before Chelsea arrives.

Geoff finally cleans up his office but leaves all his footie trophies on the mantelpiece. There is a rather tension-ridden scene with me trying to be diplomatic ('How would you feel if we put your trophies in the lounge?') and Geoff looking grumpy. Perhaps it is some deep-seated male displacement thing going on. Poor Geoff. He gets his own back by doing a load of new baby things in the wash (to make sure there are no manufacturing chemicals left on them) and waving a very tiny sock at me, which he knows perfectly well will reduce me to tears.

A tree in the back garden drops a big branch. A tree 'surgeon' (why not 'barber'?) comes and describes it jauntily as 'self-lopping', so of course now we have to cut down a perfectly charming chestnut tree full of birds and expose ourselves to the scrutiny of approximately 90 flats in the block behind because we don't want it self-lopping onto the baby. And that will be £200, thanks. Honestly, sometimes you don't know where the next bill is coming from.

Aunt Julie is now worried about dust in the baby's room.

'It's thoroughly dusted and vacuumed once a week', I reassure her. Well, that's a lie.

You don't so much reassure her as send her fleeing to another fixation.

'There'll still be dust in there', she warns ominously, as if the dust were somehow radioactive.

Then when I say I am looking for a wool rug to wrap the baby in when it's cold, she starts in about that.

'I don't understand', she says, muttering about heat stroke and meningitis and the fall of civilisation as we know it. 'Nobody I know wraps a baby in a wool rug. They might throw one onto the pram, but it's not for wrapping up.'

'Yes, okay', I finally say. 'I'll just throw it on the pram then.'

Oops. Just remembered we don't have a pram. Must ring Luke and Fatimah to claim theirs.

Buy some extra-large pyjamas to take to the hospital. Start to pack hospital bag. The top of the pyjamas doesn't even look like it will fit me now, and as they were mail order I didn't realise they were going to say 'Brand New Mum' on the pocket. How ostentatious. And I think that will be fairly obvious without anyone having to read my pyjama pocket. Especially because the bloke who designed the Brand New Mum's pyjamas didn't leave enough room for a not-yet-deflated tummy. You'd think someone in the fashion industry would know better … I must have totally lost my marbles: I could have got one of the seamstresses at work to run up a giant T-shirt in four minutes flat.

This gum nodule thing just above my front teeth seems to be getting worse. It bleeds profusely every time I brush my teeth and is clearly visible as a kind of bulge between two teeth. I have started to spit blood like a prize fighter. The only book that mentions it is *What to Expect When You're Expecting*, which says it's called a pyogenic granuloma or, in the usual deeply reassuring doctor language, a 'pregnancy tumour', which is actually completely harmless and will go away right after the baby's born. Which is not what my dentist says.

My dentist says (after inquiring whether the baby's father is my boyfriend or my husband, a question obviously essential to dental hygiene): 'It won't go away. I can just slice it off. It will bleed for an hour or so and then be all right.'

Call me crazy, but I'm going to wait and see.*

Everyone is saying how beautiful Suze's baby is. I am starting to feel a bit paranoid that our baby will have a head like a robber's dog and there will just be polite silences on the subject.

*The book was right. It went away.

I have been thinking about the birth plan and I've decided that I don't want the baby to come out the vagina, and I don't want a caesarean. I may have to do some more research. Perhaps it can come out of an elbow.

My pants have started curling down my tummy like a roller blind.

I'm too busy to have a child.

Walk to work and get completely exhausted. Business lunch follows. Try to be sparkling and feel like I'm mentally swimming in custard.

Miss my appointment with the midwife as the clinic's running horribly behind schedule, and I can't face the waiting room banked up with trillions of tired women so I wag.

I am SO huge out the front that close friends can't help just patting and rubbing my tummy – like I'm a Buddha – for luck. I don't mind. People have started to ask 'How long to go?' and 'Are you excited?' (some kind of code word for 'utterly terrified', perhaps).

The last childbirth class: by this stage all the people in the class who were going to loosen up have loosened up. Only two couples haven't lost their quiet, stunned-mullet approach to everything. One woman keeps looking at her partner as if he's a ghastly apparition and she's suddenly realised she's tied to him for the rest of her life.

The picture I'll take with me is of women bulging in the middle, with their hands crossed over their bulge and their male partner leaning towards them. The woman who wanted her birth on the internet, and her husband, the filthy show-offs, arrive halfway through the class, with their baby! It came two weeks early, on the weekend, and they're still high. Melissa confides that she doesn't let parents come if they've hit the 'baby blues' stage. You don't want a brand-new mother sobbing and falling about a class, I suppose.

Melissa shows us two videos of couples with new babies. The men all work away from home and the women at home. The couples talk about lack of privacy and personal space, their relationship as a couple, tiredness, guilt, coping with a distressed and needy baby (the gist seems to be that 'this too shall pass'). And there's footage of a woman with twins: she looks a bit like someone has hit her on the back of the head with a rubber cricket bat. You would, wouldn't you?

Melissa talks about having an unsettled baby. New ones sleep 16 hours a day, but after a few weeks or months they can cry for a few hours a day no matter how well fed and clean and cuddled they are. This is often in the early evening and is known as 'arsenic hour'.

We gallop through some different things to settle the baby, how not to expect much from your sex life until at least after the six-week check-up (one man mishears and shouts 'Six years?!'), contraception (twelve condoms at once, thank you), services available if you get into trouble with feeding, sleeping or crying, and baby safety.

Revelation: one woman in the class asks 'Shouldn't you have the baby checked out by a paediatrician before it goes home?'. Melissa says yes, this is routine with a hospital birth and you'll have a GP visit after a home birth. I haven't even thought of this. I guess the obstetrician is a mother specialist, not a baby specialist.

info

labour

The first contractions you have may be 'pre-labour' ones (sometimes called 'false contractions' or 'Braxton Hicks contractions'), rather than the earliest ones of labour. These are quite bearable – more uncomfortable than painful – and irregular, and go away if you move around, lie down or have a bath.

And when labour does start – and you're in the early, 'latent' phase (during which your cervix will dilate three centimetres) – you might or might not notice, and the Real Thing might still be up to a few days or even weeks away.

early signs and symptoms
Signs and symptoms that you may be in early labour are:

⊚ uterus cramps, like period pains, that may be accompanied by diarrhoea (frequent, loose poos)

⊚ increasing pain, aches or feeling of pressure in the lower back

⊚ unusual or persistent achiness or feeling of pressure in the pelvic floor, thighs or groin

⑥ the 'show' – a watery or pinkish or brownish discharge, possibly preceded by the passage of the thick mucus plug (euwwwwww!) that has been blocking your cervix (you may not see it as it could go down the loo without you noticing as you wipe yourself)

⑥ a trickle or a sudden gush of fluid from your vagina (your 'waters breaking'), which means the amniotic sac has ruptured and some amniotic fluid is rushing or trickling out.

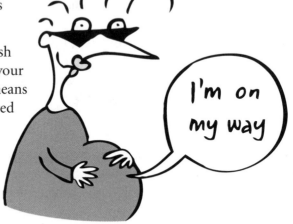

I'm on my way

STAGES OF LABOUR

A 'textbook' labour *for a first-timer* goes something like this:

first stage, latent phase – the cervix dilates to 3 centimetres (over hours, days or even weeks)

first stage, active phase – the cervix dilates from 3 centimetres to 7 centimetres (3–8 hours)

first stage, transition phase – the cervix dilates to 10 centimetres (can be up to 3 hours)

second stage – pushing, then the baby is born (average 1 hour but can be several hours)

third stage – the placenta and any other bits no longer needed are expelled (about 5–10 minutes after the birth if oxytocin is given, up to an hour if delivered naturally).

Gosh, that sounds neat. In reality your experience might be radically different. If you've done it before, it can be a lot quicker.

when to go to hospital

It's often difficult to tell the difference between pre-labour and the latent phase of the first stage of labour so don't hesitate to telephone your midwife, the hospital or birth centre or your obstetrician to describe what's happening and to find out whether to stay at home or go straight to the hospital or centre.

Call your hospital midwife or obstetrician (or your hospital if you can't get onto them) immediately if:

◎ there's a gush or trickle of amniotic fluid from your vagina

◎ you notice a green or dark stain in the amniotic fluid; this is meconium – the baby's first poo – which can be a sign of fetal distress

◎ you have bright red bleeding, which may indicate a problem with the placenta (clearish pink is probably just the 'show', but mention it anyway)

◎ you notice a significant drop in the number or strength of movements made by the baby

◎ you feel or see the umbilical cord in your vagina, which is called cord prolapse. This is an emergency. Ring an ambulance, open the door, then kneel down with your bottom in the air and head and shoulders down to take pressure off the cord until the ambulance arrives. (If you can, get someone else to make the call and open the door.)

Contractions When these start in earnest (see 'First Stage' for the details), they will usually:

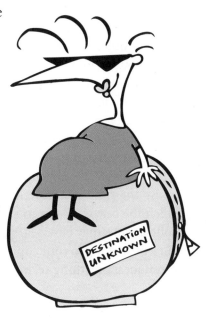

◎ be regular

◎ get stronger

◎ last for longer

◎ come closer together

◎ be increasingly tough to cope with.

Time the length and frequency of your contractions and give this information to your midwife or obstetrician, or the hospital or birth centre. They will advise you when to come in.

After you arrive   When you arrive at the hospital or birth centre (or when the midwives arrive for your home birth), you'll have a medical examination, which will probably involve:

⑥ checking your blood pressure

⑥ checking a urine sample

⑥ checking your temperature and pulse

⑥ feeling up your vagina to see how dilated your cervix is

⑥ checking the baby's heartbeat with either a handheld doppler (an ultrasound device) or a pinard (midwife's stethoscope). If a midwife or doctor wants continuous monitoring, they'll put a belt around your tummy that's connected by wires to a machine that makes a graph of the heartbeat and a recording of your contractions.

Make sure the midwife makes a note of your relevant health details or special needs.

Ideally things will now proceed according to your birth plan. But any unpredictable turns will have to be dealt with as they arise.

first stage

As mentioned, for some people the latent phase of first-stage labour – the first three centimetres of dilation – is barely perceptible. Others experience intense backache and painful contractions. For some it happens quietly over a long time; for others it may all happen in just a couple of hours. Contractions may last 30–60 seconds, and could be regular or irregular – anywhere from 5 to 20 minutes apart. You'll probably be at home and may even be able to sleep through some of this phase. Rest as much as possible and have some of the light snacks (or ice lollies) you have ready in the freezer. It can help to have warm baths, though you should keep timing your contractions.

All the following advice may fly out of your head, so get your birth support person to read it well before you might need it so that they can remind you.

By the time you're well into the active phase of the first stage, during which the cervix dilates to seven centimetres, you'll probably be in hospital. Contractions may be 45–60 seconds or longer, with 2–4 minutes between, and you'll be looking to your coping strategies: massage, TENS machine, relaxation techniques, breathing techniques. Not to mention drugs. Remember to wee frequently: the area is feeling such intense sensations from labour that you mightn't notice you need to wee. Stay as mobile and upright as possible. Try out different labouring positions for greatest comfort. Stay hydrated, taking ice chips, juice cubes or sips of water.

Try to rest completely and relax between contractions, and not expend energy anticipating the next one. Use positive visualisation and psyching techniques, such as concentrating on a mental picture of a flower opening; focus on the positive goal of seeing your baby; chant 'This will end' – anything that helps. Clenching everything up can hinder the progress of labour, so with your partner or labour support person's help use whatever it takes to go with the flow. If you can't stand the pain, or if this phase has gone on for a long time and you've had it, feel free to yell 'DRUGS!' around about now.

first stage transition

This phase, during which the cervix dilates to 10 centimetres, is generally considered to be the most challenging time of labour. Contractions are strong and getting stronger, lasting longer – up to 90 seconds – and coming at shorter intervals. Sometimes there's no time to rest between them, and you're probably exhausted. You may feel hot or shivering and cold, or alternate between temperature extremes. You may be nauseated or vomiting, and feeling overwhelmed or unable to cope. You may feel totally pissed off.

At the end of this phase your cervix will be fully dilated, and you'll be ready to start pushing. If you've hung in there without drugs, your support person can remind you that you are nearly there, that you'll have your baby very soon, and you can hit your support person. If you have the urge to push during this phase, before the cervix is fully dilated, you may be advised to blow or pant instead.

second stage: pushing and birth

About a third of labouring women have a resting phase at this point before their body starts urging them to push the baby out. The idea during this stage is to listen to your body when it comes to pushing. Contractions will still be 60–90 seconds long, but may be further apart (2–5 minutes), so you can rest between them. No need to pop the capillaries in your eyeballs or hold your breath beyond the point of comfort or turn purple. Using shorter moments of bearing down with each contraction is less stressful to the baby, and makes it easier for the pelvic floor to relax, than one big, breath-holding push, like the ones you see in the movies.

This more relaxed approach may make the second stage a bit longer than if you use the push approach, but is probably less stressful for you as well as the baby. During this phase you might be making some deep guttural grunts and moans, which many other pregnancy books seem to think will embarrass you. You'll be far too busy to be embarrassed. You might also push out a poo during this phase. No big deal.

All being well, babies are not oxygen-deprived during the birth journey; they're still getting oxygen from the placenta.

Actual, honest-to-goodness birth   There's more panting as the baby's head crowns and pushes against the perineum. You'll be asked to try not to push but instead to relax the pelvic floor, aiming to slow down the last bit to avoid tearing or the need for an episiotomy. You may be offered a bird's-eye view of proceedings with the help of a mirror: this is a fascinating prospect for some, and horrifying for others. You choose.

Mums often describe the sensation of the baby's head emerging as stinging, burning or intense pressure. A midwife may 'support' the perineum and anus (apply pressure from the outside to counter the bulging). This can help make it less painful. After the head emerges, the baby rotates so that its shoulders line up with the widest part of your pelvis and the little body slithers out. Hello there! Finally meeting and holding your baby is an indescribably awe-inspiring, emotional and happy time. (Or not, of which more later.)

third stage: the placenta and membranes expelled

You may be so engrossed in your new baby, you don't notice the third stage. The uterus continues to contract, causing the placenta to come away from the wall, taking with it what's left of the amniotic sac as it detaches; further contractions will push the placenta into the vagina, from where it can be pulled out, or pushed out with another contraction. The contraction of the muscles of your truly amazing uterus also seals off the blood vessels at the site of detachment. The placenta comes out more quickly if an injection of oxytocin is given to speed up contractions.

If the placenta doesn't come out 'by itself', the doctor will need to put their hand (and, frankly, a bit of their arm) inside your vagina to ease the placenta away from the wall of your uterus. This is not as startling as it sounds because by this stage there will already have been 'traffic in the area' and you'll probably be quite blasé about some smaller traffic temporarily going in the opposite direction. Also, it won't hurt a bit, as you'll be popped into a sterile operating theatre and have a spinal injection for anaesthetic (unless you've already had an epidural which will do the same job). Afterwards, some drugs will help the womb contract to stop any bleeding, and some antibiotics will prevent infection.

The placenta is inspected to make sure it has been delivered whole. You'll be checked to make sure you don't have post-partum haemorrhage ('post-partum' means after delivery). It's diagnosed when the blood loss is 500 millilitres or more; the usual loss is less than 300 millilitres. It happens to about 5 percent of mothers.

The 'fourth stage', hardly ever mentioned in the textbooks, is champagne – I mean getting acquainted with your baby, enjoying skin-to-skin contact and keeping them warm; the baby having a red-hot go and first drink at your breasts (the midwife will help you position bub's mouth for the best attachment), and getting the standard reflex and observation tests done by a doctor or midwife; clamping of the umbilical cord; and any stitches that are needed.

YOU MAY NEED BIGGER SHOES

WEEK 35

what's going on

That baby is taking up stomach space – smaller meals more often are easier to digest. You're probably finding it hard to get your shoes on and off. Wear slip-on shoes unless you need the ankle support of lace-ups. You've probably gone up a shoe size as well, especially in width, maybe permanently. Try to walk a bit every day until the baby arrives. To reduce the swelling in your feet and ankles, stand on your head a lot. Or at the very least sit down or, preferably, lie down and put your feet above the level of your heart as much as possible. (This can be especially effective in getting yourself extra room on public transport, particularly if you shout obscenities as well.)

Toenails are in. The fingernails may be poking over the end of the fingers. Your baby would fail that test they do at the start of netball games, and can scratch itself. Weight: about 2.5 kilos.

Average approximate baby length this week from head to bum

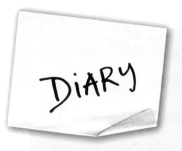

Help, it's going too fast. I'm not ready but I'm sick of being pregnant. Rosie, who does the accounts at work, says she lost 15 kilos at the birth, including the weight of the baby, and I must say THAT'S an attractive proposition. I'm wondering how long my legs will carry me. I weigh myself at a pharmacy and it says I've put on seven kilos in five days. God, I hope those scales are faulty.

Before I leave the pharmacy the assistant thrusts into my hands the chemist's special show bag to encourage me to come back and buy baby stuff there. You get your nursing pads (colostrum-and-milk-soaker-upperers), five nappy liners (whatever *they* are), twelve thick baby wipes, a disposable nappy, a sample of cocoa-butter moisturiser, a pamphlet on same, a booklet about safety, and a copy of *Practical Parenting* magazine with the cover line 'I gave birth in a petrol station!', which I don't think has enough exclamation marks, and what's practical about giving birth in a garage I'd like to know.

I take an inventory of stretch marks. Several red-purple stripes on the underside of each breast, and on each hip a bunch of marks that looks as if a hand held me too hard on each fleshy part. Nothing on the tummy itself, which has stretched more than anything. What gives? Me.

Yet another visit to the midwife for the fluid-retention check.

Jill measures the height of the baby, gives it a feel and says 'Oh God.'

First 'My, it's a whopper' and now 'Oh God'. If this goes on she'll be singing 'Oh What a Beauty! Never Seen One as Big as That Befooooore!' on my next visit. For some reason I feel resigned rather than horrified. I suspect her tactic is to soften me up and get me used to the idea of a boombah bambino.

I show her the birth plan and she reacts to each point.

Will you induce at the due date? (No. We let you go ten, even fourteen, days over.)

Ideally I would like to avoid either a vaginal birth or a caesarean. However, there do not seem to be many other options. (Ha ha. By hook or by crook the baby will come out.)

Do I have to have a Brazilian? (Only if his name is Juan.)

The labour will be attended by my independent midwife, Miss Beck, who will probably prescribe herbs and supplements after the birth. (Fine, but she can't direct what happens at the labour.)

I would like to be kept informed of what's happening. (Yep.)

I would like to avoid monitoring that might 'tether' me to the bed, and an epidural, if possible. Geoff is particularly concerned about the possible side effects of an epidural, but understands it might not be avoidable. Anyway it's my decision. (It certainly is but epidurals are much better these days, with fewer side effects.)

I would like to avoid an episiotomy, but would rather be cut than tear if necessary. (Although sometimes an episiotomy is unavoidable, we will try to avoid it. Actually it's better to tear naturally unless it looks like you're going to tear down to the bowel or up to the clitoris, or shatter the whole area, which is hard to repair.) (Me: That's enough. Fine. Shut up. That's quite enough chat about torn clitorises for one day.)

My Major Fears, in order, are:

1   possible neurological damage from an epidural (I read about it on a natural childbirth website) (About the same chance as getting hit by a jumbo jet, unless you already have a history of trouble, such as multiple sclerosis. A lot of so-called info warning against epidurals is based on older versions of the drugs that we don't use these days.)

2   episiotomy (We'll try hard not to. If you need it, you need it, but that'd probably only be if for some reason your baby really had to come in a rush.)

But generally we agree: whatever it takes to get a healthy baby out with the least amount of damage possible all round.

While we're talking I pop on the scales. At least these ones say I'm three kilos lighter than the chemist's did. I remark that it doesn't seem to be within the laws of physics, but I appear to have put on another four kilos. This means I have put on 20 kilos!!! I'm not eating crap – in fact I'm not eating a lot at all. It's spooky.

Jill says don't worry, I'll probably put on another five kilos before I give birth. I am absolutely flabbergasted.

'It's not humanly possible', I say.

'Don't forget,' she says, 'you can lose 12 kilos just at the birth, and all the fluid over the next couple of days. Of course you can actually puff up after the birth as well. You'll lose it. It's easier to lose the weight that's not junk food.'

I don't tell her I have at least three Magnums a week.

Suze has given me a book called *The New Age Baby Name Book* by Susan Browder. Could its names be worse than some of the suggestions from friends so far, including Hezekiah, Ringo or Bluey if it's a boy? And if it's a girl, geographical names such as Brittany, Devon and what's next, Grand Canyon? How about fabric names such as Chiffon, Polly Esther and Tencel?

There's some very good advice in the book, which you would already know unless you were completely brain dead, such as: if you have twin boys don't call them Pete and Repeat because the joke will wear off. It mentions a man in America who became a circus clown (natch) whose real name was Oofty Goofty Bowman. Geoff and I are thrilled and immediately rename Chelsea Oofty Goofty.

The book says American names that have fallen out of favour include Minnehaha, Amorous, Ham, Lettuce and Bugless. It also translates some names from their original Celtic meanings. Calvin Klein, for instance, means 'young, small, bald man'.

According to *The New Age Baby Name Book*, in some cultures they name kids for what time of the day or night they arrive. Luckily this has not caught on here, where not many children are called Cracko-Dawn or Half Past Three. Or you could use the Ghanaian language to name the child after the day of the week it was born on. Young Wednesday from the Addams family would have been called Ekua.

But the handiest idea of them all is just to combine the names of the parents. For example, if your names are Malcolm and Trisha, you can call the kid Militia. Or, say, if your names are Louise and Arnie, you can call it Loonie. It's easy. Paul and May Ling? – Appalling. Bathsheba and Matthew? – Bath-mat. Geoff and Kaz – Jazz?

I have learnt that we should only ever try out our suggested names on a few friends. There'll always be someone who doesn't like the name you choose because there was a girl at their nursery called that who used to put glue in their hair. Or it was the name of the first man who dumped them. Best to just hit them with a fait accompli after the kid's born, and they'll have to put on a brave face and get used to it.

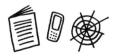

more info on baby names

The New Age Baby Name Book by Susan Browder, Workman, US, 1998

An unintentionally hilarious, American list of absolutely insanely stupid names you could give your child, as well as some definite possibilities. Good for names from different cultures. It ranges from Agnes to Zaim, meaning 'brigadier-general' in Arabic.

Naming Your Baby by Julia Cresswell, A&C Black, UK, 2007

I checked whether it has Bluey and it has Blue. Must be pretty comprehensive.

babynamewizard.com

Endless hours could be spent idling your way around here. Choose NameVoyager to see a graph of how popular a name has been (in the US) over the past 100 years. (There's no sign of any Algernons and the era of Earnests is well and truly over. Gwendolyn is gaining popularity.) Click on NameFinder to search for various criteria (must start with...) and remember to check whether a chosen name will create a problem when teamed with the last name (such as Ida Down).

info

caesarean delivery

A caesarean section operation is a surgical procedure to take the baby out of the uterus through your abdomen. It's usually called just 'a caesarean', 'a c-section' or 'a caesar'. A standard caesarean is considered to be a very safe procedure when performed by a specialist in a good hospital.

how common is a caesarean?

In the UK around a quarter of deliveries is now by caesarean, which is putting strain on the hospital system. This ratio is partly because doctors these days are much better at identifying potential problems, and choose caesareans to reduce risks to babies and mothers. It's also because in general women are older when they have their babies and statistically more likely to have complications. Read up on it because it might happen to you, even if you've had a 'perfect' pregnancy.

why would you need one?

A caesarean can be elective: you 'elect' to have one on the advice of your obstetrician and midwife and make a hospital appointment. Or it can be emergency surgery performed unexpectedly and suddenly when a problem develops during labour. If you want to avoid having a caesarean, talk to your midwife or obstetrician, but remember that there's never a guarantee you won't have one.

The basic criterion for a caesarean is whether it will be less of a risk to the mother and baby than a vaginal birth. Some reasons why you might end up needing a caesarean are:

⑥ you have a medical condition such as pre-eclampsia or eclampsia (see Week 28)

⑥ you have diabetes and must deliver early, but the cervix isn't ready

⑥ you have active genital herpes (the baby may catch the herpes from sores as it comes through the vagina, although you can take drugs earlier in pregnancy that should prevent an outbreak)

⑥ the baby is sick or isn't growing properly

⑥ the baby is in an awkward position – perhaps sideways, which is known as the 'transverse lie', or bum not head down, which is called the 'breech position' (very, very few obstetricians will agree to try first to deliver a breech baby in the normal way)

⑥ the baby's head seems to be too big to fit through its mum's pelvis; this is technically called cephalo-pelvic disproportion (CPD)

⑥ placenta praevia (the placenta is positioned over the cervix – see Week 19)

⑥ placental abruption (the placenta comes away too early – see Week 29)

⑥ an overdue baby in a deteriorating uterine environment

⑥ the umbilical cord is 'prolapsed' – coming down into the vagina, possibly cutting off the baby's circulation if the baby's head is against the cervix

⑥ the baby's lowered or erratic heartbeat during labour indicates it is distressed or in danger

⑥ 'failure to progress' during labour, which basically means nothing is happening.

what happens?

During a standard caesarean, you may have the top half of your pubic hair trimmed or shaved, and then you'll be put on a hospital trolley and wheeled off to the operating room. In this very brightly lit room all the medical staff will wear shower caps, face masks and protective smocks, and so will your support person. An intravenous (IV) drip will be put into your arm, then you'll be given an epidural injection – or a spinal-block injection (or a combination of both) – by the anaesthetist (both procedures are explained in 'Pain-relief Options During Labour' in Week 32) to numb the lower half of your body. As well as numbing all sensation in the abdomen, an epidural or a spinal block for a caesarean may also affect the nerves in the legs, making them feel very heavy, and nerves in the bladder (so you'll probably have a catheter inserted in your bladder because you won't know when you're weeing).

A screen will be put up between you and your tummy, but a mirror can be angled for you to watch the operation if you're that way inclined. A nurse or doctor will swab the lower part of your tummy with antiseptic. Your obstetrician will make an incision just above your pubic hairline, usually horizontal and about 10 centimetres long. Then the obstetrician will cut through layers of fat and muscle to the uterus wall, cut open the uterus and pull the baby out. You may have some sensation of pulling or pressure. There's a *slim* chance with an epidural that you'll still feel pain. If the incision, or anything else done to you, hurts say so loudly and quickly. Your surgical team will have extra anaesthetic ready to give you.

It all happens very quickly: the baby is generally born five to ten minutes after the first incision. The baby will be shown to you and then will be fully examined by a paediatrician or midwife standing by in the room. (The baby might also have mucus sucked from its tiny airways.) If the baby doesn't need to be taken away for special care, insist on a long cuddle and first breastfeed straight away. Measuring or baths are not important enough reasons to separate you and your baby at this crucial time, but many hospitals take babies away to suit their policy not you.

You might be too preoccupied to notice what happens next, but usually you'll hear some gurgling, slurping noises when the amniotic fluid is suctioned out. The placenta and membranes, and the swabs, are removed, then you are stitched up. This can take quite a while because it's not just one row of stitches, it's seven different wounds to be sewn, including layers of skin, fat, muscle and the inner and outer walls of the uterus.

recovery from the surgery

Probably the first thing you'll notice when you're in the recovery room or back in your own hospital room is that you're still hooked up to the drip and doing wee into a bag through a tube, which will continue for up to a day. There will be a very nice drug coming through the drip, probably morphine or pethidine. You might be hungry, but you won't be allowed to eat or drink anything until your bowel shows signs of post-operative activity (okay, farting), at which time your drip can be removed.

Over several days your pain relief is likely to be reduced in strength. Don't skimp on relief, and ask the nurses or midwives for it if they miss your due time or you are in pain. It's important not to be in pain whenever possible.

THE CAESAREAN DEBATE

Are women having unnecessary caesareans? Natural childbirth activists say that women are being scared into unnecessary caesareans, often for the convenience of doctors. Doctors and midwives say they want to avoid the risk of a baby getting stuck or for any other reason being deprived of oxygen, which means the baby could die or be brain damaged. In some cases that risk might be only 1 percent. Perhaps, or even probably, the baby would have been fine without intervention. But most women would take a look at the odds of their baby being that one in 100 who ends up damaged and say 'I'll take the caesarean, just in case.'

That means there will be some 'unnecessary' caesareans. And some of us will never know whether our emergency caesarean was unnecessary or as necessary as hell. Being 'over-medicalised' is the price some of us pay to be as sure as we can be that we've taken the safest route to get the baby out.

Elective caesareans   A caesarean is not an 'easy option'. Women who have a caesarean stay in hospital longer and need more resources. It is not 'less messy': we don't have a zip down there. It's major surgery. It has a far higher risk of infection and complications, and women who have caesareans usually take longer to recover from the physical and emotional aftermath of birth than those who have a normal vaginal birth. Because recovery is similar to that from major abdominal surgery or a car accident, it's not a good choice unless there's a medical reason for it.

Women do not have zips

Some women say they want an elective caesarean so they can be 'honeymoon fresh' – a somewhat ludicrous euphemism for keeping a tight vagina. This is more a psychological worry than a real physical issue. A vagina is very rarely noticeably changed after a vaginal birth. It goes back to about the same size it was before. As one doctor so sweetly put it, 'It's a very forgiving area.'

An elective caesarean could cause unnecessary trauma for a baby who would have been happier coming out naturally. Babies tend to get their lungs working during the process of birth. A caesarean means they're more likely to have breathing difficulties when they come out, and have more trouble getting their sucking reflex to work for breastfeeding. Caesareans can result in complications that cause trouble in future pregnancies. Most obstetricians will only perform them for medical reasons.

Vaginal birth after caesarean section (VBAC)   Some websites and women advocate that a woman who's had a caesarean should have a vaginal birth for her next baby. They're cross that too many women are told 'once a caesarean always a caesarean'. In fact, many women who've had a caesarean can try for a vaginal birth next time. Your birth team will have to make an assessment of your individual needs, based on what happened previously, the placement of the incision last time and what happens during the next labour.

If you have a natural therapist, see or call them about any vitamins and minerals that may help recovery. Make sure they're approved for breastfeeding and by your doctor.

Get up and move as soon as possible. Immediately you can feel your legs again, start flexing and rotating your feet, and doing leg bends in bed. Get out of bed and go for a walk as soon as you're allowed to. It won't be a brisk hike, mind you. It'll be more of a small shuffle round the bed. Soon you'll be going down the corridor and back. Make sure someone goes with you because you'll be a bit woozy.

Early mobility will help you to avoid complications such as pain from gas, difficulty weeing and blood clots in the legs. (You may be given anti-clotting injections once a day for three days.) And it's amazing how quickly you start to feel better once you are mobile. But DON'T OVERDO IT. Do only half as much as you feel you can, even if you're sure you can walk around the whole block on day four. Discipline yourself to increase the exercise a *little* bit each day, otherwise you'll get overtired and set back your recovery.

Laughing, coughing and sneezing in bed are less painful if you bend your knees and support your scar with a pillow. If you're standing up, bend over and put your hands over the scar. Avoid constipation, by drinking lots of water, as it will be painful. If it gets to dire proportions (four to five days without a poo) your doctor can prescribe an anal suppository.

Your tummy will look as if it's in the earlier stages of pregnancy for a while. It will be sore, but on the plus side there will be no stitches in your fanny and you can sit without pain.

Your hospital stay will be longer than for a vaginal delivery – up to a week, depending on hospital policy and how you feel. Don't be swayed by friends or staff: if you want to go earlier or stay longer, discuss it with your obstetrician and do the best thing for you, not for some bureaucrat's government policy guidelines on bed allocation based on funding cuts. After you go home, any sign of infection such as oozing or pus from the wound should of course be reported to your obstetrician.

Full recovery generally takes longer after a caesarean than after a vaginal delivery – it's about six weeks until everything is healed and several more weeks before you're up to full pre-pregnancy exercise capabilities. And of course it is harder to look after a baby and recover from major abdominal surgery at the same time. You will be very tired, and your body will be in shock for longer. Remember that recovering from a caesarean is comparable to convalescing after a serious injury: go easy on yourself.

The double burden of looking after a baby and recovering from surgery can lead to feelings of depression, and some women believe they are failures because they have not had a natural birth. Having a caesar, though, doesn't necessarily mean you'll have negative feelings about the birth – not least because the operation may have saved your life or the baby's.

You're usually told not to drive until your six-week check-up (mainly because it hurts to brake so you may brake more slowly than usual), although some doctors believe it is safe after about three weeks; if you do drive before six weeks, check with your insurance company that you are covered. You're also usually told not to reach above your head to get things down from shelves or do any similar activity, or lift anything heavier than your baby, before the six-week check-up. The rules for taking things easy still apply: only do half of the exercise you think you could do, and keep it gentle.

After a caesarean you'll usually need pain relief at home for up to two weeks. Ask your obstetrician what to take, and ignore any bossy hospital midwives who say you shouldn't need pain relief.

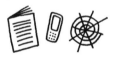

more info on **caesareans**

Many of the pregnancy websites listed in Week 1 have birth stories about natural births, caesareans and other variations.

caesarean.org.uk
> Run by the authors of the NCT book reviewed above, the Caesarean Birth and VBAC Information website includes answers to FAQs as well as more detailed articles on both medical and emotional issues. There are also book reviews, caesar birth stories, scar pictures and suggestions for compiling a caesar birth plan.

Caesarean Birth: Your Questions Answered by Debbie Chippington-Derrick, Gina Lowdon and Fiona Barlow, NCT Books, UK, 2005
> Good practical tips and sound advice based on a wealth of research evidence.

what's going on

You're tired. You've probably got sore feet, fluid retention causing swollen everything, and tingling fingers; and you could be breathless or dizzy. If you're really lucky you might even faint. You'll probably have antenatal check-ups once a fortnight from now on. You may get stabbing pelvic pains or aches – like a 'stitch' – which are probably the pelvic ligaments loosening up. The baby's head may be down low in the pelvis and can bounce up and down on your cervix giving you 'shocks', particularly if you sit down too quickly. This doesn't necessarily mean that the baby is 'engaged' (in position and ready to come out head first). You should begin to feel movements every day, even if it's only a little leg wave. Those new lungs are still not completely finished. The baby has put on lots of fat. If it hasn't turned upside down already, it may be about to. (If it's still the wrong way up by the time labour starts, you may have a breech birth – meaning bum first and hello caesarean.)

Weight: about 2.7 kilos.

EK 36

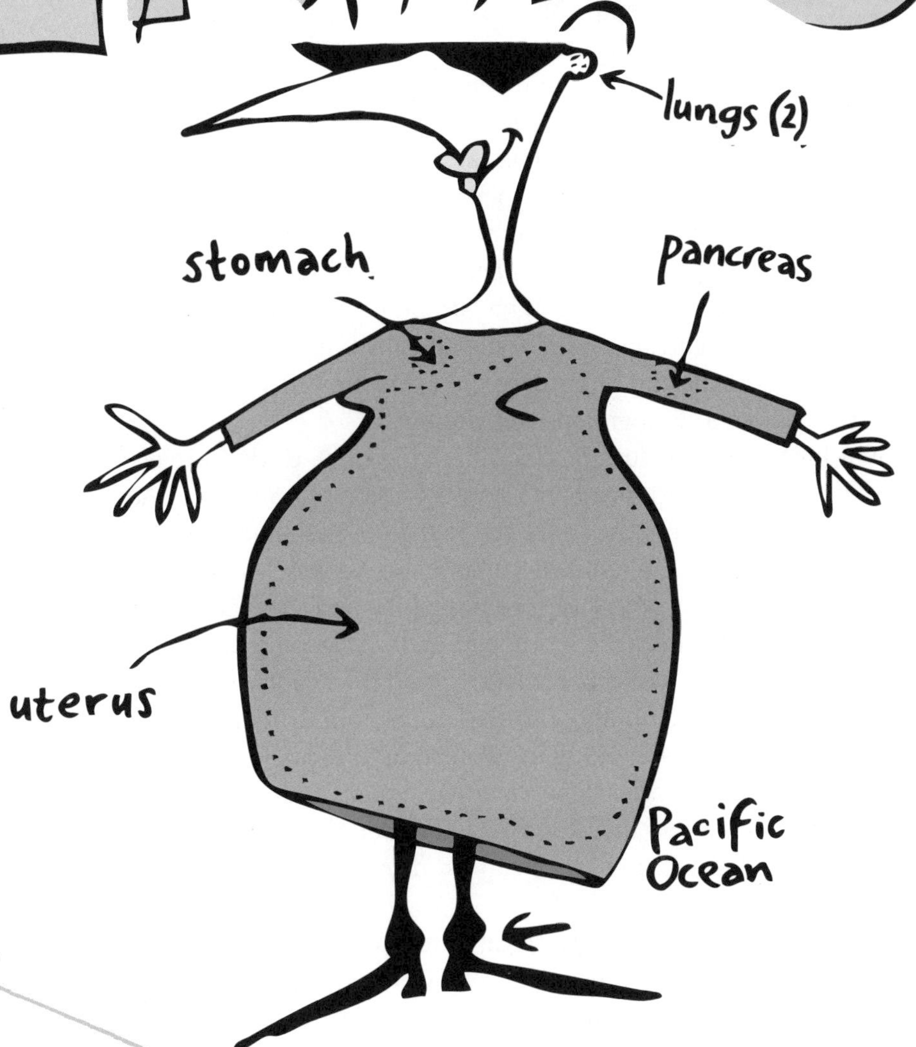

lungs (2)

stomach

pancreas

uterus

Pacific
Ocean

DIAGRAM OF KEY ORGANS
IN LATE PREGNANCY

Average approximate baby length this week from head to bum

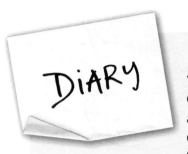
DiARY

Wish I had given up work. The boss wants me to fly to Glasgow for a business meeting. Fat chance. Ha. That would be a hollow laugh except that I feel anything but hollow. Instead of waddling, I now lurch from side to side like a drunken yeti.

On the way up to my hospital appointment (they still want to see me once a week because of my fluid retention), a woman in the lift tells me she had a one-hour labour and not to worry, it doesn't even hurt. I think she might have been at the pethidine cabinet. The obstetrician sees me with Claire and says I'm still 'carrying high' so it won't be soon, but I should read about caesareans just in case. 'I'd bet that you won't go early', Claire says. She reminds me I'll probably put on another five kilos.

The lumps that come and go in my armpit have nothing to do with deodorant, the obstetrician says. They're actually breast tissue getting over-excited about soon having to produce milk, and are called 'breast tails'. Which sounds like a stripper's speciality to me.

Aunt Julie is making cushions (don't ask me why). Uncle Mike is ringing up to see how I'm going. Just had a horrible vision of Aurelia and Aunt Julie meeting over the head of the new baby in the hospital. Must warn Uncle Mike to keep Aurelia away until we come home. Keeping Aunt Julie away would be possible only with a very cunning plan and some Semtex.

Finally surrendering to the inevitable: Geoff is sleeping on the sofa.

My old pal Simon Weaselpantz has scoured the country fêtes and sent the little nipper a knitted lamb and a knitted bunny rabbit. Thank heavens some people are keeping up the old skills. Women used to know how to do 'fancy work', showing-off sewing, crochet, knitting, tatting and heaven knows what else. Now they're lucky if they know how to order a caffè latte for themselves. Can't say I would like to go back to the old days, but nice to know somebody is keeping up appearances.

Jane is organising a nappy-wash cartel for me, and helping me compile a database for the birth announcements. We've got two versions ready to go, one that says Eddy and one that says Matilda. I think that's all the options covered. I've been thinking about the pros and cons of having a boy or a girl. Boy: won't be so bombarded with 'you're ugly' messages from advertising and film and TV. Girl: will probably find it easier to talk about emotions and be slightly less likely to play noisy war games on the roof.

Although, truth be told, it's impossible to really imagine what it will be like when this baby is OUT. The baby-being-IN thing and the getting-the-baby-out thing just take up so much brain space.

The worst part of being this pregnant, except for being uncomfortable and sort of nervous (could go any time from now), is that if you have someone to cuddle it's an exercise in geometry. It's impossible to get really close with a third person stuck way out there in the middle.

info

babies who arrive late

why do babies arrive late?

Your baby is not likely to arrive at precisely midnight on the 266th day of pregnancy. So if it isn't early, it's going to be late (duh). We don't know exactly what makes a woman's body go into labour, but it's now believed that the mum's brain somehow releases hormones or prostaglandins or a greeting card or something that doctors don't quite understand yet, when the baby is ready to be born. This unknown signal triggers the softening of the cervix, ready for it to dilate and let the baby through, and contractions of the uterus.

Only about 5 percent of babies are born exactly on their due date. Most are born within two weeks before or after the due date. Traditionally, babies of first pregnancies have been more likely to be 'overdue' than subsequent ones.

how long can you go?

You can go up to 42 weeks (14 days over the due date) with careful monitoring, although most obstetricians and midwives don't like to leave it that long. If you go beyond 14 days overdue the doctor will probably induce the birth as the placenta might start to deteriorate. Beyond 42 weeks of pregnancy, babies are at increased risk of 'fetal distress' during labour, inhaling their first poo and, as the placenta starts packing up, even dying. Some of the most common methods of checking that an overdue baby is okay are:

⊚ your obstetrician examines you to see whether the cervix is ripe – if it is not, it may be an indication that the baby is not ready to be born yet

⊚ the baby's reaction to sound or vibrations is tested

⊚ the baby's heart rate is electronically monitored

⊚ an ultrasound is done to help estimate the baby's size, the amount of amniotic fluid and whether the umbilical cord is still doing a good job.

induction methods

Membrane sweep   This is usually the first thing offered as a gentle way of increasing the chances of labour starting naturally. Membrane sweeping involves your midwife or doctor placing a finger just inside your cervix and making a circular, sweeping movement to separate the membranes from the cervix. It can be uncomfortable and may cause a small amount of bleeding, but it will not cause any harm to your baby and has been shown to reduce the need for other methods of induction.

Prostaglandin   Prostaglandins (which are like hormones) are found naturally in the uterus; some prostaglandins stimulate contractions at the beginning of labour. A synthetic prostaglandin gel or pessary (like a large pill) put on the cervix can ripen it and trigger labour. It usually takes a number of doses, sometimes spaced over more than one day, before labour starts, but it is one of the least intrusive and most effective methods of induction.

Artificial rupture of the membranes (amniotomy)   This won't be done if the baby's head isn't engaged in the ready position. An amnihook (a plastic hook sort of like a crochet one) is used to break the membranes of the amniotic sac. Often it is enough just to brush the hook against the membranes, but sometimes it will have to be inserted to make a small hole. It usually doesn't hurt at all. Once the membranes have been broken, labour usually follows quickly as the baby's head is no longer cushioned by amniotic fluid so descends, putting pressure on the ripe cervix and encouraging it to widen. Breaking the membranes also triggers the release of prostaglandins, which help to speed up the labour process.

Artificial rupture of the membranes is a very effective method of induction on its own if the cervix is ripe, and the contractions afterwards should be no more painful than normal. Amniotomy is often used during an otherwise normal labour to speed things up, and also if an electrode needs to be attached to your baby's scalp to monitor its heartbeat. It can also be used to check the colour of the amnio fluid. Dirty brown or green can mean the baby was stressed and did a poo – this can indicate it needs to come out quickly.

Oxytocin   A synthetic form of oxytocin (the hormone that causes the uterus to contract) is given through a drip to increase the strength and regularity of contractions. The membranes will always be ruptured as well. Contractions brought on by oxytocin are usually stronger, longer and more painful than normal, so pain-relief drugs are often used during labour.

Other methods

⊚ Acupuncture or acupressure (often as a course of treatments over a few days) – this must be performed by a trained specialist.

⊚ Mum's orgasm – this can get the contractions started.

⊚ Keeping moving – staying upright and moving will allow a little extra pressure to be exerted on your cervix by your baby's head, which may stimulate ripening, but remember not to overdo it.

⊚ Visualisation – some people believe that the power of suggestion can affect the body. If you're good at this sort of thing, try to relax and visualise the birth (leaving out any bits that make you anxious). Some women have found that watching films of babies being born triggers labour.

characteristic features of babies who arrive late
Late babies often look a bit different from those born on time.

⊚ They tend to have longer fingernails and more hair.

⊚ Although often skinnier, they keep growing in the uterus so they are larger all over than babies born earlier.

⊚ They are generally more alert than babies born earlier.

⊚ A longer time spent in the uterus may result in a greenish staining of the skin and umbilical cord by meconium: in very post-term babies these stains will be yellow.

⊚ They are sometimes described as looking 'overcooked' because during their extra time in the uterus they lose fat from all over their body, and their skin becomes red and wrinkly and may 'crack' as the waxy coating of vernix disappears. They don't need oils or moisturiser. The flaky skin will just fall off by itself and leave the lovely new skin underneath.

men: your instructions for the birth

Men (and lady partners): whether your partner gives birth naturally or ends up having a caesarean, you may feel useless. You're not. Here are your orders.

your duties before it starts

Set up a system so that after the birth you only have to ring one or two friends and relatives, and they will pass on the news to those who need to know. Right after the birth is the time to be bonding with your baby, not talking to other people on the phone.

Hospitals and birth centres can be very strict about the number of people allowed in during a birth, and they can alter this at the time depending on how busy they are and other circumstances. Even when the baby is born visitors may be restricted to one or two at a time. Your partner may change her mind on the spot about who she wants. Be the gatekeeper. If your partner wants you to keep certain relatives out of the labour ward or hospital, do that no matter what. Blame the hospital rules and get the nurses on side to back you up if necessary. Here's your chance to be caveman.

Keep a change of your own clothes and a shaving kit in your partner's hospital bag or in your car boot.

your duties during the birth

1   Do what the medical staff tell you. Your job is to co-operate with them to help ensure a healthy baby. Conflict and anger won't help if things don't go to plan.

2   Stay at your partner's head-end unless this conflicts with point 1.

3   Take breaks for food and fluids (NOT alcohol), and rest. This will make you less likely to faint.

4   Yes, there will be blood, whichever way she gives birth. If you think you might faint go outside and walk up and down a bit, bouncing on the balls of your feet to get the blood flowing to your head; or lie down on the floor in a corner so that you won't fall and take away some of the medical attention from the main event.

5   Let your hand be squeezed. Let your partner swear at you. Don't under any circumstances actually argue with a person in labour. Just keep saying reassuring things such as 'You're doing great', 'You're doing everything right', 'I'm so proud of you' and 'Everything's going the way it should be'.

6   Words you do not want to say, no matter what: 'Yuk', 'Euwww', 'I can't hack this' or 'That's gotta hurt'.

7   Don't ask if it hurts. Yes, it does hurt. It's not your job to stop the pain, just to support her.

8   Ask her before you take a photo.

9   Don't be amazed if a medical person puts their hand and part of their arm up your partner's vagina. They're not flirting, they're feeling which bits of the baby may be coming first, or rotating the baby's head and shoulders.

10 Yes, you can cry when the baby comes out.

your duties after the birth

You'll usually be asked if you want to cut the umbilical cord (they have special scissors – you don't have to bring secateurs). It's a pretty tough, ropey thing, so you won't feel like you're cutting a ribbon. If you reckon this will make you faint, say 'No thanks'.

Get somebody to take a photo of you, your partner and the baby as soon as it's possible. People often forget or just get mum and bub, or dad and bub.

Again, be guided by medical staff, but keep asking when you can hold the baby, especially if your partner can't because, say, she's having post-op procedures. Your job is to hold that baby as much as possible. Weighing and measuring shouldn't take long and rather than letting a staff member take the baby away for a while, hospital policy should allow you to be there.

You may fall in love with your baby straight away, or you may feel a bit freaked out by the sudden realisation that you've got to protect and nurture this little person. There's no 'right way' or 'wrong way' to feel. Be patient if your partner doesn't automatically bond or say lovey-dovey things to your baby. She's had a pretty shocking experience. Hormones, painkillers and exhaustion can all affect immediate thoughts and words.

Man up. Your partner may be feeling vulnerable. Expect hormonal tears, especially a few days after the birth when the 'happy hormones' all bugger off. Your manly, tough-but-gentle side is a good one to show now. You'll protect them, you'll look after them, she doesn't need to worry. You can do this, she can do this, you'll do it together, one day at a time. Don't tell her to pull herself together, or compare her skills to your mother's or sister's or anybody else's baby handling.

Your partner may be feeling guilt or a sense of failure if labour wasn't how she wanted it to be; for example, no drugs, minimum intervention, a natural labour. These feelings can lead to postnatal depression. If the birth was premature or difficult or your partner needed a caesarean, keep telling her what a fantastic job she did carrying that baby all those months and giving them everything they needed, and how you and she are now keeping them alive and giving them all the love and care they need. Keep encouraging her. Keep being supportive and saying that the important thing was doing what was needed to get the baby out with the least amount of risk: *that* is a successful birth.

Get in there and learn how to do stuff. Be a real partner in parenting. Don't let your partner shut you out or make you feel incompetent – you'll both be incompetent if it's your first time. She may just be a bit more scared to admit that, because she thinks she's supposed to have a 'mother's instincts'. Reassure her (and yourself) that this is a learning process.

Many people think it's good for the partner to give bottles of expressed milk to encourage the bonding with the baby and to let the mum sleep longer. Bath, burp or burble at your baby, but don't feel you have to have the experience of feeding the bub. In the early days especially it's better for the baby to stay with the breast, even if your partner has to wake up. Make up for not having bosoms in different ways and find other times to give the lady a lie-down.

Don't say you want to have sex straight away unless you want a shoe thrown at your head. Bank on at least six weeks without, and if it happens before then it's a bonus (see 'Post-baby Sex' in Week 43).

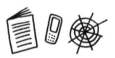

more info **for blokes**

Most of the pregnancy websites given in Week 1 have a couple of pages for men. The books for blokes often aren't much cop as 'how to' manuals for dads who are at home being the 'primary caregiver', but blokes can read the usual books and other stuff aimed at mums (see Week 43). After all, the problems and the advice are the same for all parents, regardless of gender. Here's some stuff specifically for blokes, most of it produced by dads.

dad.info

Linked to the Fatherhood Institute research and policy charity, this practical site provides loads of info on everything from expecting to parenting. Click on 'Email courses' to sign up for monthly emails during pregnancy and the early years. There's dad-friendly stuff about antenatal classes, birth plans, postnatal depression, money, divorced parenting, work, money and lifestyle, and links to useful services. Ask your midwife or birth centre to give you one of their credit-card-sized 'Dad Cards', which are packed with info and contacts, for your wallet.

greatdad.com

A huge US website for blokes expecting a baby, and for dads. Don't forget that its resources and medical advice are American.

busydadblog.com

The busy one has taken time to link to lots of other dad blogs.

Being Dad: Inspiration and Information for Dads to Be, DVD, AUUK Consultancy, 2009

Made by a private film company. View the trailer and buy a copy online at beingdad.co.uk.

A Dad's Guide to Babycare by Colin Cooper, Carroll and Brown, UK, 2008

Here's your go-to manual. With pictures! Of dads with babies! Hoorah. Practical stuff about feeding, holding, equipment and how to behave around a bub. Thoughtful stuff about seeing your partner in a new light.

Dad Rules: How My Children Taught Me to Be a Good Parent by Andrew Clover, Fig Tree, UK, 2008

Based on his observational columns in *The Sunday Times*, Mr Clover's book brings some realism, some surrealism and a story of trying to hog the gas in the delivery room.

Full Time Father: How to Succeed as a Stay-at-Home Dad by Richard Hallows, White Ladder Press, UK, 2004

Covers all the mental, emotional and practical considerations, including who has control of the finances, the negotiations with your partner, how to divide up the housework, and dealing with other people's perceptions and reactions.

what's going on Your bosoms may have developed a mind of their own and be leaking for no apparent reason or when a baby cries. (Any old baby will do.) The stuff is the colostrum, which will give your newborn baby protein and antibodies in the few days before your milk 'comes in'. The baby can't tumble around so much because it's run out of room, but the kicking and whacking can have a real force when they do happen. From here on in, try to be strict about getting as much rest and sleep as you can. Labour and recovery are much easier if you are well rested.

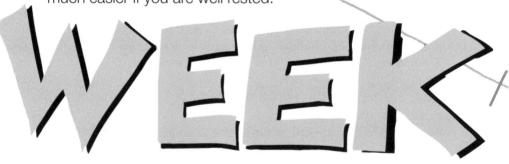

WEEK

The baby isn't doing much except putting on more weight. The tiny lungs are getting ready to work on their own. The baby has a firm hand grip and is swallowing about 750 millilitres of amniotic fluid a day. Weight: about 3 kilos.

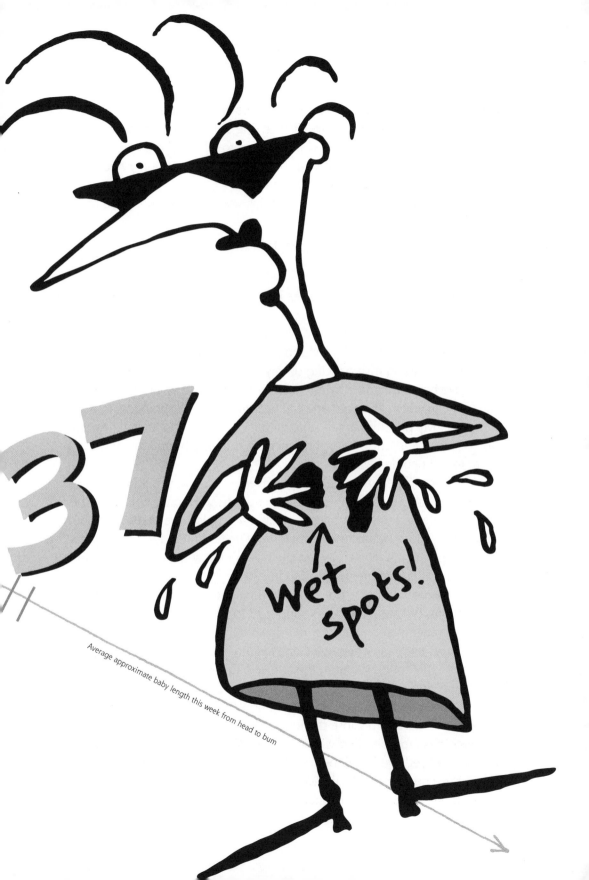

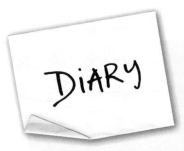

DiARy

Jill says 'Don't have the baby on Saturday.' She is going for her motorbike licence. She says her helmet is very black and racy. I say if I do go into labour she'll have to come, but she can wear her helmet. 'It's part of my mid-life crisis', she says cheerily.

It is a measure of Jill's serenity that this statement doesn't make me nervous in the slightest.

'Does your husband just laugh at you?' I ask.

'Yes he does, actually.'

I am not astonished.

Jill is still convinced that Chelsea won't come early, but on the due date or later.

'Is it engaged?' she asks.

How would I know? All I can report is that it appears to be wearing Doc Martens and doing Irish dancing on my cervix.

I have been overcome by an ineluctable torpor. In other words I lie on the sofa and watch *The Bold and the Beautiful*, and it is pointless to try doing otherwise. My priorities are all changing ('Stuff all of you at work! And the horse you rode in on!'), I am consumed by stupidity hormones, and can't seem to call people back.

I hear from Great-Aunt Zelda, the adventuress, now settled in Peru, who sends me a tiny card with twelve teensy buttons sewn onto it, each half the size of a little fingernail. 'A decent great-aunt would have made these buttons into a three-piece Lafayette or something. I've had them for twenty years', she writes. I am somehow pleased she doesn't know the difference between layette and Lafayette: neither do I.

I hit the wall and give up work. I had planned to work until the first contractions, but something has happened to my brain. I was working too hard for contemplation, and my mind was demanding space. So of course what always happens when you stop working? I get a cold.

I buy some lollies to put in the labour bag for energy and eat them all by three o'clock. I have written down the phone numbers of the hospital and Geoff's work and Beck's mobile, but if I don't pin them to the inside of my underpants I'll probably lose the lot.

Beck asks am I bonding with the baby? 'As much as I can with someone I haven't met yet', I think. Other mums have warned me a fog of ambivalence might descend after the birth. We'll see.

Nausea. Walks not. Horizontal. No verbs in sentences.

info

your newborn baby

Newborn babies can look pretty weird. Yours might have the following:

⑥ blood and creamy vernix all over them (premature babies have more vernix, late babies may have hardly any)

⑥ puffy, bruised or squinty-looking eyes

⑥ an unfocused, sometimes cross-eyed gaze; at this early stage a newborn can only focus on something very close, like a nipple in front of its face

⑥ a puffy face

⑥ a head that looks elongated or cone-shaped because it's been squeezed through the pelvis and vagina – this will normalise, often within hours, although it can take up to a couple of weeks (the bones have spaces between them called fontanelles so that they can squish up during childbirth; these harden within a few months and become one thick skull)

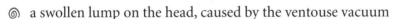

⑥ a swollen lump on the head, caused by the ventouse vacuum

⑥ temporary indentations on the face or head or a pointy-headed look from forceps

⑥ lanugo on the body – this downy hair is often on the shoulders, the back, and the face around the hairline (with more if the baby is premature); it usually rubs off within a few weeks

⑥ small white spots on the face called milia, which are caused by temporary blockages of the sebaceous glands

⑥ red blotches (often called 'stork marks' because they look as if a stork has held the baby in its bill (yeah, right)) on the back of the neck at the base of the skull, on the forehead and/or on the eyelids, which are caused by little veins close to the skin – they will disappear after a year or so and only reappear with heat and stress

⑥ 'Mongolian spots' – bluish-grey patches on the back, the buttocks and sometimes the arms and thighs, which are more common in Asian and darker-skinned babies; the spots will fade away

⑥ other birthmarks (see a paediatrician if you're concerned)

⑥ big, swollen baby genitals and breasts, a discharge from the nipples, or even some blood from a baby's vagina, due to a temporary oversupply of oestrogen

⑥ testicles that may not yet have 'descended'

⑥ jaundice – more than half of all babies become 'jaundiced' (yellow) three to four days after birth, but their liver should soon deal with this pigment, caused by the breaking down of unneeded red cells, and only a very small percentage of babies need treatment with sun or ultraviolet lights. Have newborn jaundice checked by your doctor straight away – occasionally jaundice with other symptoms (including floppiness, not wanting to feed, constant sleepiness, or spasms) means a severe health problem

⑥ 'clicky hips' – get a hospital paediatrician to check this is routine and temporary. Don't take a baby to a chiropractor.

Breech (bum-first) babies, usually delivered by caesarean, sometimes like to continue their in-utero habit of curling up with their feet near their ears. Hilarious, harmless – and temporary.

routine medical stuff

The Apgar test will be performed to assess the baby's health. Named after its originator, Dr Virginia Apgar (oh my God, something's named after a woman), it's also an acronym for the things that are checked:

⑥ **a**ppearance (colour)

⑥ **p**ulse (heartbeat)

⑥ **g**rimace (reflex)

⑥ **a**ctivity (muscle tone)

⑥ **r**espiration (breathing).

In each category 0, 1 or 2 points are given, and a score of 7 or more is considered to be good. The test is conducted one minute after birth and again five minutes after birth. A very low score will mean emergency medical care is needed.

It is common to suggest that a baby be given a vitamin K injection very soon after the birth as a preventative measure against haemorrhagic disease of the newborn (HDN). (If you're having a home birth, check whether the midwife will give it.)

A full weigh, measurement of length and medical check will include the test for congenital dislocation of the hip (CDH), which can be corrected during the first three months using braces or a harness to stabilise the legs while the hip joint develops.

The Guthrie or PKU test, routinely done two or three days after birth, involves a blood sample being taken from the baby's heel and is a screening test for the disorders of phenylketonuria, hypothyroidism, cystic fibrosis and galactosaemia, all of which are best caught early for treatment.

Paediatricians don't routinely check babies before they leave hospital if the birth was uncomplicated but it's always worth asking, for peace of mind. Your community midwife and, later, your health visitor will regularly check for health problems (see the box in Week 41).

things you mightn't know

◎ Some newborn babies don't have tears when they cry until they are one to three months old.

◎ The eye colour a baby's born with may change before they're a year old. Despite what many people say, not all babies are born with blue eyes, especially dark-skinned ones.

◎ Newborn babies often develop sucking blisters in the centre of their top lip and on their hands.

◎ Hiccups are not a problem.

◎ They may be born with teeth. Yikes! But they'll suck, not bite. Phew!

◎ The first poo, meconium, is like something out of a horror movie; thick and sticky, it looks like extruded, green-tinged tar, but once your milk 'comes in' it gives way to the characteristic little-baby poo: yellowish and liquidy, with curds. This can come out at high velocity kerrrrrr-SPLAT!, and you

UMBILICAL CORD DONATION

Umbilical cord blood is a rich source of stem cells, which can be used to treat several conditions including immune problems and blood disorders such as leukaemia. The NHS Cord Blood Bank collects newborn babies' umbilical cords donated by parents, but currently only from four hospitals, in Barnet, Harrow, Luton and Watford. The cord blood is stored and available to anyone in need of stem cells, in the UK and around the world, as a preferred treatment to a bone marrow transplant. (A suitable match of blood cells has to be established.) These donations can't be held for particular individuals or families.

Several private companies offer a paid service to store a baby's umbilical cord for eighteen years as a possible source of stem cells for a future transplant the child may need. The NHS, however, says this is unlikely to be useful because the chance that somebody will need their own cord blood cells in the future is very small.

To find out if you can donate an umbilical cord where you plan to give birth, go to cord.blood.co.uk, the website of the NHS Cord Blood Bank, which administers cord donations: from the home page choose 'How to Donate'.

quickly learn to be ready at nappy-change time to intercept a stream with the corner of a nappy. (And baby-boy wee can also travel quite a distance at short notice, in a large arc.)

⑥ The early-baby wee may contain crystals that can make it look reddish – not to be confused with the absorbent crystals of disposable nappies, which look like tiny glass bubbles and sometimes escape.

⑥ The stump of the umbilical cord drops off in about a week or two, and the hospital midwives will show you how to take care of it in the meantime.

⑥ There is no medical reason for having baby boys circumcised, except in extremely rare cases. Cutting the foreskin from the glans of the penis involves an agonising and deeply shocking ordeal and a painful recovery (babies are too little to be given anaesthetic). Few doctors will do the procedure. Some parents insist on it for religious reasons. Others want the penis to 'match' that of the baby's father. Seems like a barbaric form of cosmetic surgery on someone who doesn't even get a say in it.

hearing tests

The NHS offers all parents a hearing test for their new baby within the first few weeks of life. Most often, this will be done in the hospital maternity unit before you go home. If not, check with your GP or midwife to find out when and where you can have your baby's hearing tested. Ear experts say that, to give kids the best chance of learning language and to speak, deafness should be detected as early as possible: ideally in the first weeks or within two months, but certainly within six months.

what's going on The nesting urge is likely to be at fever pitch. Many women find themselves scrubbing underneath shelves and may have to be restrained. Don't do anything that involves standing on a chair or a ladder, no matter how much you feel that dusting the curtain rail is crucial to life as we know it. You might have aches and pains caused by your ginormous uterus. A gentle walk should help.

The baby is technically 'full term' – that is, fully developed – by the time it enters this week, although most doctors say forty weeks is full term too because that's the typical length of a pregnancy. Most of the lanugo has fallen out, but the baby's still covered in vernix. About 14 grams of fat is laid down each day from now on. The baby probably has a bowel full of meconium in a rather disgusting-looking hard rope of greeny-black stuff. Once the baby's out and starts on milk, the poo will be much more liquid. The baby still moves every day, but not very far. Weight: about 3.2 kilos.

Average approximate baby length this week from head to bum

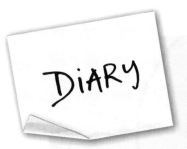

Geoff comes along to this week's midwife appointment. Claire says reassuring things about gigantic babies not necessarily being a problem because their mums' pelvises can usually handle it. Some of them simply pop out of their mothers singing a sea shanty, I'm sure. But she says they will induce ten days or so after the due date if I'm still lying around doing my walrus impressions. The only time I can sleep properly is between 8 a.m. and noon. Luckily I don't have to be anywhere.

Because it's all a bit bloody exhausting. Have taken to not returning phone calls and living in my dressing-gown. Wish I hadn't just got talked into going back to work one day a week. Hard to exercise. Shuffling about. Starting to think more about the baby coming home, and in deep denial about childbirth itself. (Surely it couldn't hurt that much. Maybe I could just buy a baby from a nice shop and avoid the whole thing.) I'm trying to focus on the advantage of having a big baby – it'll be more robust and less scary. Hang on a minute. All the advantages will come when it's out, and it's not out yet.

I try to think about what kind of person the baby will be, but get grumpy and tell Geoff off for putting the wrong things in the fridge, when it was really me all the time and I'd forgotten and maybe this is some kind of weird pregnancy Jekyll and Hyde thing, or maybe it isn't and ... Anyway, whatever. I'm all nested out. The house is getting untidy again, but I can't be bothered cleaning it. At least I know that Geoff will make the house spotless before I bring the baby home because otherwise he knows I would have him killed.

Even more chemists have started thrusting show bags at me full of pamphlets and sample-sized stuff. Heartburn lozenges, nappy-rash lotions, pads for bleeding, pads for incontinence (oh GOD), ads for safety seats and equipment, safety hats, safety pants, safety bootees, lures to get you into Toys 'R' Us, and 400 different kinds of disposable nappies. They certainly give the impression that children are (a) dangerous and (b) moist.

info

your body after the birth

immediately afterwards

After the birth of your baby you might feel shivery and shaky, ecstatic, exhausted, sore, empty, blank, numb, sleepy or wide awake: whatever you feel is okay, and certainly won't be unprecedented. (At least one woman has taken the first look at her baby and said 'Where did that come from?' or 'I don't feel anything'. Some feel an overwhelming surge of love, but even if you think 'Huh?' instead don't worry, the love will come.) If you've had an epidural you may still have a wee catheter in your urethra and an IV drip in your hand.

Putting the baby to the breast as soon as possible after birth helps stimulate the uterus to contract and to squeeze out the placenta. Your new baby might not be hungry yet, but it's nice to meet a nipple anyway.

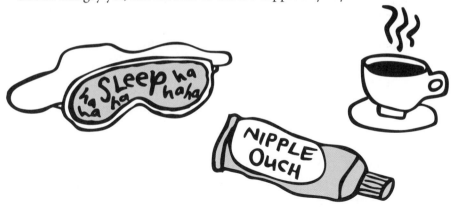

in the following days

Bleeding (the lochia)   The lochia – the discharge of blood, mucus and tissue from the uterus – will continue for two to six weeks after the birth. It is kind of like having a period at first, with some clots. It changes to a pink or brownish colour and ends as a yellow-white discharge.

⑥ Have plenty of maternity pads to hand. (Because the cervix takes a while to close and tampons can cause infection, you can't use them until your first real period after the birth, and that could be months away if you're breastfeeding.) You can use the new, ultra-absorbent, thin pads if you like, but the extra padding of the thicker maternity pads might make sitting more comfy.

◎ Tell your midwife if you have very heavy bleeding, the discharge has a yukky smell or the bleeding suddenly gets bright red. Also tell your midwife straight away if you haven't bled at all since giving birth.

'Afterpains' These usually occur for a few days or more after you have given birth, as your uterus contracts back towards its normal size. It's quite common to feel afterpains during breastfeeding. They can be worse in second and subsequent babies. If you want pain relief in hospital, make sure you get it: analgesics pass into breast milk, but not in amounts that cause a problem if you use recommended doses of over-the-counter-strength paracetamol.

Haemorrhoids and constipation

◎ Labour and delivery can give you haemorrhoids, a distension of the blood vessels at the entrance to your anus. Try not to strain when having a poo, even if you're constipated, because it will make the haemorrhoids worse. Some people don't poo for a few days, especially after a caesarean, and you might need help.

◎ If you have haemorrhoids, ask your obstetrician, midwife or the nursing staff about ice packs and ointment for relief.

◎ You may also need to eat more fruit, vegetables and cereals for fibre, and drink lots of water. See the hints on how to avoid constipation in the info in Week 8.

Your poor sore fanny There will usually be 'some level of discomfort in the perineal area', as doctors say, after a vaginal delivery, ranging from bearable to excruciating; you may need some pain relief for a day or two after delivery. If you've had an episiotomy or tear, the midwives in hospital will show you how to look after the stitched area so that it heals up well, and the site will be regularly checked for infection.

◎ Wash stitches gently two or three times a day.

◎ Regular baths in, or washes with, salty water or *very diluted* (10 drops per bath) tea tree oil can help the healing process.

◎ Dry the area well after bathing and give yourself some pants-off airing time if possible.

◎ Don't dry stitches with a hairdryer unless you have a cool setting – some people numb the area with ice or drugs and then scorch themselves with a hairdryer that's too hot or too close. It might be better to wave a paper fan or a handy copy of *Hello!*

⑥ If your stitches are sore and itchy, try dissolving a teaspoon of bicarbonate of soda or salt in warm water, then sitting in it after a wee.

⑥ Try leaning forward (with your hands reaching towards the floor) when you wee so that wee doesn't get onto the stitches.

⑥ Splash out (so to speak) on some thick, soft toilet paper.

⑥ While having a poo in the first couple of days post-delivery, you might find it more comfortable if you support the perineal area firmly with a pad or wad of toilet paper.

⑥ Avoid constipation by keeping up your fibre intake and drinking plenty of water.

⑥ Don't sit on a rubber ring – it will direct more blood to the area, creating more pressure.

⑥ Sit on a rolled-up towel or a pillow.

⑥ Fill a condom with water and freeze it, and then wrap it in a hanky or tea towel, so it doesn't stick to you, and pop it in your knickers (for no more than 10 minutes at a time).

⑥ Ask your doctor to prescribe safe anti-inflammatories or painkillers.

⑥ Ask your natural therapist for suitable healing ideas.

⑥ Pelvic-floor exercises (see the 'Pelvic-floor Exercises' box in Week 15) will stimulate circulation in the area and assist in the healing process. The first few times the area will feel very tired and trembly, and you may have some numbness, but do as many as you can as soon as you can.

⑥ Attack any urinary infection quickly by taking an alkaline powder recommended by your GP or chemist, so that weeing doesn't sting the wound.

⑥ Most doctors say no bonking until the six-week check-up at least – possibly *after* the six-week check-up would be better (*during* might be viewed as a little inconsiderate).

Getting back to your old self (sort of) See 'Your Post-baby Body' in Week 43 for info about self-image and realistic exercise.

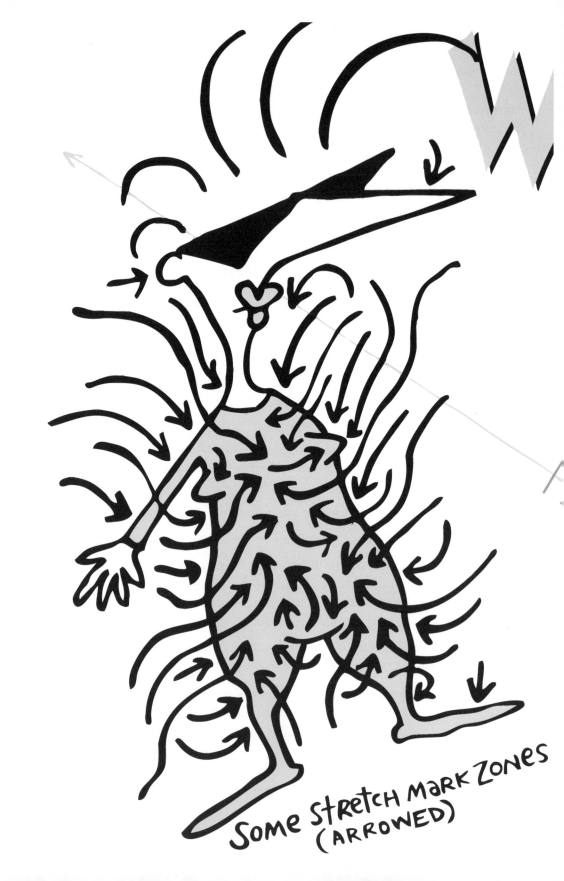

SOME STRETCH MARK ZONES (ARROWED)

EEK 39

what's going on

The cervix gets softer and thinner, ready to open wide enough for a baby's head to come through. Any time from now it could release the mucus plug, which will end up on your knickers or down the loo and is a sign that labour could start within hours. The uterus is still practising contractions; in fact that pesky Mrs Braxton Hicks may be visiting rather too often and possibly confusing you about whether it's actually labour or not. You are probably completely fed up with being pregnant and have forgotten what your feet look like.

Your baby's genitals at this point have been over-excited by all your extra hormones and will be very large indeed in comparison to the rest of the body. They will return to a more seemly size a few days after the birth. Overall, the baby's growth slows down this week in preparation for birth. Weight: about 3.3 kilos.

Average approximate baby length this week from head to bum

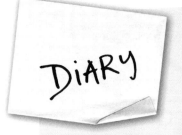
DiARY

Latest inventory of body changes: gigantic, veiny boozoombas with brown nipples; new, brown, flat moles on them, and heaps of skin tags under each one; huuuge tummy; purple, stripey stretch marks on bosoms and hips. And I can't see my legs or pubic hair. For all I know they've been stolen.

I know why whales beach themselves. THEY JUST CAN'T BE BOTHERED ANY MORE.

Having a baby is a preposterous proposition. How can this huge, hard thing possibly come out of a vagina? I hear about a woman whose first words after labour were 'What a completely shocking thing to happen'. I've also heard so many stories about people looking blankly at their newborn baby and wondering what on earth to do with it. I'm determined not to panic if I don't bond straight away.

I ask Suze 'Is it like an out-of-body experience?'

'No', she says. 'It's a get-out-of-my-body experience.'

I still can't tell what my body wants – am I hungry, tired, nauseous, getting a cold? I have no idea. Walking is hard now, the damn groin pain never goes away: those ligaments must be under so much strain the anchor points are constantly stressed.

The word 'deliver' is sexist, says one pregnancy book, because it indicates a male doctor does the work of 'delivery'. For heaven's sake. The mum's delivering – just like a postie with the mail. How about 'de-mummed', or would the mum be 'de-babied'? One person has already asked if I have been 'unsprogged'.

At this week's visit Jill looks exhausted – she's been up all night delivering babies. I didn't sleep much either.

'Is anything worrying you? Is there anything you want to ask?'

'No. Except don't go off duty, and did you get your motorcycle licence?'

Turns out she didn't do it a fortnight ago, so now she's going for the test this Saturday.

'I want to roar up next to some of the other midwives at the lights and see the looks on their faces', she says. (Apparently some of her doctor colleagues were shocked when she dyed her hair red. They sound pretty easy to shock. Maybe she should deliver the next baby wearing a peek-a-boo bra and a pair of wellies.)

People are so different about babies. Attitudes range from the clucky to the disbelieving, through to distaste and secrecy.

I told my accountant 'I feel stupid and tired.'

She was horrified I'd said it aloud. 'Don't tell anyone!'

There is a conspiracy of working mothers to hide the effects of pregnancy and motherhood so as not to be discriminated against.

I look up 'pregnant ladies' on the internet and the first eleven matches are hardcore porn sites.

info

breastfeeding your new baby

You may as well read this now because you won't feel like reading it straight after your baby's born! It's hard to think past labour at the moment, but when it's over you'll be preoccupied with your bosoms.

Breastfeeding is the best way to feed because breast milk is perfectly designed to nourish your baby with all the right nutrients and to supply antibodies to boost the baby's immune system, which formula milk can't deliver.

In the past, babies were weaned onto plain old cow's milk, which wasn't any good for them, being designed for calves, not human babies, but now infant formulas are specially designed to give as many of the nutrients in breast milk as possible. Formula still runs second, but it's a much better second than it used to be.

hooray for bosoms

Because breast milk is so fabulous for babies, because it helps you to bond with your baby and because it's on tap and free of charge, it's really worth persevering if you have initial trouble breastfeeding: very few babies and mothers can get their act together straight away.

Stuff to know about breastfeeding in the early days

⑥ For the first few days after birth the baby will be drinking the creamy yellow pre-milk, colostrum, which has evolved specially to nourish a baby and provide it with antibodies before it gets the milk. Most babies will lose a bit of weight until the milk 'comes in', and then start to gain again.

⊚ At first breastfeeding might be painful, especially if your baby is having trouble latching on properly (latching on is often called 'attachment') and chomps on the nipple or can't seem to stay 'on' and suck. The baby needs to take most of the areola as well as the nipple in its mouth and the nipple goes to the back of the mouth. Different mothers and babies find different feeding positions suit them best.

⊚ When your milk comes in (usually after three or four days), you can expect your breasts to feel full and hard. Your midwife will be able to give you advice on how to ease this, such as applying hot cloths and expressing a little milk before each feed, or using cold packs or cold (not frozen) cabbage leaves, to relieve engorgement. You might need a cream to keep your nipples supple: lactation consultants recommend different things, from pure lanolin, which you don't have to wipe off before the baby drinks, to camomile-flower ointment. You don't need tough nipples, you want pliant ones.

⊚ You might be asked if you can feel your milk coming in. This is like a shiver, a prickle or even a stabbing pain in each breast, although sometimes you don't feel it for days or even weeks after the birth – or ever. All the same, the 'let down' of your milk will be happening before each and every breastfeed.

⊚ Exposing your nipples to very mild sunlight for short periods (three to five minutes) after feeding will dry any excess moisture, and the ultraviolet light helps them to heal if they're sore or cracked. When you can, let them air dry after feeding.

⊚ Nipple shields can help protect sore or cracked nipples during a feed (see 'Feeding Gear' in Week 26).

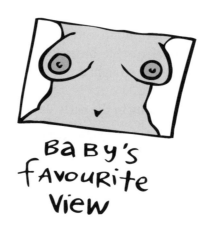

BaBy's
fAvouRite
View

If you're having trouble   The thing to remember is to try to relax (I know it's hard at the time when you've got a hungry, crying baby and you can't get it to attach properly). Take a deep breath and lower your shoulders. It takes time for you and the baby to learn breastfeeding together. Even managing six days or six weeks of breastfeeding is a big bonus for your baby.

A middle road if you're having difficulty could be expressing your milk and putting it in a bottle to give your nipples a rest. You can also supplement a low supply with formula. And if breastfeeding really doesn't work, you have a fine back-up with formula: your baby will not starve. So give it another go.

It's more convenient to get the feeding sorted out before you leave hospital than it is to figure it out at home. Because of short hospital stays, that may not be possible, though when you go home you'll get visits from a midwife, which is some help. Use the time you do have in hospital to get as much help and advice from the staff as possible. If you like, say you want to watch other mothers feeding their babies. (Your midwife will help you if you've had a home birth.)

If you're having problems breastfeeding and feel that the staff have done all they can to help you, or don't have the time, ask them to get the hospital's lactation consultant, or a private one, to come and see you.

Quite often mothers get conflicting advice from hospital midwives about how to hold their baby and how to position themselves while they feed. If all the advice is putting your head in a whirl (you'll be madly sleep-deprived, which doesn't help), choose to listen to ONE of the staff – the lactation consultant, for example – and don't be swayed from their advice if it's working. Choose someone who clearly likes babies, is encouraging and gentle, and takes the time to help you, sit with you, watch your technique and try different ways to help. (Don't choose anyone who grabs your breast in one hand, the baby in the other and brings them together like a clash of cymbals.)

There are a number of specialist charities in the UK offering breastfeeding support (see the 'More Info' section coming up for helpline numbers and other details), and these can be a marvellous help. All claim to listen, support and offer up-to-date information, rather than simply urging you to stick at it. But some are more evangelical than others, and you may find their advisers put more emphasis on the WHY than the HOW of breastfeeding. If so, try a different helpline, and ask for practical advice, not just encouragement to continue. Or get a visit from a trained lactation consultant or try one of the books listed below.

You may find that in their zeal for breastfeeding, some people gloss over the real problems you're having, with the advice 'Just keep trying'. If you think breastfeeding is 'taking too much out of you', it probably is – don't accept that this is 'nonsense' or inevitable: get some nutritional and coping advice. If you're finding it impossible to juggle work and breastfeeding, don't just accept that 'Many other women do it and you can too': make sure you get practical help on how to continue.

BREASTFEEDING BASICS

Sit comfortably with a drink to hand (preferably non-alcoholic), answering machine on or phone off the hook, and take a deep breath…

⊚ Rest the baby on a pillow so that it can come up to the breast and make eye contact with you.

⊚ The baby should be lying on its side facing you (you can remember this as 'tummy to mummy').

⊚ The baby's nose should be in line with your nipple ('nose to nipple').

⊚ Support your breast by placing your fingers flat on your ribs at the junction of your breast and the ribs, keeping your thumb uppermost.

⊚ Support the baby's head and shoulders in such a way that its head is free to extend slightly as it is brought to the breast – so that its chin and lower jaw reach the breast first.

⊚ Move the baby towards the breast so that its nose and upper lip touch the nipple, causing its mouth to gape wide open.

⊚ When the baby's mouth is wide open, move the baby quickly to your breast and aim your nipple towards the top of the back of its mouth. Its lower lip should be as far from the nipple as possible.

⊚ The baby is then ready and with a wide mouth and a strong tongue it will suck rhythmically, taking short breaks every so often but still remaining attached.

If the connection is painful, break the suction the baby has on your nipple gently, by first sliding your little finger into the baby's mouth next to your nipple, and then pulling the baby off gently. Otherwise it will be very hard on your nipples.

more info on **breastfeeding**

Your health visitor can help you with breastfeeding, and you can also see the chapter on breastfeeding in the sequel to this book, *The Rough Guide to Babies and Toddlers*. Don't forget that US websites and books will say 'nursing' instead of 'breastfeeding'.

National Breastfeeding Helpline
0300 100 0212 (9.30 a.m. to 9.30 p.m.)
Government-sponsored helpline staffed by volunteers from two charities, the Association of Breastfeeding Mothers and the Breastfeeding Network.

National Childbirth Trust
Helpline: 0300 33 00 771 (8 a.m. to 10 p.m.)
nctpregnancyandbabycare.com
The helpline will give immediate advice, or put you in touch with a local breastfeeding counsellor for a personal visit. On the website, click on 'Info centre' then 'Feeding your baby' for detailed info and advice, or visit the online shop for books, DVDs and other products.

NCT: Breastfeeding for Beginners by Caroline Deacon, Thorsons, UK, 2002
Great little book from the National Childbirth Trust covering all the basics, with practical advice from trained counsellors and answers to common questions. Also offers help with expressing breast milk and advice on going back to work.

breastfeedingmums.com
Extensive site with instructional videos which can be viewed online (by 'VideoJug', but we won't snigger about that). Blogs, Q&As, and community forums with an approachable, non-evangelical tone. (Okay, I sniggered a bit.)

The Breastfeeding Book by William Sears, MD, and Martha Sears, Little, Brown, US, 2000
They're really into breastfeeding, but also have a great troubleshooting section, a guide to products (remember it's meant for the US, although a lot is relevant here) and a chapter on mums and babies with 'special needs'.

BREAST WRANGLING

Remember to have your bra size re-measured after pregnancy and when you finish breastfeeding: your breasts *will* change and may not go back to their original size.

not breastfeeding

If the worst comes to the worst and you can't breastfeed your baby or breastfeeding is not for you, it's nowhere near the end of the world. The way people go on about it, you'd think not breastfeeding was the equivalent of making the baby drink gin and wheeling it across motorways during blizzards in a war zone. Plenty of bottlefed babies grow up to be strapping, robust, healthy adults. Look at the adults around you. Look at the kids around you. Can you tell who was bottlefed? 'Course you can't. Many other factors affect a child's development and immune system, including the chemicals in an environment, access to fresh, healthy food, and exposure to germs to build up resistance.

It would be lovely if you could breastfeed, but you can't. Instead you can enjoy the relaxed feeling of bottlefeeding your baby while making eye contact, and the freedom it gives you because you can always get somebody else to feed the baby if you'd like to go out for an hour or so and have an affair with a couple of firemen. Now crank up the steriliser, tweak those teats – not those, the ones that fit on the bottle. And get on with it.

A midwife or your health visitor (see the 'Child Health Clinics' box in Week 41) can help you with all the stuff you need to know about sterilising equipment and storing and heating bottles.

GOOD MILK, BAD MILK

All babies must be fed breast milk, or a baby formula based on cow's or other milk, or a combination of both. Babies who are fed just cow's milk or soy milk or rice milk, by parents wanting to be 'natural', have died. Always check what you're feeding your baby with a midwife or your health visitor.

stuff to tell nosy people

⑥ I have an illness controlled by medication, which mustn't be passed through breast milk to my baby.

⑥ Both my nipples blew off during a storm.

⑥ I have an antibiotic-resistant form of infected bosoms, and either of them could explode at any moment.

⑥ It's easier to get the gin into a bottle.

⑥ Both my bosoms were removed years ago.

⑥ I can't breastfeed, and I don't want to talk about it. Gosh, that's a lovely blouse.

⑥ So far five lactation specialists have told me I'm one of those women who just can't breastfeed. In the old days I would have had a wet nurse.

⑥ Oh, just BUGGER OFF.

more info on **bottlefeeding**

The websites of the major brands for formula and bottles have info.

nhs.uk/conditions/bottle-feeding
Covers the pros and cons of bottlefeeding and advice on sterilising and choosing the right formula milk for your baby. Much emphasis, though, on breastfeeding being preferable if possible.

ivillage.co.uk/boards
Search on 'bottlefeeding support' for friendly and sympathetic advice from other bottlefeeders. As always, things internetty can get internutty in chatrooms and forums so don't take any advice as gospel and always check info with your doctor.

babyfriendly.org.uk
While the United Nations Children's Fund (UNICEF) supports breastfeeding wherever possible it also provides instructions for safe bottlefeeding. From the home page, search 'Bottle Feeding' to find an info sheet and other useful stuff.

what's going on This is the magic week when your baby is due, unless somebody has cocked up the dates. But this is based on averages, so don't expect to give birth on the due date. If you do, it is simply showing off.

The baby is rounder and fatter and probably ready to be born. It is now nearly 200 times heavier than it was at twelve weeks. Weight: 3.3 to 3.5 kilos. Boys are often bigger than girls.

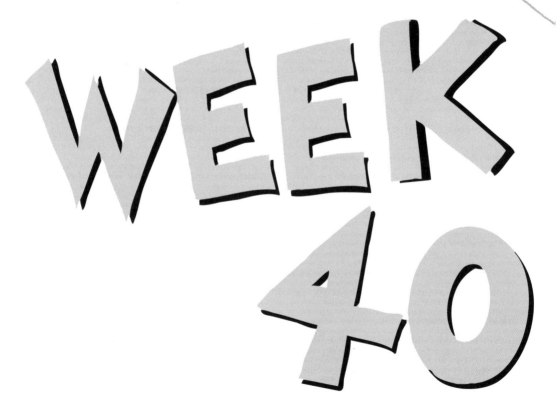

WEEK 40

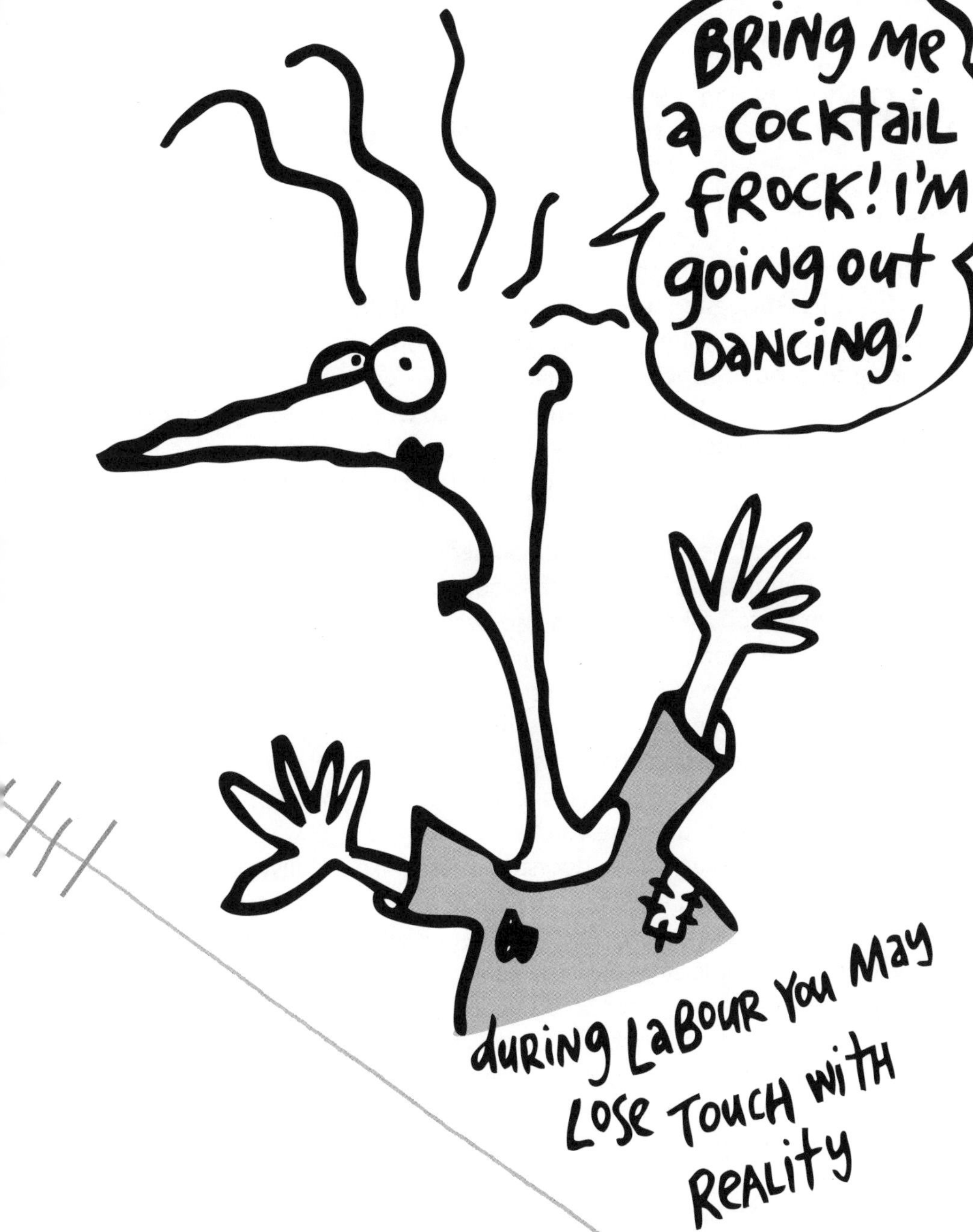
BRING ME A COCKTAIL FROCK! I'M GOING OUT DANCING!
DURING LABOUR YOU MAY LOSE TOUCH WITH REALITY
Average approximate baby length this week from head to bum

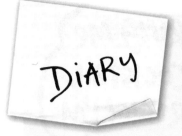

DiARY

I'm due. And I am nothing but a limbo-living, dimply-arsed, stoned giantess. When I go to see the midwife the women in the waiting room who are only a couple of months pregnant look at me with very contemplative expressions: 'Surely I couldn't get THAT big', I hear them saying in their innermost thoughts.

Geoff has suggested we change the name of the baby to Godot, and I am like a cat waiting to have kittens, prowling around the house looking for a good cupboard to give birth in – or tidy up. I'm finding it harder to drink Beck's herbal uterine tonic concoction – I'm just sick of it, but I persevere because she says I have good uterine tone, which I am immensely proud of, it being the only part of my body that HAS ANY TONE.

Obsessed with the idea of labour. Someone reminds me of writer Kathy Lette's description of a post-caesarean vagina as 'honeymoon fresh'. If I didn't laugh I'd sob m'self silly. It's also becoming clear to me how many pregnant women worry about pooing during labour. I'm just surprised your lungs don't come out your bum considering all the pressure.

Have left a message on the answering machine saying nothing's happened yet. People ringing and asking all the time. All the ones who are already mothers say 'Good luck', 'Take the drugs' and 'You're not going to try and have a natural birth are you?'

Uncle Mike turns up on the doorstep dressed like a Hollywood B-movie costume designer's idea of a part-time pimp: opaque, yellow-lensed, concave, wraparound sunglasses, ankle-length leather jacket, high-heeled boots and grey beard. I try not to stare. Aurelia is always waiting in the car, usually taking advantage of the mirror on the inside of the passenger sun visor.

He hands me a bunch of organic mangos and remarks casually that he and Aurelia are going on holiday next week to a commune.

'So', I venture, 'you won't be here when the baby's born?'

'Leave a message on the answering machine!' he cries gaily as he heads for the gate.

Family support. What would you do without it? Get along all right, is my guess.

My dream birth: I am lying on a sexy, dusky-pink, satin-quilted four-poster bed reading a magazine full of photos of gorgeous clothes I could afford that would look quite nice on me (I *said* it was a dream) when a man in a leopard-skin suit comes past with a cocktail trolley on wheels full of

excellent cakes, bottles of attractively coloured
alcohol, an icebucket and some syringes.

'Martini?' he inquires politely. 'Or would
modom care for an epidural?'

Just at that moment a perfectly charming baby
pops out of my vagina.

'Ow', I remark, absent-mindedly. 'Why, thank you, I'll take a gin and
lime. And a small colostrum for my new young friend.'

Just in case this doesn't happen, Jill has arranged with the hospital
doctors for me to have an induction. I am scheduled to go into the
maternity hospital next Monday at 5 p.m. to have my cervix annointed with
a prostaglandin that mimics the one in the body that basically says 'Lady,
start your engines for labour'. I have to stay in hospital, and they might put
some more in the next morning. Then I should be able to start on my own
without the oxytocin drip, although in some cases the membranes have
to be broken by the doctor if the waters don't break by themselves. This is
scary.

Had a problem sleeping last night, thinking about bringing a baby home,
and caesarean, and pain...

Beck's given me acupuncture twice to try to move the baby along a bit.
The baby finally 'engages' (goes into firing position). Jill says she thinks it
would have happened anyway. So TIRED. Some anxiety attacks, but mostly
sort of numb.

Everyone is ringing up saying 'Has anything happened?'

'NO!'

info

your hospital stay/early days

Midwives will be assigned to you in hospital (or at home, if you've had a
home birth). Their job is to take care of you as you recover from the birth.
They are also there to help you learn how to feed and look after your baby.

Ask them anything you want to know, and take full advantage of their time and knowledge. You can ask to be discharged when you feel ready to go home, providing you and your baby get the all-clear from medical staff. Most women spend 24–36 hours in hospital after giving birth (or three nights, following a caesarean). You can go home sooner if both you and the baby are doing well. Equally, if you feel you need more time in hospital – either because you don't have the hang of breastfeeding yet or feel ready to cope with the baby on your own – talk to your midwife and explain that you need to stay a couple of extra days.

food

⑥ Nutrition and beating hunger are important issues for breastfeeding. Ask a lactation consultant, hospital dietician, midwife, health visitor or natural therapist for suggestions.

⑥ It may be nutritionally sound, but hospital food is usually, at best, pathetically boring. Get friends to bring you decent food such as fresh fruit. Most wards have a fridge and access to a microwave so you can have a stash of your own.

visitors

⑥ Don't feel obliged to see everyone who wants to check out the baby while you're in hospital (or in your early days at home). In hospital, make the most of this time when your meals, cleaning and other needs are being taken care of by other people to recover from the birth and to prepare yourself for when you go home.

⑥ If you like, ban all but a few close friends and family from visiting for the first few days so you can rest and spend time with your baby.

⑥ Hospital visiting hours are not as strict as they used to be, but you can pretend that they are. If you don't want people dropping in outside the set hours, enlist the help of the midwives and ward staff.

⑥ If you have a phone, you can ask the switchboard to take messages for you so that you can ring out but the phone doesn't go all the time.

⑥ Ask people to phone you before they come to visit. If you're too tired or don't feel up to seeing anyone, you can ask them to come another time.

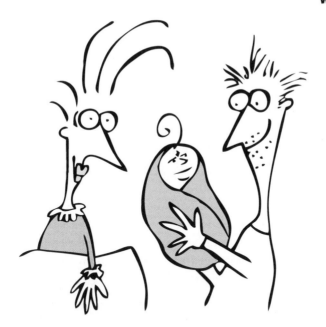

⑥ If masses of flowers get in the way and cause allergies, ask people who are coming to visit you not to bring them. Instead, have one or two close friends bring you a small bunch to brighten things up.

time out

Some families encourage new mums to go out for an evening with their partner or another companion, leaving the baby in the care of rellies or friends. This can be a real treat, but you may find that your first separation from your baby just makes you think about the baby non-stop. If you don't feel like it, don't go.

paperwork and other nitty-gritties

Birth notice   You might want to write a paragraph for the classifieds in the newspaper and keep that edition for the baby when they grow up.

Registering the birth   Legally, you're supposed to register the birth of your baby in the first six weeks after the birth, unless you live in Scotland where you have only three weeks. At some hospitals the registrar comes to the maternity unit each day so that you can register the baby before you go home (assuming you've thought of a name). Elsewhere you'll have to make an appointment at the local registry office and go along in person. If you're married, only one partner need go. If you're not married and want two parents' names on the birth certificate you'll both need to go along together, or the parent who doesn't go must fill out a 'statutory declaration form'. Don't ask me why being married has anything to do with it, you're in Bureaucracyland now, and you'll just have to wait until it moves on from the top of the Magic Faraway Tree. Until your child starts childcare or school this is probably about as legalistic and bureaucratic as it gets. A word of warning: whoever does register the birth and the name should not be plastered lest the temptation prove too great to officially call the baby Aston Martin.

If you're not sure what involvement the father wants with the child, or the father isn't around, get legal advice from a community legal centre or your own lawyer about whether to put his name on the certificate. It's quite okay to leave the father bit blank if you need to. Don't let anyone write 'unknown' or anything judgemental for the kid to read when they grow up and get a copy.

Once your baby is registered you will be given their birth certificate. This is a short form stating the child's name and sex, and the date and place of birth. If you want a copy of the full certificate (a nice paper job with details in writing rather than computer-printed) you will need to pay a small fee. Your baby will also be issued with a National Health Service number, which will enable you to register your baby with a doctor.

Registering for benefits You need your baby's birth certificate to claim the benefits that are due to you. You should find a child benefit claim form among the mountain of leaflets you're given while in hospital; if not, phone the Child Benefit Helpline on 0845 302 1444. Child benefit is usually paid either weekly or monthly directly into your bank account, though it can be paid to you by cheque if needed. See the 'Money for Mums (and Dads)' box in 'Getting Ready' at the start of the book for more on benefits available to new parents.

Health cover If you have private family health insurance, you will need to add the baby to your policy. Usually you have about eight weeks to do this after the birth, but check to be sure.

WRAP PARTY

Wrapping new bubs securely in a muslin square or swaddling blanket is the key to getting them to sleep: it makes them feel all snug and as if they're still in the womb. Most babies like to stay wrapped for sleep until three or four months old, although some are too wriggly after a month and others are happy to stay bundled until six months. For the next stage you can move to a sleeping-bag suit without a hood, which is safest.

Get a midwife or health visitor to teach you how to wrap, and practise on a teddy. Both Mum and Dad will get very good at it with practice!

more info

sidsandkids.org/sa/documents/wrappingbrochure.pdf
This downloadable brochure has info on why wrapping is good and how-to instructions with cute pics.

tinyurl.com/babywrapping
One of a number of YouTube demonstration videos.

what's going on If your pregnancy has been 'average' (forty weeks long), your baby is out in the world and perhaps sleeping off the shock. After your baby is born a whole bunch of hormonal activities happen, quite suddenly. Your body expels the placenta, which has been pumping out huge quantities of hormones. Suddenly you're bereft of the 'happy hormones' and getting a boost of hormones such as prolactin to help breastfeeding. Your body looks less pregnant, but your tummy is still very big. You're bleeding from your vagina as the body expels all that nice uterine surface the baby needed. Your body is recovering from the massive shock of childbirth – whether natural or surgical. Give yourself a break. Don't do anything but recover and be with your baby.

The baby may have some characteristic newborn marks, such as 'stork marks' (red, rashlike shapes on the forehead, eyelids and/or back of the neck) or temporary marks from forceps. Your baby is sucking colostrum because your milk probably won't come in until day 3 or 4.

The bub will be down a bit from its birth weight before the breast milk kicks in. Don't worry about this: too much scientific measuring and talk of weight-loss percentages can make you worried for no reason. Lost weight in those first few days is expected in all babies and the loss can be made up in just a few days.

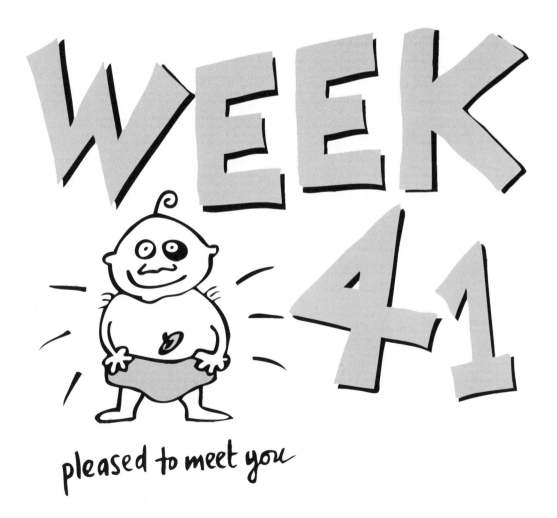

WEEK 41

pleased to meet you

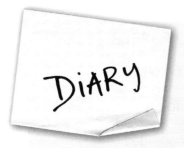
DiARY

It's time. We drive to the hospital for the prostaglandin-on-the-cervix induction, with the bag neatly packed with all the things we'll need for labour, feeling nervous but excited. Luckily Maternity isn't busy so I get my own room.

I'll have the induction, sleep a bit, then in the morning, when contractions will probably start, I'll ring Beck and tell her to come in sporting her best midwifery hat.

Jill comes into our room wearing a lovely frock and some Issey Miyake perfume on her way to a movie, and she puts the gel on my cervix. What a charming bedside manner she has – she chats away about something else and one could almost be at a dinner party if she didn't have her hand up your fanny.

A second midwife arrives in a white jacket and navy trousers and puts a piece of electronic equipment on wheels next to the bed and attaches a belt around my tummy. This is the monitor. It continually rolls out a graph of any contractions and a graph of the baby's heartbeat, which is usually up around 150 beats a minute. Geoff and I start to play cards, pretending that we can keep our mind on Snap! instead of all the machinery.

A long time later I write this: Suddenly I noticed that the baby's heartbeat had dropped to 80 beats a minute and the graph line was plunging down like a sheer cliff face. And so began the worst two hours of my life.

Geoff tried to reassure me that it was probably normal, but when the midwife came back she got a look on her face I never want to see again and rang for an obstetrician, who, it transpires, was just about to have his first meal in 24 hours in the canteen. Within five minutes he was in the room, looking at the graph.

'I'm just going outside to consult with someone, and I'll be back in a moment to tell you what we're going to do', he said calmly.

Left alone, Geoff and I held hands and tried not to look as frightened as each other.

'He's going to do an emergency caesarean. I guess Beck's not going to make it in time', I thought suddenly.

The doctor came back in and sat on the bed, and held my hand and said – oh dear, I still can't write these words without crying – 'Your baby is distressed, and if it's this distressed because of a little Braxton Hicks contraction, we won't risk going through labour.'

Behind the scenes an anaesthetist, a paediatrician and another obstetrician were rushing in from elsewhere in the building. The midwife marched Geoff off, which was awful, and they quickly wheeled me out on one of those cold, gleaming trolleys and into the white, shining operating theatre, where there were people with blue paper masks, shower caps and gowns. ('Nice to see some fashion co-ordination', I thought, ages later. At the time I wasn't thinking much at all, I was just frightened.)

The anaesthetist put an IV drip in my left hand, and then gave me a spinal-block injection into the lower back, with me curled in a fetal position while a nurse held my hand. It was really scary staying perfectly still so he didn't get the wrong bit of the spine. As the anaesthetic started to work, Jill (who had been paged at the cinema) came in with her midwife colleague, a paediatrician, two obstetricians and – thank God! – Geoff, who looked like he was playing an extra in a TV medical drama. They put up a blue fabric screen over my chest so I couldn't see my tummy. Everyone fussed around behind the screen for a moment.

'Let me know when you start', I said to Jill.

Everybody laughed.

'We've been in for three minutes', she said.

When I looked up at the huge light with the flat globe cover, I could see the reflection of my insides, yellow and pink and purple. These were the things I was thinking: 'Please let my baby be all right', 'Thank God I live in a First World country', 'Thank God I'm not having a home birth', and large stretches of blank that probably had something to do with shock.

'There's your baby coming out', said the second midwife, taking a Polaroid photo.

'Is it Eddy or Matilda?' I asked.

'It's Matilda!' everyone chorused.

And suddenly Jill held up a silent, purple, slimy creature with a screwed-up, tiny little face and a smudge of dark hair. A sob caught in my throat as I reached out and gently touched my baby's leg with the back of my hand. I didn't know if any other contact would hurt Matilda or be the wrong thing to do.

Instantly she was whipped away to a table by Jill and the paediatrician, who gave her a rub down with a warm towel and then a few puffs of oxygen with a plastic face mask.

'She's just fine', said the paediatrician. 'She's got all the right things in all the right places'.

And then Matilda started to cry. All the experienced people in the room broke into huge smiles.

'That's a good cry', they said simultaneously, and you could feel the relief in the room.

Jill and the paediatrician did some tests on Matilda over in the corner of the room. Meanwhile, the two obstetricians were doing their downstairs needlework on what Geoff would later refer to as 'the tummy smile': my curved red scar. When they were finished, Jill brought Matilda, wrapped in a rather fetching white swaddling cloth, for me to cuddle in bed, and showed Geoff how to hold her, with his hand supporting her head. We were both shaky and in tears and I of course was drugged out of my mind. In fact I couldn't believe any of this was happening.

After a while, Jill and a nurse wheeled me and Matilda and perhaps Geoff too (though he may have walked) out of theatre and off to the maternity recovery ward, where three other mums'n'bubs were already installed. I drifted in and out of sleep while Geoff sat vigil, holding Matilda in his arms in a kind of trance. When I came to, I was really worried that Matilda was all right, but I didn't feel an immediate surge of overwhelming love. Mostly relief that she was okay, and confusion about how to get her on the breast for a snack of colostrum. Matilda just looked tired and tiny, and slept a lot. And guess what? She wasn't even a whopper: 3.6 kilos. Damn. All the rest was Magnums.

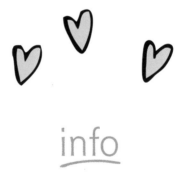

info

coping when you get home

getting organised

⑥ To stop people dropping in at all hours, insist that friends and relatives call before visiting or set aside particular times (say, certain mornings a week).

⑥ If friends or relatives offer to help with cleaning, cooking or shopping, ACCEPT IMMEDIATELY!

⑥ There will be days when preparing dinner will seem impossible or unbearable. Prepare for these on days you do cook by making extra, large batches of things that can be frozen, such as soups and casseroles. If friends and relations offer to bring you meals, ACCEPT IMMEDIATELY! Keep takeaway menus from a few decent local places.

⑥ Instead of flowers and fancy baby accessories, ask friends to contribute to getting you a nappy service for the first month or so – you'll have enough to cope with without spending hours soaking and washing dirty nappies. Instead of lots of outfits, ask a couple of friends to buy bibs. You'll soon find out why: it's much easier to whip them on and off than to change a whole sicky outfit.

⑥ If you can afford it, get a cleaning service in for a few hours every one or two weeks so that the basic housework, such as cleaning the bathroom and kitchen, is always done.

⑥ If you can't afford a cleaning service but can't stand being in a messy house, just keep one room tidy. This will give you somewhere to relax or see visitors.

⑥ If you live by yourself, try to organise a roster of friends to come by each day for the first few weeks so that you can have an uninterrupted half hour to take a shower or bath, sit down without the baby or get out of the house briefly.

looking after yourself

⑥ Use the time when your baby is sleeping during the day to have a nap or relax. Put your needs ahead of visitors, housework and other chores.

⑥ Try to get out of the house every day to help keep yourself sane.

⑥ Try to get time each day to do your postnatal exercises (especially the pelvic-floor ones) – you'll find you have more energy for them in the mornings. If you enjoy exercising with other people, a postnatal class after a few weeks will also give you a chance to talk with other new mothers. (Also see 'Your Post-baby Body' in Week 43.)

⑥ Ask someone you trust to look after your baby while you do something relaxing such as going for a walk or seeing a friend.

KEEPING A RECORD

If you're living in a fog and you want to keep a record of stuff such as when your baby feeds and from which breast, how many nappies they've gone through, when they slept and other things, you can buy special booklets to fill in, or you can just use an exercise book. Record keeping can be a good idea if you share care with each other or with relatives or friends, so that everyone can see what's been going on. It is especially good for noting symptoms or medicine doses if there's a health problem. A record can also be a help when you see your health visitor or doctor. Most people lose interest in record keeping after the first six weeks or so.

⑥ Congratulate yourself. You're keeping a human being alive. Also the baby.

⑥ If you're going somewhere like a shopping centre, check out the parents' facilities and whether there are lifts or escalators. If you have to negotiate a lot of stairs, next time you may be better off with a baby sling than a pram. (Also see 'Early Outings' in Week 43.)

⑥ If you have a partner, make time to go out alone with them, even if it's just for coffee.

⑥ Make sure your partner understands that most women don't feel like flinging themselves into chandelier-swingin' rumpy-pumpy for a few weeks at least. It might be nice to break this more gently than placing a sign saying 'Off Limits' over your fanny. (Also see 'Post-baby Sex' in Week 43.)

⑥ Don't pretend you're coping if you're not: share things with your partner or friends.

⑥ Do confide in your health worker or GP if you think you need some extra help (and see the helplines coming up over the page).

⑥ Many families who can afford it hire maternity nurses and nannies to help with the first few weeks at home, often just at night. If this sounds like your sort of thing make sure you get one whose philosophy is like yours – and don't let yourself be bullied or bossed about. And don't let it interfere with you bonding with your baby.

a crying baby

Babies often cry for mysterious reasons and aren't good at settling. Crying is not your fault.

If your baby is crying and not settling, try changing their nappy, feeding them, popping them on a rug on the floor to have a look at the ceiling, having a chat to them, and then wrapping them up and putting them down for a nap (see the 'Wrap Party' box in Week 40). If this doesn't work and you are sure they are not hungry, tired, hot, cold, wet or in pain from wind, you could try:

⑥ curling up together in bed in a warm, dark, quiet room, tummy to tummy for maximum skin contact

⑥ giving them a warm bath and baby massage (although some babies hate both until they're a few weeks old) – ask a midwife or health visitor for a demo; basically be gentle, use any sort of edible oil, and stop if it makes the baby cranky

⑥ rocking with your baby in a chair or rocking them in a baby hammock

⑥ playing soothing music, making rhythmical noises like a washing machine, or singing (you might feel like a wally but even if you have to make something up or you 'can't sing' your baby won't notice)

⑥ walking up and down a hall about 5000 times with the baby over your shoulder or in the pram

⑥ distracting the baby by holding them level with your face and nodding your head, while making an interesting (not freaky) noise or grinning – this can give them such a surprise that they forget what they were crying about

⑥ going about your business with the baby in a sling

⑥ giving them an approved dummy for newborns

⑥ accepting there's nothing you can do, and getting someone else in to hold the baby while you walk around the block.

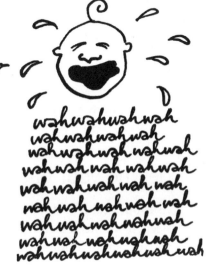

wahwahwahwah
wahwahwahwah
wahwahwahwahwah
wahwahwahwahwah
wahwahwahwahwah
wahwahwahwahwah
wahwahwahwahwah
wahwahwahwahwah
wahwahwahwahwah

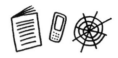

more info on **a crying baby**

'Parenting Support' in the Contacts and Resources chapter at the end of this book gives other advice lines and help info. Also see the Crying chapter in this book's sequel, *The Rough Guide to Babies and Toddlers*, for lots more.

Cry-sis

Helpline: 08451 228669 (9 a.m. to 10 p.m.)
cry-sis.org.uk
A shoulder to cry on (excuse the pun) and good advice for parents of babies who are crying or sleepless. The operational hours of the helpline won't give you comfort in the dead of night. The website has an extensive checklist for identifying reasons for crying and sleep routines for different ages.

babycentre.co.uk/baby/sleep

This baby-care website page has many links to fact sheets and soothing help for you (and your bub). Everything from why babies cry and coping with crying to how to get twins to nod off at the same time.

Understanding Your Crying Baby: Why Babies Cry, How Parents Feel and What You Can Do About It by Sheila Kitzinger, Carroll and Brown, UK, 2005

Characteristically caring from the lovely Sheila. Practical hints for mums, and importantly dads, with insightful explanations.

The Fussy Baby Book: Parenting Your High-Need Child from Birth to Five by William Sears, MD, and Martha Sears, Harper Thorsons, UK, 2005

The 'attachment parenting' duo weigh in. But you may want to wait and see if you need this book because you may not have a 'high-need' baby, just a new one.

getting your baby to sleep

Ask your health visitor how you can recognise when to put your baby down to sleep; if you need a 'routine'; and how to wrap your baby if you haven't learnt already – as mentioned, this is the secret to a sleeping bub.

⊚ Try to get into a settling pattern when your baby is due to go down so that they start to associate certain things with relaxing and going to sleep (most of the hints given earlier for settling a crying baby are relevant here). Some people even take their baby for a ride in the car, but that's an expensive habit to get into and not great if you're exhausted.

⊚ Use a dimmed light or a soft lamp to feed by at night-time, and avoid talking to or stimulating the baby or they'll think it's play time.

⊚ Try stroking your baby's head or tummy, patting their back rhythmically, or making soothing hushing sounds if they are overtired (you can do this when they're in their cot). Overtiredness is a common cause of crying, and paradoxically can make it harder for the baby to get to sleep. A baby can seem 'hyped up' when really they're overtired. Soothing methods that involve walking, rocking or singing may end up stimulating the baby more, so that it is harder to get them to sleep.

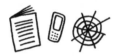

more info on **getting your baby to sleep**

See 'Parenting Support' in the Contacts and Resources chapter at the end of this book for contacts. And also see the Sleeping chapter in the sequel to this book, *The Rough Guide to Babies and Toddlers*.

Sleep Right, Sleep Tight: A Practical, Proven Guide to Solving Your Baby's Sleep Problems by Rosey Cummings, Karen Houghton and Le Ann Williams, Doubleday, Australia, 2008
> Written by hands-on staff at an Australian parenting centre. A wonderful book it covers how to develop a sleeping pattern, settling techniques, and steps and strategies that are easy to follow even if you're exhausted.

The No-Cry Sleep Solution: Gentle Ways to Help Your Baby Sleep Through the Night by Elizabeth Pantley, McGraw-Hill Contemporary, UK, 2002
> A third way between letting babies cry themselves to sleep and becoming a sleep-deprived martyr. Helps you review and choose sleep solutions and create your own sleep plan, and gives you a few tips for better sleeping yourself. With sleep charts, plans and routines.

sudden infant death syndrome (sids)

The cause of SIDS (formerly called cot death) is not known. Basically what happens is that the baby stops breathing. Eighty percent of SIDS deaths happen in the first six months. SIDS is now even rarer than it used to be because there is general agreement on how to lower the risk, and continuing research.

◎ Sleep your baby on their back, never the tummy. Newborn babies who tend to vomit can be firmly propped on their side with some rolled-up hand towels on either side, or tucked in firmly with a swaddling blanket, so that they can't roll onto their back. Ask the hospital midwives to show you, if you're unsure. Roll the baby's head to the side if that is comfortable.

◎ Place your baby in the 'feet to foot' position (that is, with their feet at the foot of the cot) to prevent them wriggling down under the covers.

◎ Don't cover your baby's head when they're sleeping or have soft toys, bumpers or bedding such as duvets and pillows in the cot or crib, which could cover a tiny face during a sleep.

◎ Don't smoke during pregnancy or your baby's first year or allow anyone to smoke in the house or the car where the baby is.

After about the age of six months, babies may stop sleeping in exactly the position you place them in and put themselves into all sorts of positions (bum up in the air is a particularly entertaining one). Some older babies roll onto their tummies during sleep, and by this age they should be able to move themselves if they get into any breathing trouble.

A few younger babies who are always placed in the same position to sleep may develop a flattened or unusual head shape. In most cases this does no harm and 'fixes itself' before school starts. Current SIDS research still indicates babies should be put to sleep on their backs, but you can change the head positions for each sleep, turning the face to one side, then to the other, then to looking straight up. (If your baby always seems to turn its head to face out into the room, you can alternate putting the baby at different ends of the cot, so their head isn't always in the one position.) And if your baby's head seems to be oddly shaped or crooked, have it checked out by a paediatrician for your peace of mind.

There is NO link between childhood vaccinations and SIDS.

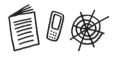

more info on **sids**

fsid.org.uk
The website of the charity the Foundation for the Study of Infant Deaths. Click on 'Looking after your baby' for oodles of info on safe sleeping positions and sleepwear (see also Week 40's 'Wrap Party' box). There are useful FAQ and Ask the Experts sections, plus an online video.

CHILD HEALTH CLINICS

Somewhere near you is a child health clinic. You may not have noticed it, but it's about to become a part of your life. Depending on where you live, it may be found at your local Health Centre, it may be attached to your GP practice or it may be a completely separate building just down your road.

The health visitors are based at the child health clinics and are required to visit you when the baby is eleven days old. They usually ring and make an appointment to visit you at home. Your hospital or home midwife will have notified them of your birth.

After that first home visit, you will go regularly to the clinic for appointments with the health visitor to check on your baby's general progress (and how you're doing yourself), to weigh and measure your baby, and to ask a ton of questions about baby care.

You should be able to contact your health visitor at any time during the day and they are generally supportive and helpful with any problems or queries you have and are trained to pick up any problems you may not have noticed. If you have a personality clash or a problem with one particular health visitor ask to see one of their colleagues. They'll probably be as relieved as you are.

Child health clinics usually run new parent postnatal programmes, and can put you in touch with parents' groups, mothers' groups and playgroups. They are good places to find pamphlets or posters about local toy libraries, babies' and children's activity groups, and other services, and they often have noticeboards for people to advertise baby clothes or equipment and babysitting.

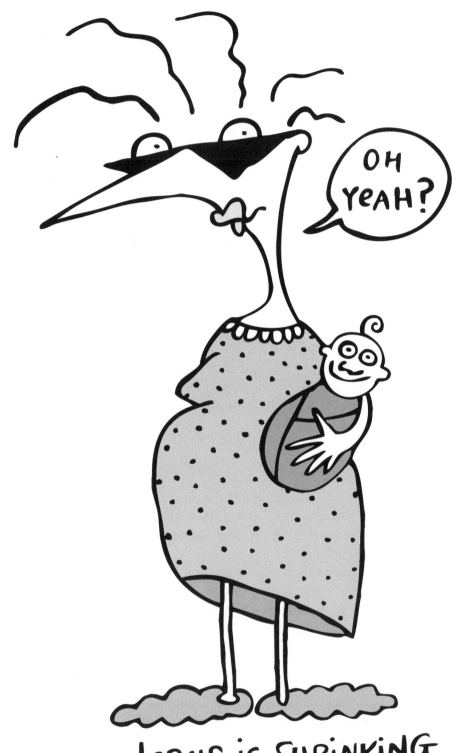

what's going on

Your uterus is slowly shrinking, contracting each time you breastfeed, or a little more quickly if drugs are administered to shrink it because you're not breastfeeding – it will be back to its right size in about six weeks. Your muscles and ligaments are all adjusting to the loss of relaxin. Retained fluid may still cause puffy ankles and sore joints, especially the knees, and the problem may stick around for some weeks.

Your baby will be starting to grow at a very fast rate. Sometimes it will seem as if you can notice the difference in a day. Your baby can't see very much because their eyes only focus on things within 30 centimetres, and probably isn't smiling yet: this can make a baby seem very passive and not much fun. But before you know it they'll be staring at you with eyes on full-beam, and within about five weeks you'll be seeing gorgeous gummy grins.

WEEK 42

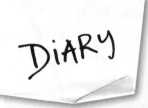

DIARY

I'm writing all this down later, as the week after Matilda's birth was a hideous haze of drug-addled fatigue and incomprehension. I know I'm supposed to say it was a wonderful, joyous time full of relief and the tinkling laughter of well-dressed parents overwhelmed with a sense of achievement, and that sort of palaver, but it was a bloody nightmare.

Poor old Matilda, the least experienced of us all in the ways of the world, was plonked into a room with two sleep-deprived, deeply gobsmacked parents, one of whom was on drugs and a trolley, wired up to a drip and in pain, and the other of whom didn't have any bosoms. Not that we weren't happy to see Matilda. But I kept looking at her through a veil of painkillers that seemed to deaden brain feelings as well as pain.

I just couldn't connect Matilda with the baby who used to be inside me. At first she just didn't feel like mine – maybe it was because we hadn't gone on the journey of labour together, and I hadn't felt her being born. Maybe it was because of the drugs or the shock, or because having a real live baby actually felt hyper-real.

Matilda looked exactly like Geoff without the five o'clock shadow. She had fists that could be gently opened into small starfish, and mother-of-pearl fingernails, and a very serious expression. She was so tiny and lovable, and so mysterious and passive. It felt like we were constantly doing things TO her – trying to breastfeed her, changing nappies, wrapping and unwrapping her. Her vulnerable 'littleness' made me feel very protective and scared at the same time.

Geoff was in shock for days afterwards, I think. He kept trying to make everyone cups of tea and explain footy to a very deadpan Matilda. We spent ages looking at Matilda's little face, wondering what she was thinking. 'Probably "get me another bosom"', said Geoff.

I was in a room with two other new mums and their bubs. Matilda's bed was a plastic tub on a trolley next to mine. The midwives were mostly wonderful, especially the ones who would change the sheets and help tidy up around my bed. They'd come round and lift Matilda up and help me try to breastfeed. But this was way tougher than I'd expected, even with a supportive midwife by my side, and with one of the less sympathetic ones it was pretty traumatic. The gruffer types would grab Matilda with one hand and my breast with the other and bring them together with the force of somebody applauding heartily. After this tense-making and confronting behaviour, often accompanied by barked instructions, they would push down on my shoulders and command 'Relax! You're supposed to enjoy it!', or pull me into a position a previous midwife had insisted was completely wrong.

One midwife was so bad we held our breath when she came into the room. Literally bursting through the door like Cranky Bart in a bad Western, she stomped across to turn off the call button and jabbed her finger at the wall so hard she injured herself.

Shaking her finger and glowering, she stood over us and asked 'What do you want?'

'My painkiller was due an hour ago', I said.

She reached into her pocket for the tablet, slapped it into my palm and stomped off again. 'Just call if you need anything', she snarled, and slammed the door.

Yeah, right. Maybe if I were on FIRE.

After two solid days of Matilda waking up to be breastfed every four hours, a feed which would take about an hour or more each time, I hadn't had more than two hours or so of sleep in a row. And as a person who needs nine or ten hours' sleep a day, this was taking its toll. I did what I always do when I'm tired. I cried and cried.

It just felt like I couldn't cope, couldn't function with the immobility and pain and feeding the baby, if I didn't get some proper sleep. If they took Matilda away for a few hours, to give me a chance to sleep, they would bring her back when she was really hungry and screaming her head off – so she would be all worked up and unsettled and harder to feed and full of wind afterwards, which meant more crying.

Anyway, it all culminated in me weeping uncontrollably after a bumbling attempt to feed Matilda with razor-painful nipples (one had a crack nobody could see except me) and watching a couple of midwives taking my baby away and telling me to sleep as they closed the door behind them. I was almost hysterical thinking 'What's the point of sleeping? It will only be two and a half hours at the most! I may as well stay awake and go mad.'

And then I said to Geoff 'They're all standing outside the room saying I can't cope and I've got postnatal depression. It's not the blues, I'm just overtired!' (Not to mention a touch paranoid.)

Well, they sent for a lactation consultant, who turned up looking starched and sympathetic, and I decided if she was the specialist I would just listen to her advice and ignore any conflicting info from each shift of midwives. (By this time I was wearing a rather firm maternity bra as my bosoms kept swelling up like melons.) This turned out to be the best move to make, as the things she suggested really did seem to help. AND what's more, she could see the nipple crack. Well, she said she could.

So many people are getting rushed out of hospital long before their milk even comes in, and having trouble when they arrive home with nobody to help. As far as breastfeeding goes, the only advice that you ever get is people saying 'persevere', in different ways – this doesn't always help if you don't know HOW to persevere.

I rang Beck every day I was in hospital (three days) to tell her how tired and incompetent I felt. She sent in vitamin B, herbal tonics and stern instructions to get out into the fresh air.

Matilda just lay wrapped up in a blanket looking at everything as if she were trying to memorise it. 'Well, sunshine', I said to her, 'I'm sure I'll get better at this caper.' Matilda presumably was thinking 'I'd like some more of that bosom business, if it's all the same to you, Leaky.'

info

postnatal depression (pnd)

what is it?

Most women experience what is known as the 'baby blues' – feeling weepy and sad – often on about day 4 after giving birth, when the 'happy hormones' go and the prolactin kicks in for real milk production. For most women these blues last only a few days, but some find that the depression stays, or returns, and gets worse. It's hard to decide where the baby blues end and postnatal depression begins, so figures for new mothers experiencing PND vary from one in ten to more than half of all new mums. Recently there has been some research into the incidence of PND in the partners of new mothers, with early findings suggesting that it could affect some men in the same way.

what causes PND?

No one knows why PND affects some women more than others, but hormones seem to be the main culprits. Oestrogen and progesterone levels drop rapidly after childbirth, which may trigger depression in a similar way to fluctuating hormone levels causing PMS (pre-menstrual syndrome). There's some evidence that it runs in families. The following are all recognised as contributing factors in PND and logical reasons why you may feel down.

⊚ A traumatic birth – this can cause shock and disappointment.

⊚ Exhaustion – childbirth wears you out; so do visitors and trying to follow any kind of schedule once you have a baby. One of the reasons for exhaustion is that your volume of blood has suddenly been cut by 30 percent so a lesser volume is reaching your muscles than they have become used to, making them tire easily and feel weak. It takes a few weeks for your body to readjust to this. Sleep is one of the first things to suffer once the baby is born, and if you are depressed you can suffer from insomnia so you're unable to take advantage of even the ludicrously short sleep periods available.

⊚ Frustrating or bad hospital experiences – you might feel you need to get away from all the prodding, the unfamiliar cramped surroundings and the artificial air.

⊚ Anxiety about coping – whether this is your first baby or you have other children to look after, going home can seem overwhelming and terrifying when you think about how much you have to do.

⊚ A sense of failure – this can arise from feeling unable to cope with all the things you think you 'have' to do to be a good mother; disappointment if the birth didn't go according to plan; or feeling that you have somehow failed as a woman if you are having problems feeding and settling your baby. In reality, almost EVERYONE has a problem at some point.

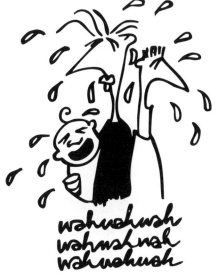

⊚ A health problem – most new mothers will suffer from at least one following the birth: backache, fatigue, mastitis (infection of the milk ducts), painful episiotomy stitches, massive sleep deprivation. Feeling physically unwell adds to depression.

⊚ Ennui – after spending nine months on the high of anticipating seeing your baby for the first time, you may find yourself feeling underwhelmed by them. It is quite common to think that your baby is less than gorgeous or scintillating company until you have had time to bond emotionally. Tiny, new babies are very passive – there's none of the cooing, extended eye contact and sticking their heads up out of flower pots we associate with babies (and greeting cards) for a few weeks or months yet. The guilt you experience when you feel bored by, or distant from, your baby only adds to the depression.

⊚ Loss of individual identity – before the birth, everyone is focused on the pregnant woman and how she is feeling, and afterwards many women feel that they are less important to their family and friends as all attention is on the baby. You may feel as if people have stopped seeing you as an individual and now see you only as a mother.

⊚ Perfectionist or anxious approach to life – PND appears more in people who tend to worry or are perfectionists. Many women feel disappointed in themselves if they have always dealt with things to exacting standards in their professional and social lives and suddenly feel unable to reach that level of 'perfection' in motherhood.

⊚ Subsequent pregnancies – PND is more common in women who already have children. Having to look after older children as well as a new baby is likely to place even tighter constraints on the time you have to yourself and to get enough rest. It can be scary wondering how you'll cope.

⊚ Loneliness – if everyone you know is busy with their own lives and yours revolves around the baby, you may feel as though you are missing out on other things.

⊚ A feeling of being trapped in this lifestyle for the rest of your days – 'Why on earth did I have a baby?'

Signs and symptoms:

⊚ the blues persist for more than a couple of weeks, and there are few or no good feelings

⊚ sleeplessness

⊚ lack of appetite

⊚ low self-esteem

⊚ confusion and/or panic attacks

⑥ sadness or feeling 'flat'

⑥ feeling angry or aggressive towards yourself or your baby

⑥ feeling wildly out of your depth.

strategies

⑥ Set up a support network of family, friends and professionals – accept help from others rather than feeling as if you have to prove you're capable by doing it all yourself. Remember that in sensible cultures babies are looked after by an extended family or even a whole tribe of people from the moment they're born. We weren't meant to do it alone.

⑥ Look after yourself – use the time when your baby sleeps to rest instead of catching up on all the things you think you should have done such as the housework; treat yourself to things that help you feel pampered and relaxed such as a massage or haircut.

⑥ Get some fresh air – gentle exercise such as walking or yoga, with or without the baby, is calming and releases energy. Try to spend a little time each day realising it IS day, and not just sleeping, eating and feeding the baby in a twilight, indoor world.

⑥ Get together with other new mums – contact the women in your childbirth class, join a postnatal exercise class or ask your health visitor about groups for new mothers.

⑥ Ask your GP to rule out a thyroid problem that could cause similar symptoms to PND.

⑥ If you feel your depression is a deeper problem or that you cannot cope any longer, discuss your feelings with your GP. If you have a partner, they should come to the GP with you. If not, you might like to ask your mum, sister or a friend. Before you go, write down a list of all the symptoms that you are experiencing. Your GP will be able to offer various treatments that may help, such as counselling, cognitive therapy, oestrogen or progesterone supplements, or perhaps antidepressant medication. For most mothers, this will be enough to set them on the road to recovery: the bad days will get fewer and less upsetting and the good days become more numerous. However, occasionally postnatal depression may be unusually difficult and not respond to treatment, in which case you may be referred to a specialist team who will be able to offer you more intensive talking therapies, or you may be admitted to hospital or a clinic. Depending on whether they feel it will help you recover, you may be able to take your baby with you into the clinic.

⑥ Be aware that your partner, if you have one, might also have the blues. They might benefit from counselling or special help as well, and it's a good step for the baby's sake too.

Any thoughts that you might self-harm or hurt the baby or that you are hearing voices should be reported to your doctor straight away. Help and treatment will sort this out.

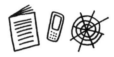

more info on **postnatal depression (pnd)**

You can recover from PND; you need to reach out. See 'Parenting Support' in the Contacts and Resources chapter at the back of this book. Any of these servives can help you. Your GP will also be able to refer you for help. (Special info for dads is at the end of the list.)

Parentline
0808 800 2222
The Samaritans
08457 90 90 90
Both helplines have 24-hour counselling services.

Association for Post-Natal Illness
apni.org
Helpline: 020 7386 0868 (Mon–Fri 10 a.m. to 2 p.m.)
The Association for Post-Natal Illness has a phone hotline, information leaflets and a network of volunteers who've been through it and can help you on the phone or by email.

mama.co.uk
Helpline: 0845 120 3746 (Mon–Fri 7 p.m. to 10 p.m.)
Founded by Esther Rantzen, the Meet a Mum Association aims to help mums who are depressed or isolated, or have moved to a new area, find other mums for support. The network is patchy as yet, but the site has some useful information on postnatal depression: from the main page, click 'About PND'.

mind.org.uk

Helpline: 0845 766 0163 (Mon–Fri 9.15 a.m. to 5.15 p.m.)
The National Association for Mental Health is the leading mental health charity in England and Wales. Phone counsellors can talk to you about PND, and recommend a support group in your area. On the main page of the website, search 'postnatal depression'.

mythyroid.com

Postpartum thyroiditis is often misdiagnosed as PND. From the main page, click 'Post Partum Thyroiditis' for information, including the latest scientific research.

Feelings After Birth: The NCT Book of Postnatal Depression by Heather Welford, NCT, UK, 2002

Useful little book with clear explanations, treatments, case studies and suggested resources for further help.

dad.info

Click on 'Health', 'Your health', then 'Post-natal depression: dads' for info about postnatal depression in dads, what you can do about it, and links to other support services.

My Journey to Her World: How I Coped with My Wife's Postnatal Depression by Michael Lurie, Grosvenor House Publishing, UK, 2007

An English author tells his story. For men who want to read about the bloke's experience and for women to understand a partner's point of view.

what's going on You're tired. You're still trying to get breastfeeding to be smooth and easy for both of you. Your body has started to heal. You're trying to cope with visitors as well as looking after the baby. You're in a dreamworld. FORGET THE BLOODY HOUSEWORK.

You'll find that the tiny outfits that fitted in the first week start to get too small (the baby's outfits, not yours). Your baby's eye colour may be changing, and the baby hair may be falling out, to be slowly replaced by a new lot. After another couple of weeks the shrivelled, stumpy bit of umbilical cord will come away from the navel and you'll see what your baby's tummy button looks like. The hands will stay curled in fists for a few weeks yet. Length and weight? Oh who cares.

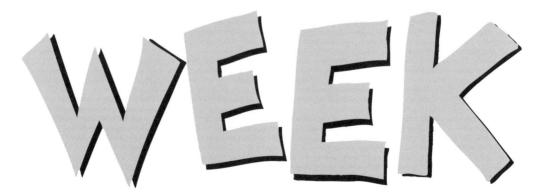

Forget the statistics for a minute. Every day your baby's getting closer to becoming a social being who sleeps more and doesn't cry so much (although the amount of crying reaches a peak at about six weeks old). So every day you're getting closer to the time when you can get some more sleep. Live in the moment, as babies do. Forget about what you have to do tomorrow or next week. Take it one day, even one hour, at a time, sister.

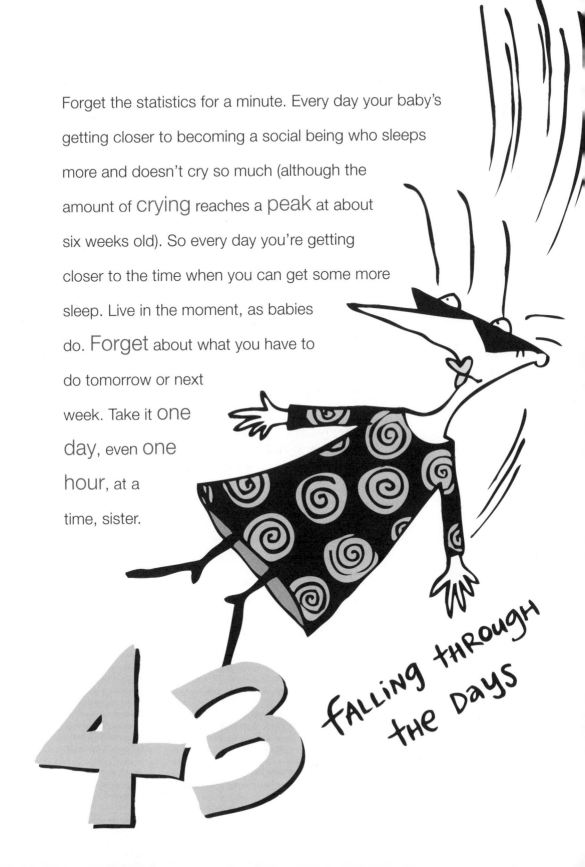

43 FALLING THROUGH THE DAYS

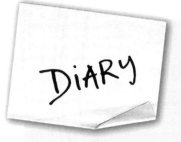
DIARY

The only thing that really helped me to get a grip on the blues was getting home into an environment with fresh air, and the chance to sit outside even if I felt like a zombie and was not at all sure what to do with a tiny baby. It was kind of comforting having the hospital midwives nearby, but nothing like being at home. Besides, Jill came every day for a visit.

I was so tired in those early days I thought it would never end. I cried towards the end of every day when fatigue started to overwhelm me. We discouraged visitors because, rather than offering help, so many seemed to need attention. The visitors who were really helpful were the ones who would pick up the baby or otherwise make themselves useful around the house.

Aunt Julie has forgotten about tiny babies. I remember that Julie didn't get hold of me until I was three months old, when Mum died – so she's all at sea with such a small bundle as Matilda and convinced that every snuffle means malaria, the plague or convulsions.

All at once I felt lonely, but too tired to make the effort to reach out to friends. It seemed like I was living in a fog of fatigue, robotically waking, feeding the baby and trying to sleep again; like some kind of demented wet nurse on Valium. Beck told Geoff to make me go outside for a walk in the afternoons so at least I would feel like I knew which was day and which was night, and that there was an outside world. This helped a lot.

Matilda was sleeping in the pram every night because she seemed so TINY in the cot – until this morning when Geoff goes in to see her and this weeny, supposedly immobile baby has wiggled her way to the top end of the pram and is millimetres away from sticking her head down into a dangerous gap. This gives us a big shock, so from now on Matilda will be in the cot at night: the rate she's growing, she'll soon fill it up.

Every time I think about how I told everyone I'd start work part-time in eight weeks, I'm overwhelmed with stress and anxiety. I've got to try to go with the flow. Matilda is waking up every four hours, which is not too bad compared with some babies, but I am still absolutely stonkered from lack of sleep. Not only do you have to live day by day, but sometimes hour by hour, without looking forward or back.

Suze described the first few weeks as 'falling through the days', and she had her sister and mother to help. Geoff and I don't have any help, but at least there's two of us. Even so we're lucky if one of us has had a shower by nightfall and somebody can make the dinner. For a while there the washing machine and dryer seemed to be going all day long and there were mountains of nappies...

Why didn't I think of it before! We've swapped to disposable nappies and are using the cloth ones as essential, all-purpose shoulder drapes, wipes, bum cleaners and nummy folded surfaces for the changing table. Matilda sleeps up to an extra hour or two at night with a disposable nappy on, and I decide she might as well be more comfortable in the daytime as well.

There is a certain guilt in this, and we expect to be raided by the Baby Police or the Environment Squad at any moment. I listen to a caller who rings up a radio station and says that women who use formula baby milk and disposable nappies are 'lazy'. About 100 people rang and said they'd like to kill her. Hurrah! I do feel guilty about the environment, so I've joined Greenpeace in Matilda's name.

Breastfeeding is easier than it was at the beginning, but Matilda still has a lot of trouble attaching, especially to the left nipple (which is odd because it has always been her father's favourite). The scar and pain from the caesarean make everything harder, including finding a good position for breastfeeding. I need two pillows to balance her on, and how to feed her insouciantly and – arrgghhh – in public is a complete mystery to me.

Her 'wind' is still bad and she cries and cries inconsolably after all the daytime feeds, really screaaaaaaming in the ear of whichever parent is holding her: it's extraordinary how loud a baby can yell. It's so hard not being able to take the pain away, and hard to remain patient with the crying. Yesterday I found myself raising my voice in frustration and saying angrily 'Shut up!', which is about as useful as saying 'Act your age' and as soothing as a lovely death-metal song. Luckily I got hold of myself, stopped raising my voice, and just ended up crying as well. I've read the stuff on crying in books and websites over and over. But nothing really helps. I just have to keep saying 'This will end, this will end.'

I ring a breastfeeding organisation's local contact and ask 'How do I tell, when the baby cries three hours after a feed, whether she's hungry or there's something else wrong?'

'Just feed her when she cries', she says.

'But it may be too soon and she isn't hungry', I reply, knowing full well from experience that if I feed Matilda after two hours she'll projectile vomit. Which, by the way, is such an extremely shocking moment it makes you draw your breath in and open your eyes really wide like a pantomime actor called Dame Chortlepants.

'Some women feed their babies every hour, 24 hours a day', she says.
'But how do they do that without going mad?' I ask.
'Oh,' she says airily, 'they just do.'
How very marvellous.

I'm supposed to be doing all these exercises to help the post-caesarean body, but I might as well be told to read a couple of novels a day – there is just no time at all. And when there is, I'm afraid I need to be horizontal, usually with ear plugs in, my head under the pillow, an eye mask on, dreaming of getting stuck into a big fat glass of chardy.

early outings

Baby excursions in the first few weeks can be a tad gruelling, and you should never feel you have to go anywhere. It's good just to take your time at home, gradually getting to know your baby, apart from going for short walks in the fresh air, or sitting in the park.

One of the worst things about the early forays out the front door is that you are giving your first public performances as a new parent. Heaps of new mums cry with frustration the first few times they try to collapse that damn new pram into the car or get off a bus with a baby AND some shopping. After a few days they can do it backwards and upside down in the dark with one foot. It's just a matter of practice.

If you're still getting the hang of changing nappies, breastfeeding and working out why the hell your baby is crying, going out can be a bit stressful. Also, the virtually full-time nature of new-baby care doesn't change just because you're out. Your baby will still need to feed, be burped, have their nappy and maybe clothes changed, be settled down to sleep, feed some more, sleep – or whatever happens at home – while you're trying to have a cup of tea, stay awake and sound intelligible, or get home before dark.

Don't worry: it gets easier every time.

so what's in the bag?

The big bag that all parents haul about with them contains whatever you need to change and feed the baby. Its exact contents alter as the baby grows older, reaching peak capacity during toddler years, when it includes all the nappy-changing equipment plus sundry snacks, drinks, security blankets and can't-leave-the-house-without-Binky-type toys.

The newborn-baby bag will need to contain:

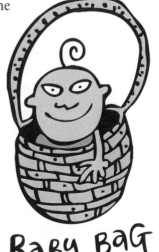

BaBy BaG

◎ nappies (and snappy fasteners, and maybe plastic over-pants, if you use certain cloth ones) – usually three or four depending on how long you plan to be out (even those who prefer cloth nappies and a water wash at home can find it more convenient to use disposable nappies and commercial baby wipes for excursions)

◎ one or two changes of outfit in case the going-out clothes get poo on them, which is more likely if you have cloth nappies

◎ a surface to change the nappies on – some bags have a built-in changing pad; if yours doesn't, a swaddling blanket with a folded nappy on top or a waterproof-backed changing sheet on the floor works just as well

◎ whatever you use to clean your baby's bottom at changing time: a container of water or a bottle of nappy-change lotion, and some cotton wool balls or a packet of baby wipes

◎ nappy-rash cream to form a barrier between wee and skin

◎ a few plastic bags to bring dirty nappies and clothes home in – re-using supermarket bags is ideal, but check they're not ripped, and tie a knot or two in them for safety until you use them (then tie them up firmly again) in case another baby or a toddler gets hold of them

◎ swaddling blankets or muslin squares to wrap the baby in, depending on the weather

◎ maybe a sun hat if it's hot, or cap if it's cold

◎ a couple of clean cloth nappies or muslin squares to drape over the shoulder of anyone holding the baby as a vomit guard or chin wiper

◎ a couple of toys suitable for little babies – because newborn babies see mostly contrasts rather than colours during the early months, black and white toys are good, and they also like those plastic rings in a chain that you see dangling on prams, which pharmacies sell

☺ bibs if you are already using them

☺ sterilised bottles of freshly made up but cold formula with protective sterilised caps if you are bottlefeeding, kept in an insulated bottle-carrier. Better still, take the right measurement of cooled boiled water in a sterilised bottle (with a sterilised cap on) and add formula from a sachet to it (follow sachet instructions) while you are out, then heat it up. This prevents bacteria forming. Never take bottles of hot formula out and never try to keep them hot. Bottles should be drunk within an hour of being heated. Formula sachets are more expensive than bulk formula, and check the instructions because you may have to make up a larger amount than your baby usually drinks.

The main thing about the big bag is this: have it packed and ready to go at all times. Getting around sleeping, feeding and changing times and actually out of the house is a finely tuned exercise in time management. There is no time for delay while you hunt about looking for things to put in the bag. The exception to this, of course, is if you are bottlefeeding, in which case you need to take freshly prepared bottles in an insulated bottle-carrier.

To have the bag ready, you need duplicates of nappy-change items – probably in smaller, more portable-sized containers or packages than you use at home. You also need to remember to restock the bag when you're home from an outing. Get used to bringing it in every single time in case the car goes away with it, or you need to restock before you go out in the car again.

As well as the big bag, you may need somewhere portable for the baby to sleep (although if it's a short visit newborn babies can be just as comfortable sleeping in their parents' arms as anywhere). You can take a carrycot (the body of some prams converts to a carrycot, which is handy for visiting), or a quilted baby bag, or a lambswool, or a Moses basket. If you set the baby on the floor, don't forget to draw everyone's attention to this, so the baby doesn't get trodden or sat on. And remember that babies not sleeping in their own (safe) cot must be kept in sight at all times. Be very aware of other people's toddlers and pets as a potential danger: they may not be used to babies or take any notice of warnings.

You can wear your baby in a sling as a charming fashion accessory, with optional vomiting feature, so long as the baby is not going to be in a smoky environment, and someone can help you when the baby gets too heavy.

Leaving the house gets easier when feeding and sleeping turn into something resembling a routine. About when they're asking for their first pocket money, maybe.

your post-baby body

You've either had a major body shock (labour), or surgery akin to a serious injury in terms of damage and bruising (a caesarean). People can be jailed for making workers sleep as little as you are. You're keeping a new baby alive. This is no time for star jumps. You don't need a strict exercise regime, or a demanding plan, or a personal trainer who wakes you up before dawn and shouts at you.

dos and don'ts for new-mum exercise

⊚ Realise that your body may never be the same again. It's less likely to 'go back to where it was' the older you are. Big tummies can last for weeks, for months or forever. Post-caesarean tummies can continue to have a double 'bump'.

⊚ Understand that pregnancy changes breasts especially forever, whether or not you can breastfeed.

⊚ Acknowledge that it takes weeks to lose the extra blood volume, fluids, fat tissue and other reserves you needed for pregnancy. Breastfeeding helps some women lose weight, but not everybody.

⊚ Accept that the key goal is fitness and vitality, not slimness or a magic weight or dress size.

⊚ Don't compare your body with a celebrity's. Or with your sister's or your mum's or a friend's. Everyone is different. And celebrities lie through their whitey-white teeth about what they did to lose weight and how healthy it was. They are demented.

⊚ Don't obsess about what your body looks like.

⊚ Don't plan to exercise when the baby is asleep. In the early days, sleep when the baby sleeps.

⊚ Ask your GP at the six-week check-up about any activity you plan to get into.

⊚ Wait until you feel ready to start.

⊚ Get fresh air and sunshine whenever possible – much better to get out and walk than to watch TV aerobics or be inside a gym.

⊚ Consider free or cheap exercise: walking, dancing in the lounge, swimming at the local pool (maybe on a season's pass), joining a fun sports team with other mums or locals.

⑥ Organise a walking group with friends or a new-mums' group: you're more likely to go. Get an off-road three-wheel pram if that will help.

⑥ Keep things moderate. Vigorous or high-impact, high-energy gym routines or running can make you sore and haggard. Fatigue is a special risk if you're breastfeeding.

⑥ Don't feel you have to pay for a special programme with a special baby- or mum-relevant name. It's better for your baby to go on a walk with you and hear you chatting to them. These 'programmes' can give you unrealistic expectations about how quickly your body will recover. You still have a lot of the hormone relaxin, and this can cause back and pelvic pain or other stresses and strains.

⑥ Don't give up if you can't do an hour a day – do half an hour a day, or an hour three or four times a week or whenever you can.

⑥ Don't give up because you have to wrangle toddlers as well as a baby. Get a double pram for walks, or ask for babysitting help so that you can get active and have some fun.

⑥ Keep up the calories. You need to eat well if you are convalescing from childbirth, breastfeeding or exercising – and here you are, possibly doing all three. Eat.

⑥ Don't dismiss your needs. If you feel you can't take 'me-time', look at exercise this way: a fit mum with a healthy immune system is good for the kids.

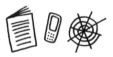

more info on **your post-baby body**

The Body Shape Bible by Trinny and Susannah, Phoenix, UK, 2008
>   It can be far less stressful to accept you can change your style a bit, than to expect to retain the dream of your pre-baby body. The TV tough-talkers speak sense about dressing to flatter your body shape. And there's lots of helpful pics.

An Unfit Mother: How to Get Your Health, Shape and Sanity Back After Childbirth by Kate Cook with Lucy Wyndham-Read, Collins, UK, 2005
>   Funny, and acknowledging that tiredness is the death of good intentions, this book gives suggestions for simple exercises and healthy and organic eating rather than dieting. It's realistic about what you can hope to achieve in the early weeks.

post-baby sex

Because the doctors say 'No sex until after the six-week check-up', a lot of chaps think 'Whacko, that night my sex life will resume and go on like it used to!' Oh dear.

Well, some people do resume energetic and regular rumpy-pumpy pronto, but a great many women (yes, it's more likely to be the women) are feeling too leaky, bulky, sick of their body being required on demand for feeding and seemingly everything else, and desperate to adjust to hideous broken-sleep patterns and the draining, droning tiredness, to be able to find any clean knickers, let alone put on lingerie. Generally. Not. Up. For. It.

Hormonal contraception or ordinary old post-baby hormone changes can also throw a woman's libido down the loo. Vaginal bleeding can go on for up to six weeks after the birth, so most women don't feel all that frisky after a six-week-long 'period' sitting on maternity pads.

Even with a straightforward birth, or one that didn't require stitches for a tear or cut to the vagina, the general area needs time to heal. Perhaps if men could imagine their penis being stretched to ten times its normal size, then being torn down the middle, having an orange being passed through it and being sewn back up again, they might empathise with their partner and understand that some rest and recuperation is required.

Some women who've had a traumatic birth or a long labour and stitches are frightened of having sex. Please talk to your doctor to make sure everything's physically ready, and wait until you're mentally ready. Gentlemen may have to be a little patient. (Of course they may be a bit knocked around themselves in the sleep department.)

Misunderstandings can crop up if you and your partner don't discuss this stuff openly. Here are some she says/he says (or thinks) examples:

He only wants me for sex, so when he kisses and cuddles me I wriggle away because I'm not up for it. (I'm just happy with the cuddle and the kiss.)

He couldn't possibly want sex with me. He saw something come out of my vagina, and I haven't had time to doll myself up for weeks, and I haven't lost my baby tummy. (She doesn't realise she still turns me on.)

She doesn't want me any more. She just wanted the baby. (Of course I still love him and find him attractive. I'm just too exhausted to feel sexy right now.)

I want it to be like it was before. (Things change. That doesn't mean it's bad. Just different.)

Oh my God, I'll never have sex again. (This is temporary.)

Are you awake? (ZZZZZ.)

Are you awake? (ZZZZZ.)

Are you awa— oh forget it. (ZZZZZ.)

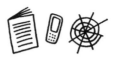

more info on **post-baby sex**

The dad blogs and sites listed in Week 36 have questions or articles on sex during pregnancy and after. So do the pregnancy sites in Week 1 and the parenting sites coming up.

And Baby Makes Three: The Six-Step Plan For Preserving Marital Intimacy and Rekindling Romance After Baby Arrives by John Gottman and Julie Schwartz Gottman, Three Rivers, US, 2007

> Oh My God, I'd rather find the energy to have sex twice than read a book with the phrase 'marital intimacy' in it. But it could be very useful if you're looking to sort out the issues in your head and look for a future together that involves some underpants-off action. American, with suggested dialogue to use when talking to each other. It's quite a sensible and comprehensive relationship manual, at its core.

Love In the Time of Colic: The New Parents' Guide to Getting It On Again by Ian Kerner and Heidi Raykeil, Harper Collins, US, 2009

> Two relationship and lifestyle authors get together (but don't get it ON, as they're married to other people) to suggest why no sex might be happening. There's some elementary female and male psychology, plus a few raunchy options for getting over the exhaustion and into some other positions. It's American, so be warned, you'll get references to Billy Crystal rather than Billy Connolly and 'date night' rather than popping out to the pub.

WHAT WILL YOU DO WITH ALL YOUR FREE TIME?

One survey of new mums showed that they spent on average, per week, 16 hours less on personal grooming, got 8 hours less sleep and had 20 hours less for socialising than before; and that they fed their babies eight or ten times a day, for an average of half an hour each time. A new mum is usually the person primarily responsible for the household's cleaning, cooking, washing and any other children. The only reason she doesn't eat her husband's head after sex is she doesn't have the time.

and btw – stuff that's good to know

⑥ Say it loud and say it proud: IF THE CHOICE IS BETWEEN SLEEPING AND THE HOUSEWORK, SLEEP.

⑥ If a certain website, book, theory or person is making you feel guilty, avoid it or them.

⑥ If your baby screams blue murder when you do the bath thing, avoid the stress. It can be much more restful to get in the big bath together and cuddle while you wash, or to just wash bits of your baby with a flannel. And you don't have to do it every day.

⑥ After a few weeks your bosoms will stop being so hard and full before each feed, and be much floppier, but they are actually producing more and more milk for your growing baby. Don't assume you're running out because your bosoms are softer between feeds: your body's just getting more efficient. And it's common for one breast to produce more milk than the other – or be easier for the baby to 'draw on'.

⑥ If you have committed yourself to other projects and you find that looking after a baby is harder than you thought, try to get out of everything you can, without damaging your work prospects. Or decide which prospects you're prepared to sacrifice, or find ways to get more help with the baby.

⑥ Show friends and family how they can help. Many people, not only blokes, will be feeling inexperienced and tentative, and scared of hurting a small baby. Show them the way, and everyone will have a better time.

PARENTING AND BABY-CARE WEBSITES, MAGAZINES AND BOOKS

parenting websites and magazines

As well as the websites listed below, check out the ones in Week 1, including babycentre.co.uk, askamum.co.uk and the sites of magazines *Babyworld* (babyworld.co.uk) and *Practical Parenting and Pregnancy* (practicalparenting. co.uk).

Mags range from fashion-fussy glossies such as *Junior, Mother and Baby* and *Practical Parenting* to local mags such as *Angels and Urchins* (London) and *ABC* (free in six south-eastern counties).

netmums.com

Type in your postcode to be redirected to a local version of the site that has info about nearby groups, places to go with kids and family-friendly events, as well as nearly-new listings and message boards. There's lots of general parenting info and advice too.

parenting styles

I'm not going to get into the debate here about which parenting approach is best. Be guided by your own philosophy, your needs and the results.

attachmentparenting.org
askdrsears.com

These two websites are starting points for the attachment-parenting philosophy, which advocates a go-with-the-flow style with lots of one-on-one care.

Sleeping Like a Baby by Pinky McKay, Penguin, UK, 2007

Australian Pinky McKay is big on the philosophy of attachment parenting, and this book has her kindly tips and ideas for all things sleep-related, up to the toddler years.

If you want info on how to do 'controlled crying' with an older baby, the stricter and more routine-loving folk such as British authors Gina Ford (*The New Contented Little Baby Book*, Vermilion, UK, 2006), the late Tracy Hogg (*Secrets of the Baby Whisperer*, Ballantine, UK, 2005) and TV's 'Supernanny' Jo Frost (*Confident Baby Care*, Orion, UK, 2007) have what you're looking for.

baby-care books

The Rough Guide to Babies and Toddlers by Kaz Cooke, Rough Guides, UK, 2009

My sequel to *The Rough Guide to Pregnancy* has the same style of info and cartoons. It delivers up-to-date, reliable info on getting through the first weeks; bosoms; bottles; sleeping; crying; coping; the blues; what dads need to know; immunisation; safety; dealing with common illnesses; first food; teething; family food; using the loo; teaching kids how to behave; childcare; exercise; emotional and physical development 0–5; games, toys and activities; being at home; paid work; birthday parties and presents; travel; getting ready for school; and lists of where to go for extra help.

The Great Ormond Street New Baby and Child Care Book by Tessa Hilton with Maire Messenger, Vermilion, UK, 2004

A comprehensive reference from the UK's leading children's hospital that starts at conception and takes you to age five. All the practical info on lookin after a new baby, growth and movement, language development, common medical concerns and why play is important.

The Philosophical Baby by Alison Gopnik, Farrar Straus Giroux, US, 2009

At last somebody has pulled together the latest from the worlds of science and psychology to show us what we know about how babies and little children think. Ms Gopnik, a mother who's also a philosopher, a psychologist and a great writer, explains why 'babies are actually smarter, more thoughtful and more conscious than adults'. All about how although they come with their own potential personalities, their development has to do with how babies learn to love, learn and relate by watching and interracting with us and the world around them.

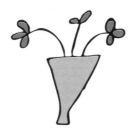

medical and health advice

The following websites and books will give you fast general info on illnesses, health problems, allergies and the like, but remember that they are no substitute for advice from your own doctor.

Baby and Child Health Care by Dr Miriam Stoppard, Dorling Kindersley, UK, 2001

Dr Miriam again – and this really is a book you will want to have on your shelf, hopefully little used and read. The core of the book is an A–Z of common and not so common complaints, first-aid crises ('Nose, foreign body in'), and childhood illnesses: how to spot the symptoms, what you should do first, when you should consult the doctor and what the doctor will do.

ich.ucl.ac.uk

The joint website of the Great Ormond Street Hospital and the Institute of Child Health, University College London, includes fact sheets on various common childhood health problems, handy hints on bringing a child to hospital, a round-up of support groups for families with kids who have certain conditions, advice from child health experts (including an alphabetical archive of 'Dr Jane's' down-to-earth advice on everything from pigeon toes to hayfever) and a glossary of terms you may need to understand.

nhsdirect.nhs.uk

Helpline: 0845 4647

Contact the nurse-led phone line for information or queries on all child health matters. The website has self-help information too. Also useful is the NHS's main portal, nhs.uk, which has masses of relevant information on all aspects of health care.

nhs.uk/planners/birthtofive

Basic guidance from the NHS on various baby essentials, health and development and other key issues for parents.

A NOTE ON 'NATURAL' BABY CARE AND PARENTING

While many of us are interested in natural remedies and solutions, sensible natural therapists understand that some problems will require medical solutions. Especially with small babies, it's always important to get a medical opinion about anything that worries you. In particular, if a baby is listless and floppy, is not putting on weight, or is constantly crying, swift medical advice is very important.

Some of the 'natural' advice given on vaccination can be dangerous. Many websites continue to give information that is outdated by decades, misleading or just plain wrong, such as that childhood vaccinations have mercury in them (they don't); breastfeeding or homeopathic remedies will protect against infectious diseases (absolutely untrue); and a child should only be vaccinated after six months or two years of age (this is dangerous because it leaves babies open to diseases at the very time when they're most vulnerable, and there's no evidence that delaying has any benefit).

Many links on immunisation are to virulently anti-vaccination activists. Many of the claims in like-minded books and sites have been totally discredited or disproven. Also see 'Immunisation' in the Contacts and Resources chapter at the end of the book (and for full info see the Immunisation chapter in *The Rough Guide to Babies and Toddlers*).

more info

thegreenparent.co.uk

The website of *Green Parent* magazine, with articles, forums and blogs on environmental parenting. Has info on organic gardening and ethical shopping but be aware that its blog includes the dangerous suggestion that homeopathy and general health is an alternative to immunisation in preventing certain diseases (it isn't, as the British Homeopathic Association agrees), and it links to an anti-vaccination website which contains wrong information.

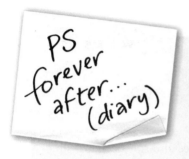

Months down the track after Matilda was born I look back at those first weeks and wonder how anyone does it without going completely mad. Before I had Matilda, when people used to talk about 'lack of sleep' I thought of it as an inconvenience – like staying up too late and having a bit of a hangover. Now I can see why they use sleep deprivation as a method of torture. Good old Matilda is finally sleeping for eight hours straight a night.

'We got a good one, la la la', sings Geoff.

I can't remember a thing about being pregnant but I still look about six months 'gone'. You know how they say you automatically lose weight when you breastfeed? Nope. And you know how they say you'll lose it when you stop breastfeeding, instead? Not me.

Took me about nine months to feel robust again after the caesarean.

I breastfed for three months, then my endometriosis problem started again and I had to go on the Pill. And the Pill goes through into breast milk and that's no good for Matilda. Sadly, she no longer regards my bosoms as something special, but don't get between her and a bottle of formula. She loves the stuff, and she's thriving on it. She also likes to 'chew' rice cereal, severely distressed banana and, well, anything else she can reach.

Some friends have disappeared over the horizon, but I've made new ones among my antenatal classmates and other mums. Thank God for the childless pals who still ring and ask me out. I've hired a lovely young woman called Anna, from a nanny agency, to come and look after Matilda on Mondays and Tuesdays when I'm working part-time from home. I tried to make her wear a French maid's uniform with a white lace cap, but she says she prefers jeans and to get over myself. Matilda chats away happily in baby language to herself and everyone else, and we've weathered our first ear infection (which crept up and clobbered us while we were waiting for the much-warned-about teething that happened later than most people expect). I'm afraid gummy old Matilda is a little backward in the teeth department. At least she's a gifted vomiter or we couldn't hold up our heads at playgroup. (And she's a champion dribbler, I'll have you know.)

Sometimes I just want to stop the clock and have a week off. Sometimes it's fascinating, sometimes it's dead boring. Sometimes I yearn for a few hours just to myself and yet sometimes it's so lonely. And then there's that moment when she smiles and laughs and reaches out for a cuddle and I think it's the most gorgeous feeling I've ever had.

I suppose the next thing I know Matilda'll be crawling, and going to school, and designing a titanium spaceship, or cooking a dinner party for six. But until then there's a lot of cardboard books about duckies to be read, a lot of ludicrous baby headgear to be worn, a lot of walks in the park to be had, and a lot of hurtling round the garden being a fairy-seeking missile. And there's a little indent on the back of her neck that's just perfect for kissing, and if you whisper 'Oofty Goofty' in her ear she might giggle again. So. If you'll excuse me...

The End. (And just the beginning...)

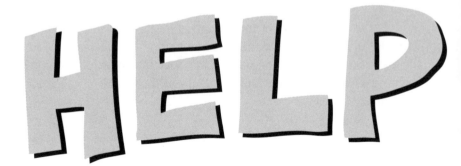

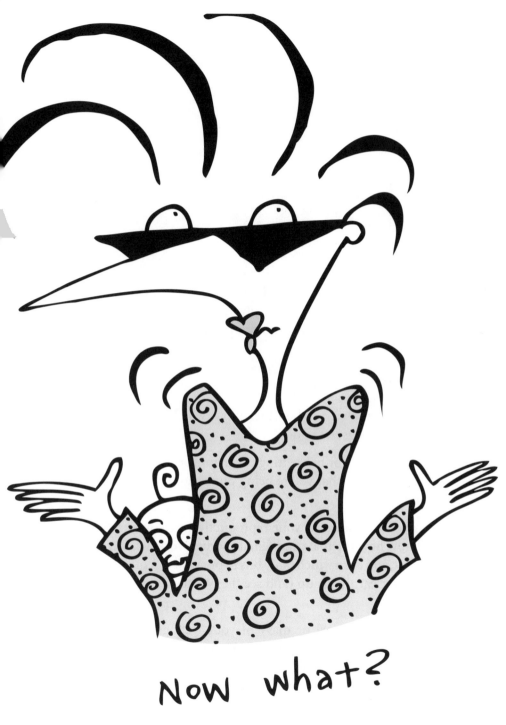

Now what?

FERTILITY TROUBLES

If you seem to be having trouble getting pregnant, don't assume that you or your partner is infertile, meaning physically unable to do your bit to conceive. There are lots of reasons, including random chance, why you might not be pregnant yet.

trying to boost fertility

There are some common ways to boost fertility – which may or may not work for you – and some things *not* to do.

◎ Don't blame yourself for not getting pregnant (or see it as your partner's 'fault'); and don't assume that you're being punished for something you did or didn't do in the past.

◎ Educate yourself about how your reproductive cycle works. Some of us need help to know how the male and female bodies work, when you can and can't get pregnant, and even which body bits to put where. A quick explanation from your GP can clear things up (and see the 'What's Going On' sections of Weeks 1, 2 and 3).

◎ If it helps, keep a journal or diary of your feelings, but don't get too hung up on detailed entries about everything you eat, how much you weigh or your vaginal temperature and the other possible signs of ovulation or pregnancy – that way lies obsession and unhappiness.

◎ Check that you and your partner have a healthy lifestyle and eat well (the first chapter, Getting Ready, has the lowdown on this), but don't start strictly weighing, counting or 'dieting'.

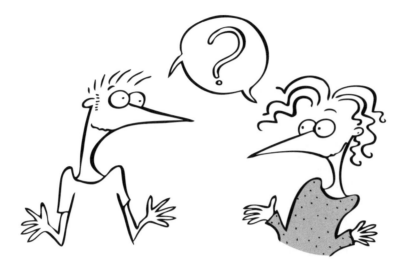

◎ Don't attempt to increase your fertility by doing something drastic such as adopting a vegan, vegetarian or all-organic diet, eating only one kind of food, or fasting or 'detoxing'. This could stress your body and cause ill-health, making it harder to get pregnant.

◎ Stop worrying about getting pregnant (I know, easier said than done). Have sex when you want to, not just when you 'have to'. As long as you're having sex at least two or three times a week you don't need to think about your 'fertile time'.

◎ Cultivate a new, less stressed approach to life: make the time to talk to your partner and friends about your feelings, take a long, hard look at whether you need a new job or fewer jobs – and possibly tell a few people to propel themselves vertically into the nearest body of still water (jump in the lake).

◎ Try some relaxation techniques: yoga and meditation can be really helpful for reducing stress. Choose a popular class with an experienced, accredited yoga teacher who can move you to a pregnancy class if you get lucky.

◎ You could investigate natural therapy treatments such as vitamins and minerals, herbal concoctions or acupuncture from a recognised herbalist, acupuncturist or other practitioner specialising in fertility – these have increased overall health and the chance of getting pregnant for some women. Many medical fertility experts are linking up with respected natural therapists for a combined approach. Always tell your doctor and natural health practitioner (or your chemist) what the other one has recommended you take or do. And don't self-prescribe or automatically follow the advice of friends and family about what to take.

Remember that your herbalist should be a member of the National Institute of Medical Herbalists and your natural therapist should be registered with the Complementary and Natural Healthcare Council (see the Contacts and Resources chapter); your acupuncturist should be a recognised fertility or gynaecological specialist; and your gynaecologist should not wear white shoes (I just think that's plain weird).

if you haven't conceived

If you've been trying to get pregnant without success (after a year when you're under 35, or after six months when you're older) see your GP. They will arrange some basic tests and may refer you to a gynaecologist who specialises in infertility. You won't know if you have a medical problem unless you have it diagnosed. Sometimes doctors don't know exactly what's causing a fertility problem, but they're pretty good at ruling out some things, confirming if you have a problem and suggesting what to try next – so don't stay at home guessing. 'Some (But Not All) of the Possible Causes', coming up, gives some of the reasons researchers have found for fertility troubles.

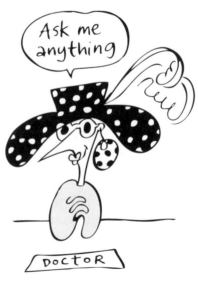

choose a doctor you like.

TALKING TO OTHERS ABOUT FERTILITY

It's important to acknowledge that not having kids is a legitimate choice for some women, which they're happy to live with. For others, 'no kids' can be a reason for regret or grief. Some women go along with their partner's decision not to have children, or they try to get pregnant but don't get lucky or find they have left it too late.

We shouldn't assume that not having kids is a choice, or a problem, for somebody else. We all need to be a bit careful not to make judgements or blundering comments. Whether they're a woman or a man, if you're about to ask somebody a question that relates to their fertility, first ask yourself:

 Do I know this person well enough?

 Are we in an appropriate place? (Over coffee and alone might be okay, but at work in front of others at a meeting isn't.)

 Will I read signs of reluctance to talk about it? (It may be better to say 'I'd love to hear your feelings about having kids, if you ever want to talk about them.' This signals caring interest but not pressure or prying.)

 Am I prepared to become this person's trusted confidante about an otherwise secret matter? Or am I just making conversation?

How to support a friend with fertility troubles

 Let them know you're there if they want to talk about it. You don't have to solve the problem; you just have to be their friend.

 Respect their feelings if they want to avoid major child zones, full-on family events such as Christmas and Easter, or functions such as baby showers.

 If you become pregnant or want to let them know that someone else is, tell them privately and be sensitive about their reaction. They can still be happy for you but grieving for themselves.

 Be prepared for their medically and emotionally induced mood swings if they're undergoing treatment such as IVF.

 Ask them to let you know when and if they want to be involved in your child's life by being invited to events or asked to babysit. Be understanding if this changes.

some (but not all) of the possible causes

Researchers believe that the reasons for infertility are probably fairly evenly divided between a problem caused by the male equipment; trouble with the female equipment; both of these; and an unknown cause. Many couples never find out the reason why they're having problems: nothing is medically obvious. They may even strike fertility trouble after already having a child together, or go through IVF and later conceive naturally.

You're not ovulating This could be because of misbehaving hormones. You may have no hint of this, but warning signs can include very erratic, unpredictable or missing periods, or a cycle longer than 35 days. Not ovulating can be due to stress, not eating well, over-exercising, being above or below a healthy weight, or having an illness such as polycystic ovary syndrome (PCOS).

Age The figures given for the number of eggs you have at different times in your life vary widely, but here's one rough estimate that provides the general picture. As a fetus in your mother's womb you have 6 or 7 million eggs in your ovaries. By the time you're born this has fallen to 1 or 2 million, and by your teens you have about 300,000 eggs to play with: of these, 400 or 500 are used for ovulation during your life. (Each monthly cycle one of your ovaries, usually in turn, releases an egg.) A steady decline in numbers continues to occur, and this really accelerates after the age of 35. By your early forties you may have only a handful of 'good' eggs left, or none.

Misbehaving sperm They could be weak swimmers or badly formed. Or there might not be enough of them, they might be blocked from getting out, or there might be none at all. Most blokes produce about 40–60 million sperm each time they ejaculate. Which frankly is just showing off. Sperm tend to hold up a bit better than eggs as their owners get older – that's why craggy old rock stars in ill-advised leopard-skin pants can have babies with young women.

Because of the truly unfriendly language of the medical world, you may be told your little swimmers are 'abnormal'. It's very common for men to freak out at this point, feel a failure and lose their sex drive. But an 'abnormal' result could have absolutely nothing to do with whether your sperm are fertile or not. Eighty to 90 percent of your swimmers can look irregular but be perfectly good for fertilising eggs. It could just mean they wriggle in an individually funky way. It may not affect your fertility, your 'potency' or your health in any way.

RECURRENT MISCARRIAGE

If you've had one miscarriage it doesn't necessarily mean you'll have more. A miscarriage is pretty common: the rate is given variously as between one in five and one in ten or fifteen pregnancies. It can happen in the first few weeks without anybody knowing, because it feels and looks like a normal period (see 'Miscarriage' in Week 6). But some women have repeated miscarriages for an unknown, or only eventually diagnosed, reason.

You may have heard about women who need to take daily aspirin while pregnant in order not to miscarry. It's only useful in a few individual situations; in others it can cause problems. If you are pregnant or 'trying', only take aspirin if it is prescribed for you by a doctor who knows your situation.

Sneaky problems Ovaries and fallopian tubes can be damaged by some disorders, including pelvic inflammatory disease (PID), a known complication of the common sexually transmitted infections chlamydia and gonorrhoea. Most women with PID don't know they've got it or have had it: usually there are no recognisable symptoms, such as pain or discharge, that they could have picked up on. (Sometimes surgery can correct PID, or you can choose in-vitro fertilisation to bypass your tubes entirely – see the next chapter for details on IVF.)

Endometriosis, which lots of women suffer from, may reduce fertility and require treatment even if mild. More severe endometriosis may affect fertility so much that IVF is required.

Fibroids These are knots of tissue, or benign tumours, in the wall of the uterus; if they protrude into the uterus space they can make it harder for an egg to implant. They are quite common and don't always cause problems. A symptom can be heavy periods. (Fibroids can be hard to remove, and unless they're inside the actual uterus space, or very large, surgery is not usually recommended.)

Stress This could come from your relationship, from work, from relatives who keep asking 'WHEN ARE YOU GOING TO GIVE US SOME GRANDCHILDREN?', and even from worrying about whether or not you'll get pregnant.

a diagnosis of a fertility problem or infertility

The diagnosis can be rather a big shock so make sure you understand your individual situation: if you're not sure what was said, because of the emotional overload, go back to the doctor, ask questions and take notes. It may mean that you're going to have difficulty in getting pregnant rather than that it's impossible.

◎ Allow yourself and your partner some time to absorb the diagnosis and to feel sad.

◎ If you're the partner whose 'problem' it is (of course it's a problem for both of you) you might feel especially guilty, ashamed or confused about it. But ask yourself whether you would have blamed your partner if it had gone the other way? No. So treat yourself as you would your partner in the same situation, or say to yourself what you'd say to your best friend going through this.

◎ Don't feel 'defective' if you're the one who has the problem or if a cause can't be easily found. You're as much of a real natural woman, or man, as anybody else. It's just that life randomly gave you this problem, instead of, say, strangely large feet. (Okay, if you have strangely large feet let me say they look fine. Really.) Getting stuck at the 'poor me' or 'I'm weird' stage won't help in the long run. Get help to move through it if you need to (see 'More Info' at the end of this section).

◎ Make sure you fully understand what you could do next (see the options listed later in the chapter). Having a fertility problem or being infertile doesn't necessarily mean you won't be parents.

◎ Choose who among your family and friends you want to tell. Saying nothing can avoid endless questions and bizarre folk 'remedy' suggestions, but can also make you feel lonely. Web chat rooms can be good, but as you know, info on forums and some websites can be a bit bonkers, so keep a look out; be especially careful of ratbags of various persuasions.

◎ Men may need to talk to a relative or friend as well as their partner. Feel free to choose a woman: sometimes other blokes aren't quite as good at talking about things or listening. (Many IVF clinics have support groups for men, and see also the box 'IVF Info for Blokes' in the next chapter, Assisted Conception.)

DEALING WITH UNWANTED QUESTIONS

Here are some possible replies to those thoughtless and sometimes infuriating or upsetting questions you don't want to answer.

When are you two going to start a family? (Well, when we have something to tell you, we'll let you know *or* You know, we're trying but I'd rather not go into it.)

Isn't your biological clock ticking? (Isn't your social radar telling you that's an overly personal question?)

You should start trying before it's too late. (Yes, I've heard *or* Tell you what, let's agree not to talk about it. It's pretty personal.)

I heard you can't get pregnant. What's wrong with you? (Get away from me, you thoughtless troll.)

Hey! What's up with you and babies anyway? (Excuse me, I've just realised I should be somewhere else. *Say this quietly, maintaining eye contact, and then walk away calmly – where you go may be the toilets to have a cry, but they don't need to know that.*)

Who's the sperm donor? (Why do you ask? *or* George Clooney.)

I know you're trying – are you pregnant yet? *or* **How are things going with IVF?** (Actually I find it pretty stressful to be asked about it, and our doctor's advised us to avoid stress, so let's change the subject *or* I really appreciate you being interested, but it's probably best if you don't keep asking me what's happening. We'll let you know if we've got any news to share.)

I know somebody who said 'Well, I did get pregnant once but then I gave birth to an umbrella. I'm not going through THAT again'. It was certainly surreal, but it worked brilliantly as a conversation-stopper. People were too confused to keep up the interrogation.

Always have a new conversation-starter ready, such as 'Tell me, where do you get your hair done?' or 'What would you call the colour on these walls? I've always wanted to be one of those people who named the colours on the paint charts. I'd call this Frighty Mauve'. Then everyone has moved on.

◎ Prepare to feel baby yearning. This can make you feel jealous of friends with babies, and all the others who seem to conceive easily. If it's affecting your ability to be around them or at functions where there are babies, you may want to let friends and relatives know you're working on adjusting your feelings as well as trying to get pregnant.

◎ Remember that you aren't alone. One in six couples has problems conceiving.

the next step

Depending on your individual situation, the next step might be:

◎ hormonal drugs or herbs prescribed to correct misbehaving hormones and boost ovulation – these drugs can cause severe mood swings

◎ surgery to see what's going on in there, and to try to repair a problem such as blocked fallopian tubes

◎ assisted conception (see the following chapter) – IVF is the most commonly chosen way. Other assistance includes an egg or sperm donor (because sperm quality tends to decrease with age, donors need to be aged 25–45, and egg donors need to be under 35), or a surrogate (a woman chosen to carry the fetus through pregnancy).

You'll want to talk the options through with your partner. Doing something to try to overcome a fertility problem could be a simple, happy process or the first step on a long, difficult road. Do you want to leave things to chance, or explore all the medical assistance available – and for how long if you still don't conceive? (The next chapter has more on this.) Are you both on the same page about what you'd like to do next?

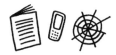

more info on fertility troubles and infertility

'More Info on Assisted Conception' at the end of the next chapter has good websites and other books for you.

infertilitynetworkuk.com
Helpline: 0800 008 7464
The UK's premier infertility charity has loads of info on treatments, details of support groups and plenty of fact sheets.

Pink For a Girl: Wanting a Baby and Not Conceiving by Isla McGuckin, Hay House, UK, 2006
A very personal story from a woman who longed for a baby and 'tried everything' but had to take a long and difficult journey through organic obsessions and psychological self-examination, the heartbreak of miscarriage, the kindness or idiocy of strangers, and hard yards of grieving, to final acceptance. It's lovely to see that her book is dedicated to the children in her life, 'children I would have chosen for myself'.

The Stork Club by Imogen Edwards-Jones, Corgi, UK, 2007
Another memoir, well-written, realistic and very funny, based on all the fertility treatment and IVF palaver she went through, starting with earnest sex that was as 'sexy as a lard sandwich' and moving through sperm delivery to scary scans and hard decisions and … well, to cut to the chase, having a baby. There's something determined about a woman who refers to her husband as 'Less Attractive' the whole way through a book. I so wanted things to work out for them. Hurrah.

ASSISTED CONCEPTION

In-vitro fertilisation is the most well-known method of assisted conception. It involves eggs being fertilised outside a woman's body, in a laboratory.

IVF and how it works

It's important to understand that IVF is not automatically successful – it's not a guaranteed 'cure' for any cause of infertility.

IVF uses eggs from a woman who wants to become pregnant or from a donor, and sperm from her partner or a donor. The sperm is usually produced by the man going into a room at the IVF clinic and reading raunchy magazines with titles such as 'Phwoarrr' and 'Get a Load of That' while giving himself a hand, so to speak.

The basic process is as follows:

1 Releasing eggs To prepare for IVF many women take hormonal drugs, usually as injections and/or nasal sprays, perhaps complemented by doctor-approved herbal treatments and acupuncture at another clinic. The aim is to boost ovary activity so that more than one egg 'ripens' at a time. The drug treatments can cause mood swings and bloating. In rare cases the ovaries go into overdrive, causing symptoms such as severe nausea, tummy area pain and shortness of breath.

2 Getting eggs A pain-relief drug (by intravenous drip) is given, or a sedating anaesthetic, and then the eggs are collected over about 15–20 minutes, during an ultrasound procedure (the 'Having an Ultrasound' box in Week 11 explains how this works). The doctor uses a vaginal probe, which looks rather like a large pen, to help focus the ultrasound waves that create the on-screen picture showing where things are inside you. A needle attached

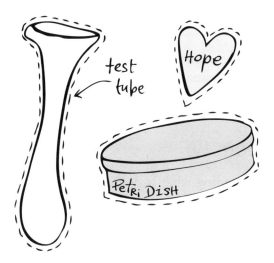

to the probe is then pushed through the vaginal wall (local anesthetic numbs the area), to each ovary in turn, from which it draws up some eggs. You can go home an hour after the procedure, but you need to take it easy for the rest of the day.

3   Getting sperm   Meanwhile, your partner is standing by, ready to produce sperm on-site in a private room (or a donor will have provided sperm in the same way). Sometimes sperm is frozen and used as needed but doctors tend to prefer 'fresh'.

4   Mixing eggs and sperm   Soon after the eggs are collected, sperm will be introduced to them in a little glass dish (*in vitro* is Latin for using glass), or the sperm will be injected directly into the eggs. If an egg is fertilised it will start dividing into new cells and in a day or so become a teeny pre-embryo, much smaller than this full stop.

5   Delivering the embryo (it's called an embryo from day 2)   Sometimes embryos are frozen, then thawed and used later. But most doctors prefer to pop them into an incubator for two to five days and then deliver one (usually only one nowadays) into the uterus, using a long tube like a very fine drinking straw, which goes up through your cervix into your uterus. This can feel a little odd and uncomfortable, but shouldn't hurt – a bit like a routine smear test. Everyone hopes the embryo will attach itself well to the wall of the uterus, after floating around for a couple of days, and keep dividing and growing.

6 Waiting Usually you're advised to go home and take it easy for a couple of days and not get stressed. This can be hard for people who have so many hopes riding on a pregnancy test that will be done a couple of weeks later. Most people on IVF say the hardest part is waiting.

thinking about IVF

As well as understanding what happens during IVF, before you decide to have the procedure you'll want to know some details of what you might be in for.

downsides and upsides
Downsides

◎ It may not work.

◎ It's expensive – if you are under 40 and you and your partner have no children, you are likely to be eligible for NHS funding for your first cycle of treatment at least, but private treatment will set you back several thousand pounds per cycle.

◎ Some of the procedures and drugs cause pain or mood swings.

◎ Couples may disagree on ethical questions such as what to do with any leftover fertilised eggs.

◎ There appears to be a slightly higher rate of birth defects, including minor ones, in IVF babies (2.6 in 100, compared with about 2 in 100 naturally conceived babies). Research is continuing to find out why this happens.

◎ Some religious groups oppose IVF, saying that it is not God's will.

◎ The most common phrase used by former IVF patients is that it's an emotional roller coaster, with ups and downs that are sometimes severe as hopes and disappointments and side effects take their toll.

◎ Sometimes people expect success straight away, when in fact it often takes a few goes over a year or so. If you know this you can relax a bit more.

Upsides

⊚ For some people it's their only chance of conceiving.

⊚ You could end up with a healthy baby or babies.

It's a short list of upsides, but for many it far outweighs the downsides.

chances of a multiple birth

In the early days of IVF multiple fertilised eggs were often transferred to the uterus to provide the best chance of at least one 'taking'. In fact sometimes more than one 'took', resulting in twins, triplets and even quads. A multiple birth, although a boon for the manufacturers of people carriers, is harder on the mum's body than a single one and may create problems for the babies.

To avoid this, British IVF doctors have now agreed to recommend very strongly to a patient that they transfer only one fertilised egg, providing it is

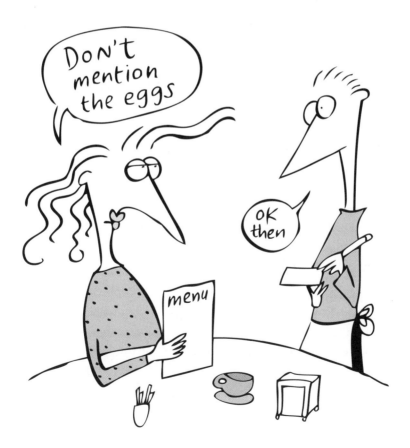

IVF INFO FOR BLOKES

Men, you can wear cotton pants or boxers every day but wool or nylon underdungers may warm up your testicles too much, which makes sperm less useful. (That's why you've evolved to carry them in a little bag out the front of your body instead of having them warm up inside your body.) Go commando if you must but don't pretend there's a medical reason, and please do not sit legs akimbo in your shorts at a barbecue. It is not couth. We love you more when you cultivate a sense of scrotal mystery.

You won't wear out your sperm. You're good to go again the next day or whenever you want to. You don't need rest days.

Feel free to bring your own magazine in a plain brown wrapper to a sperm-producing session at a clinic. You can probably take your partner with you instead to … erm … 'give you a hand' in some way.

You may be embarrassed, but they're blasé about it all at the clinic.

Yes, you can still have sex with your partner, although be sensitive about her moods. Sure-fire romance tips include candlelight, sweet nothings, doing some housework and begging.

If your partner asks you what you do when getting a sperm sample alone, the correct answer is 'I always think of you, darling', not 'I had a picture of Angelina Jolie' or 'I was reading a phwoarrr-filled men's magazine'. For heaven's sake, man, tact!

more info

Ask your IVF clinic counsellor for recommendations of bloke-friendly blogs, books or other resources on male infertility and how to cope, and on how to go through IVF and support your partner. (Also see 'More Info' at the end of this chapter.)

PS: A cheering thought

Remember, you never 'waste' your sperm. You can have sex with your partner (ahem, or yourself) as many times as you like, and don't have to 'save yourself' and only have sex on fertile days or produce sperm on a 'sample day'. In fact, it's now official medical advice to give yourself a damned good going over once a day whenever you feel like it – if anything it will improve your sperm quality. But please … not on the bus …

of good quality, especially if the woman is under 40. A maximum of two pre-embryos should be transferred into women older than 40. Doctors have to balance giving a woman the best chance to conceive and avoiding a multiple birth if possible.

where to go

To choose an IVF clinic ask friends or family or discuss it with your GP – and web forums may be of some help. Most teaching hospitals and some district hospitals have IVF clinics. Or you may prefer to go to a private unit. They'll be under 'IVF' in phone listings.

Before you visit an IVF specialist use websites or books to get an idea of how it works (see 'More Info' at the end of the chapter), and familiarise yourself with the terms that might be used.

Sometimes it's hard to remember everything that happens in a consultation: feel free to take specific written questions with you and to jot down the answers at the time.

trying again

If the first time isn't successful, many people try six to eight times more before deciding to give up. Statistically women younger than 37 have about a 25–30 percent chance of pregnancy with each embryo transferred. Women aged 37–40 have about an 18 percent chance. After the age of 41 the chance of pregnancy with each embryo is less than 10 percent. But of course you never know whether you'll get lucky in that cycle.

Since 1978, more than 100,000 babies have been born in the UK using IVF – more than 2 million worldwide. About 1.5 percent of babies born in the UK are the result of an IVF pregnancy.

who to tell

You may want to tell a supervisor or boss that you're undergoing IVF because you'll need a few days off each month when you're having eggs collected or transferred. Or you may want not to flag your intention of getting pregnant and instead use up sick days or holidays owed. Most IVF clinics have pamphlets or website downloads about what to expect, which can be given to friends, relatives and workmates. You may want to warn people that you'll need some understanding about the mental and physical side effects while you're undergoing treatment.

medical, legal and emotional aspects

For some people, assisted conception can be logistically and emotionally complicated. They may need or want assisted conception because they're single or gay or lesbian. Some women won't need fertility treatment or IVF but will want some sort of sperm donation, and will try to use it to get pregnant without involving a clinic.

There are medical and legal requirements concerning IVF and donations (it's illegal to discriminate on the grounds of marital status or sexuality). There are rules about using eggs or sperm donated by somebody else, about who has to be told, about guardianship, and about confidentiality arrangements. There are also laws covering surrogacy (when a woman carries a baby for someone else).

There are also regulations about what access children can have to information about their biological, donor parent. Usually access is legal once the child turns 18 even if the legal parents or guardians are against the idea.

Then there are plenty of permutations in the emotional department, particularly around what happens if somebody changes their mind before or after the birth, and whether the child will be told about all the aspects of their parentage.

Many other questions may not be medical or legal, but could be even more important to think through before you start. Who will be the biological parents? Who will be the child's legal parents? If a child has two mummies and two daddies (say, because a gay couple donates sperm to a lesbian couple and both guys want to be part of the child's future), will they have eight grandparents? Who will be financially responsible? What if a donor decides halfway through a pregnancy or after the birth that they want to have a say in the child's life instead of being anonymous? And of course a question for anybody: who will look after a child if the parents no longer can? If you need or want to explore these possibilities, the websites and books listed in the 'More Info' section at the end of the chapter will give you a head start. And all IVF units will offer counselling to help you explore these issues.

fertility and your future

Whatever methods you try in order to conceive, there are only two possible results: they'll work or they won't. Here are some things to consider for both possibilities.

if fertility treatment works

Yes, you finally got your baby but you may still have problems. Life isn't perfect and neither are you or your new arrival. That's okay.

You still have as much right or likelihood as any other mum or couple to panic about whether you'll be a good parent or a good provider. You may feel less able than other mums to admit to it when you're sleep-deprived or confused about what to do, because you wanted this baby for so long and thought it would all be so wonderful.

You may be too scared to complain now to the people you'd previously told this was all you ever wanted. But hey, being a mum is not a competency competition (if it was there'd be plenty of us bringing up the rear). Everyone gets better at it or feels better about it as time goes on, although many of us need some help to do that. That could mean talking to a health visitor, your GP, a parent group found through your local council, or an anonymous helpline. Don't be afraid to get help from any of the resources listed in this book.

In the meantime, pick a wacko, rehab-bouncing celebrity who clearly can't work out how to be a good parent and compare yourself with them. I think you'll find you feel soooo much better.

if fertility treatment doesn't work

Only you can decide whether you've exhausted all the avenues you want to go down. You can agree to say 'Enough now' or 'It wasn't meant to be for us' at any time. Some people can decide quite suddenly that they've had enough, feel they've given it their best shot, and now want their life back and for it not to revolve around fertility any more. Others may recognise that their relationship is under strain. And some look to adopt, if they can.

Most people will come to the decision to stop trying after thinking everything through thoroughly. The really important thing is for both partners to have those conversations together, as well as in their own head. If you have tried IVF your IVF clinic should have counselling services you can use and be able to recommend further resources. There are many website forums and books available on the difficulty and grief of finding yourself in this position.

It's a matter of fascination to doctors that some people who tried for years and are then unsuccessful with IVF go away and come back in a few months amazed to find they're pregnant naturally. You never know what the future will bring.

It may not be what you want to hear or accept at the time of acknowledging feelings of tremendous loss, but you can still have children in your life in some way. After absorbing the reality, lots of generous and giving couples who are devastated by finding they can't be biological parents together become more involved at some point in the lives of other people's children. So many mothers and fathers need help with their children, and so many children need – not just want – special non-parents in their lives. There is something unique and precious about fun uncles and role-model career-girl aunties (whether or not you're related by blood), and about those who have 'special godparent' status, with or without the god part.

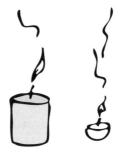

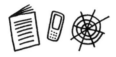

more info on **assisted conception**

Make sure you check any medical info from books or websites with your specialist doctor. There is misinformation out there, and even correct information can become out-of-date very quickly in this field.

hfea.co.uk
> The Human Fertilisation and Embryology Authority is the UK's independent regulator for fertility treatments. From the main page of its website click on 'For Patients and their Supporters' for lots of info about infertility and treatments, donor issues, sources of emotional support, and eligibility for treatment on the NHS. There's also advice on choosing a clinic, plus details of all clinics in the UK, including success rates.

donor-conception-network.org
> A useful site covering all the issues, from the viewpoint of the parents and the child.

The Complete Guide to IVF by Kate Brian, Piatkus, UK, 2009
> Kate Brian, a trustee of Infertility Network UK, became a mum with the help of IVF. Great explanations of freaky-sounding medical procedures and terms, with good advice about how to get and understand a diagnosis, where to go for help, what it's like to go through IVF, how it works, the maelstrom of feelings you may have, and how to balance medical and alternative treatments.

CONTACTS & RESOURCES

Contact details and website addresses may change. If in doubt, try your web search engine, or phone directory enquiries or the relevant government departments.

CONTRACEPTION

Family planning clinics
To find details of your local family planning clinic, phone the relevant number below:

England: fpa helpline
            0845 122 8690
Wales: NHS Direct
            0845 46 47
Scotland: NHS 24
            08454 24 24 24
NI: fpa helpline
            0845 122 8687

Alternatively, from the main page of the website of the Family Planning Association (fpa.org.uk) click on 'Find a Clinic' to search by postcode. Phone a clinic before visiting, as many have limited opening hours.

Family Planning Association
fpa.org.uk
Helplines: 0845 122 8690 (England)
              0845 122 8687 (NI)
Provides advice by phone or via the web. The helplines (currently only available in England and Northern Ireland) can answer questions about contraception, as well as a range of issues such as women's health, sexually transmitted infections and pregnancy termination (see also 'Termination of Pregnancy' later in this chapter). Or use the site's Web Enquiry Service (type 'Ask WES' in the search box on the main page): you'll receive an email within three working days.

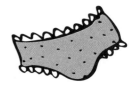

DISABLED PARENTS

disabledparentsnetwork.org.uk
Helpline: 0300 3300 639
Email advice: supportservice@disabledparentsnetwork.org.uk
The Disabled Parents Network offers pregnancy, childbirth and parenting support. Contact them for advice or to get in touch with other disabled parents in your area.

FAMILY AND PARTNER ABUSE AND VIOLENCE

24-hour National Domestic Violence Helpline
0808 2000 247
Immediate help and practical advice, run by Refuge and Women's Aid (see below).

Women's Aid
womensaid.org.uk
The excellent site of national charity Women's Aid offers fact sheets on what to do if you or a friend needs help, answers to frequently asked questions, lots of information about violence and abuse, and how to get help in your area. Make sure you include 'UK' at the end of the address.

Refuge
refuge.org.uk
This charity site offers help for women and children in a violent or abusive situation. Links pages, plus info on prevention, how to work to change a family situation, and where to go if you need to get away.

National Centre for Domestic Violence
ncdv.org.uk
A free service that helps domestic violence victims secure legal injunctions or non-molestation orders to protect them from further abuse.

National Society for the Prevention of Cruelty to Children
nspcc.org.uk
Adult helpline: 0808 800 5000
The NSPCC's adult helpline can offer advice about protecting your children from abuse.

carelineuk.org
Helpline: 0845 122 8622
Confidential telephone crisis counselling service.

respect.uk.net
Helpline: 0845 122 8609
Help for those who want to stop being the abuser or violent partner.

mankind.org.uk
Helpline: 01823 334244
Advice and help for men suffering from domestic violence.

GRIEF AND LOSS

It is rare, but some babies die in the last weeks of pregnancy and are induced stillborn. Some babies die soon after birth, or in the following weeks. Often the general baby books are no help to the grieving parents, and often you can't remember what you've been told by medical staff because of the shock and grief. During these terrible times there are lots of experts who may be able to offer you a great deal of help:

⊚ midwives and doctors

⊚ hospital social workers

⊚ counsellors (through the hospital or your GP).

A friend or relative who can take notes of what is said by these people, and your options, can be invaluable.

There are support groups for parents and siblings affected by the death of a baby, or those trying to deal with a baby who has special needs. Ask your hospital to put you in touch with them.

People react very differently to grief – some don't want to talk about it, and this can seem to others who grieve differently as if they do not care as much. This is not true. Grief counsellors can help a couple or a whole family, including brothers and sisters, understand what has happened. Your hospital or doctor should be able to help you find one who specialises in the loss of a baby (that's important). Or see contacts below.

Stillbirth and Neonatal Death Support (SANDS)
uk-sands.org
Helpline: 020 7436 5881
The helpline offers immediate support and understanding and can also direct you to support groups in your area.

Foundation for the Study of Infant Deaths (FSID)
fsid.org.uk
Helpline: 0808 802 6868
From the main page of the website click on 'If you are bereaved', or phone the helpline for sympathetic advice.

An Exact Replica of a Figment of My Imagination by Elizabeth McCracken, Jonathan Cape, UK, 2009

A great writer's wrenching but beautiful memoir of her first pregnancy and her first baby, who died just before birth without warning. Her writing is loving and respectful; she does not shy away from the terrible grief, or the things that help to acknowledge her loss, the things she can still find funny or wonderful, or the good feelings she has about her baby who is no longer here. She writes of welcoming her second child, a healthy boy she joyfully greets not as a 'miracle' but as exhilaratingly 'ordinary'.

IMMUNISATION

Immunisation is not compulsory in the UK, but the medical profession and the government strongly recommend it. The UK has very low rates of infectious diseases, and to maintain this all kids should be immunised. All immunisations given to children are logged in the Personal Child Health Record (the 'red book'), which is issued at birth for all babies and kept by the parents. Nurseries and schools in the UK do not usually require proof of immunisation, but you may be required to show some record when entering another country.

You can get 'scheduled' immunisations for free at your health centre or GP's surgery. There are routine vaccinations and boosters for diphtheria, whooping cough, polio, measles, mumps, rubella, pneumococcal infection, tetanus, *Haemophilus influenzae* type b (Hib) and meningitis C. Sometimes several are given in one 'cocktail' injection. Children considered 'at risk' may be given extra, free vaccinations against, for example, hepatitis B. If you need other vaccinations for travel, you will probably have to pay for these.

Common side effects following immunisation are minor fever, soreness where an injection has been given, nausea and irritability. These should not be too severe or last for very long. Some of the newer vaccines show far fewer side effects. Anti-vaccination websites present out-of-date and disproven information as 'fact'. Another view is often held by older people who remember the days before vaccinations when thousands of babies died from whooping cough or measles, and several kids in each school had polio and started wearing the callipers and using the walking sticks they'd need forever. A very large majority of parents in the UK choose to have their children immunised.

Immunisation schedule Check with your GP or health centre for your schedule. Sometimes they adjust the recommended schedules, so keep in touch with them as your child grows. Usually there are injections, including vital boosters, scheduled for when the child is aged 2 months, 3 months, 4 months, 12 months and 13 months, with another just before primary school starts, and a final top-up of some things at secondary school age.

Helping your baby through it Also find out from your GP or health centre what side effects to look out for after particular injections. Don't worry – the injections are no big deal. Usually babies just look horrified and accusing for a moment when they get them and cry a little until they're distracted, perhaps by a breastfeed or a bottlefeed.

The whole rundown on immunisation for kids up to the age of five is given in the sequel to this book, *The Rough Guide to Babies and Toddlers*.

immunisation.nhs.uk
The official NHS immunisation website gives the current immunisation schedule and explains the diseases and their vaccines. There's a comprehensive FAQ section.

LESBIAN AND GAY PARENTS

pinkparents.org.uk
Helpline: 01380 727 935
Information, advice and support for lesbian and gay parents or children of lesbian and gay couples.

MIDWIVES

You will be referred to an NHS midwife by your GP, or you can contact your local midwife team direct: ask at your health centre or write to the Supervisor of Midwives at your local hospital.

Independent Midwives UK
independentmidwives.org.uk
If you are considering hiring an independent midwife, visit this website for info about fees, insurance and other considerations, plus a directory of independent midwives.

MULTIPLE BIRTHS

TAMBA (Twins and Multiple Births Association)
tamba.org.uk
Helpline: 0800 128 0509
The website has FAQs and fact sheets. Members get a quarterly magazine, discounts, access to a web forum and the opportunity to join local twins clubs.

twinsclub.co.uk
Despite the name, this specialist parenting website is for all numbers of multiple births. It has a busy forum, details of local twins clubs, and a classified section where you can buy and sell equipment and clothes for big broods.

twinsuk.co.uk
An online shop for twin and tripletty things, it includes a good resources section with tips on a range of relevant topics.

Birmingham Registry for Twin and Heritability Studies
www.genepid.bham.ac.uk/births.shtml
Families expecting twins are invited to register with this project from the University of Birmingham, which aims to study genetic and environmental influences on children's development.

Double Trouble: Twins and How to Survive Them by Emma Mahony, Thorsons, UK, 2003
> A twin herself, and the mum of twins, Ms Mahony gives helpful info and advice on pregnancy and parenting, including bosom wrangling, sleeping and getting in extra help.

NATURAL HEALTH CARE

Check that your practitioner has the right level of qualification, or find one that does.

National Institute of Medical Herbalists
01392 426022
nimh.org.uk

Complementary and Natural Healthcare Council
0203 178 2199
cnhc.org.uk

PARENTING SUPPORT

Your health visitor, local health centre or doctor's surgery should be your first port of call if you are struggling. If necessary, they can make referrals for other help available on the NHS. The services listed below may also be useful in helping you move on from a bad patch.

Parentline Plus
Helpline: 0808 800 2222
parentlineplus.org.uk
Call the 24-hour helpline for confidential support and understanding. The volunteers can also refer you for one-to-one local support, and give you details of local parenting groups and workshops. The website has advice leaflets and a useful links page listing other support services.

National Childbirth Trust
nct.org.uk
General enquiries: 0300 3300 770
Breastfeeding helpline: 0300 3300 771
In addition to its popular antenatal classes, the NCT runs postnatal courses, giving practical parenting advice and helping you adjust to the reality of parenthood. Local

branches offer friendship and support to new parents, including breastfeeding drop-in sessions and a range of social activities. The website's 'Info Centre' also has lots of pages of useful advice on parenting problems.

Home-Start
0800 068 6368
home-start.org.uk
Home-Start offers support to parents struggling with isolation, illness, bereavement, multiples or other challenges. You are matched with a volunteer who'll visit you in your home each week and offer practical and emotional help.

Parents Advice Centre (Northern Ireland)
parentsadvicecentre.org
Helpline: 0808 801 0722
The Parents Advice Centre has a helpline, and runs parenting courses.

bbc.co.uk/parenting
The BBC's parenting portal has heaps of info on caring for kids, plus links to other useful online resources.

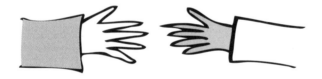

SINGLE, SOLE, SHARED AND STEP PARENTS

One Parent Families/Gingerbread
oneparentfamilies.org.uk
Helpline: 0800 018 5026
This newly merged outfit is now the organisation of first resort for lone-parent families in the UK. Its helpline can offer advice on benefits, employment and other financial and practical issues. It also publishes a *Lone Parent's Survival Guide*, a useful downloadable resource. Call the helpline or search online for details of your local group and activities.

One Parent Families Scotland
opfs.org.uk
Helpline: 0808 801 0323
Offers advice by phone and outreach projects, with a particular emphasis on helping lone parents with employment issues.

Children and Family Court Advisory Support Service (Cafcass)
cafcass.gov.uk
Cafcass's website provides information about the family courts' involvement when parents separate.

Child Support Agency
csa.gov.uk
08457 133 133
A government agency that runs the collection of child maintenance payments.

Single Parent Travel Club
sptc.org.uk
0870 2416210
A club which puts single parents in touch with one another, for holidays, outings and other activities.

separatedfamilies.info
The Centre for Separated Families has lots of info on all the relevant issues including divorce, support groups, even prison. Click on Families to get info for parents, children and grandparents.

The Guide for Separated Parents: Putting Your Children First by Karen and Nick Woodall, Piatkus, UK, 2009
> Written by two of the founders of the Centre for Separated Families, this is smart and soothing. It lays out the common feelings of children of both genders and at various ages and gives practical advice on how to reassure them. It covers negotiating shared custody, respecting your ex and building a relationship that's about parenting, not being together. There's also a bit about new partners.

Shared Parenting: Raising Your Children Cooperatively After Separation by Jill Burrett and Michael Green, Finch, Australia, 2007
> Info on how to communicate, shared care plans and timetables, hand-over suggestions, and avoiding court if both parties want to.

The Single Parent's Handbook by Rachel Morris, Life Publishing, UK, 2007
> Loads on the development of kids at different ages (up to teens), how their feelings are shown in behaviour, not words, and how to help reduce their stress

in break-ups and custody disputes as well as ongoing life apart. Lots also on avoiding martyrdom and dealing with prejudice, the relationship with your kids, grandparents who interfere or are terrified of losing access, and practical help with finances, work and reducing stress in the family. Less on what to do if ex-partners are proving difficult or unwilling to subscribe to the civilised co-parenting ideal (for that, see relate.org.uk, below).

relate.org.uk
0300 100 1234
The UK's biggest counselling organisation has a free service for people who are separating or divorcing, but will also help if you are already apart. Ask for help with trying to establish a working co-parent arrangement. You can have counselling or attend courses (you can go to different sessions, rather than together) and there is special info (and services) for kids. There's also online help and the phone advice service, above, which can help directly or put you in touch with local services.

bonusfamilies.com
For separated parents and others with so-called 'blended families', this is a useful US website. You'll have to dodge Halloween questions, but this non-profit site answers lots of questions on etiquette, step-parenting dilemmas and more.

Stepfamilies: Living Successfully With Other People's Children by Suzie Hayman, Vermilion, UK, 2001
> Part of the counselling charity Relate's series of books, this is a straightforward and useful book which addresses issues of making friends with your partner's kids, dealing or building some sort of relationship with 'the ex', discipline, and 'blended families' when some kids are 'theirs' and some are 'yours' and what difference that makes.

The Step Parents' Parachute: The Four Cornerstones to Good Step-parenting by Flora McEvedy, Piatkus, UK, 2009
> I feel I can break a confidence and tell you the four cornerstones are 'You and Your Partner Are a Team', 'Know Your Role', 'Keep Rejection at Arm's Length' and 'Your Step Children Need Your Love' – but there's lots more useful stuff in between. Written by a step-mum whose step-daughters 'did her head in' by not liking her at first. She has a blended family, including three children of her 'own', and her approach is kind and sensible without being unrealistic or Mary Poppins-lite.

SPECIAL NEEDS AND HEALTH PROBLEMS

Many babies are born with health problems or special needs, ranging from a routine, temporary problem to a serious and dangerous one requiring intensive care and very hard decisions.

You will be able to derive some comfort from knowing that the UK has some of the best-trained and most dedicated hospital midwives, doctors, paediatricians, specialist surgeons, hospital social workers and counsellors in the world. Keep pushing until you feel satisfied that everything that needs to be done is being done, and vote for and put pressure on people who you believe put medical care as a high priority.

Immediately there is a problem, take notes or bring a friend to take notes of your conversations with doctors and other relevant people – it can be a time when shock causes everything to go in one ear and out the other.

There are several parent support groups for specific conditions such as Down's syndrome and spina bifida. Some possible starting points for finding them: your doctor, your nearest children's hospital, searching a key word on the NHS website (nhs.uk), and asking your local council what help is available. Also see 'Women's Hospitals' later in this chapter.

When using a search engine on the web, remember that large international sites are often good sources of information but local sites may have links, contacts and resources more relevant to you.

TEENAGE PREGNANCY AND YOUNG MUMS

Your doctor should put you in touch with a health centre or hospital with special information, classes and support groups for you. Or ring your closest major hospital and ask to be put in contact with whoever looks after young mums: they will have books and videos you can borrow, as well as clinics and confidential advice.

The health centre, hospital or clinic will be able to help you work out plans for your pregnancy and birth. They can also help you plan for the future, such as getting back to school or into work, and give advice on how to look after the baby (or suggest organisations that will teach you). They'll arrange financial help if your family is not being supportive, as well as helping you with any other worries you might have, speaking to your parents if that's difficult for you, and even helping you find accommodation.

The websites and book listed overleaf may be helpful. Also see the 'Contraception' and 'Termination of Pregnancy' sections in this chapter.

brook.org.uk
Helpline: 0808 802 1234
The non-profit-making Brook Advisory Centres offer free, confidential advice, info and counselling to young people, including under-16s. Choose 'The facts', then 'Pregnancy' for information, or 'Find a centre' to get help in your area.

ywca.org.uk/youngmums
The brilliant Respect Young Mums campaign site has stories by real girls who've had babies, a quiz on myths and facts, and lots more. From the main page, choose 'Links and help' for a jump-off point to other great websites with support for young mums.

sexetc.org
A US site by and for teens. Choose 'Teen Parenting' for stories and FAQ.

The Rough Guide to Girl Stuff by Kaz Cooke, Rough Guides, UK, 2009
My book for teenagers has a chapter on pregnancy.

TERMINATION OF PREGNANCY

Termination is legal and free through the NHS in England, Scotland and Wales, up to 24 weeks of pregnancy. Termination later in pregnancy is allowed for various medical reasons. In Northern Ireland, termination is only legal in very exceptional circumstances, so most women from Northern Ireland wanting a termination will need to travel to another part of the UK or abroad for a private termination (they are not entitled to a termination on the NHS).

To get a termination on the NHS you'll need a referral from a GP or family planning clinic (see the 'Contraception' section at the start of this chapter). Or you can contact a private abortion clinic direct.

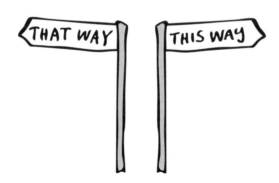

Surgical termination is safe if performed by qualified medical staff. It should not cause future fertility problems. Within the first nine weeks, a pregnancy can also be terminated with drugs that cause an early miscarriage (this looks like a period); note that this is different from the 'morning-after pill' for emergency contraception, which is available from pharmacies but must be taken within 72 hours of unprotected sex (and is not guaranteed to work).

Be aware of pregnancy counselling websites and phone services that have been set up primarily as anti-abortion centres run by religious or other organisations (their bias may not be at all apparent at first glance, as they often have innocuous, mainstream-sounding names). Many of these give information to try to dissuade you from having a pregnancy termination: some of it can be false and disproven (such as 'abortion causes breast cancer'). There are other, independent pregnancy counselling services that will talk about and help with all options: having the baby, adoption and pregnancy termination (see the listings below).

See also the Family Planning listings in 'Contraception'.

Family Planning Association
fpa.org.uk
Helplines: 0845 122 8690 (England)
0845 122 8687 (NI)
The Family Planning Association offer confidential, non-biased info and advice. Download their booklet 'Pregnant and Don't Know What to Do', phone the helpline or choose 'Find a Clinic'.

Marie Stopes
mariestopes.co.uk
Helpline: 0845 200 80 90
Has information and offers termination and other services related to contraception and family planning.

British Pregnancy Advisory Service
bpas.org
Helpline: 08457 30 40 30
A registered charity, BPAS offers counselling on all your options and a termination if that is what you choose.

TRAUMATIC BIRTH

Birth Trauma Association
birthtraumaassociation.org.uk
The Birth Trauma Association campaigns to raise awareness of birth trauma and supports women who've had a difficult birth, or trouble dealing with their experience. Though there's no dedicated helpline, there's a list of volunteers willing to correspond by email or phone. There's also a glossary on the website to help you make sense of your maternity notes, and advice for those afraid to go through childbirth again.

WOMEN'S HOSPITALS

There are two dedicated women's hospitals in the UK:

Birmingham Women's Hospital
Edgbaston
Birmingham B15 2TG
bwhct.nhs.uk
(0121) 472 1377

Liverpool Women's Hospital
Crown Street
Liverpool L8 7SS
lwh.me.uk
(0151) 708 9988

All other major hospitals have women's health departments and many also have maternity units and obstetric and gynaecology departments. To find a hospital in your area, check out one of the following websites.

nhs.uk/servicedirectories
An online search facility where you can look up your local health-care practitioners, from GPs, dentists and opticians to walk-in clinics and hospitals.

drfosterintelligence.co.uk
Run by a joint NHS-private venture, this site offers up-to-date info on hospitals, birth centres, and medical and alternative health specialists. Click on 'Information for the Public' to use the search facility but remember, the details will have been provided by the centre, doctor or practitioner themselves: this is not an independent review or recommendation.

WORK (PAID)

Find out what policies your employer has on flexible and family-friendly work practices and hours. Ask your union about your rights in this area, and check whether entitlements such as sick pay and holiday pay would be affected.

Ask at your local Jobcentre Plus (see listing below) about schemes or retraining programmes that might help you ease back into the workforce if you've been out of it for a long while.

Jobcentre Plus
jobcentreplus.gov.uk
Click on 'Contact Jobcentre Plus' then 'contact your nearest Jobcentre Plus office' to search for your local branch. Or click 'Looking for a job' and then 'Parents' for information about childcare, training and other support available to parents looking to re-enter the workforce.

direct.gov.uk
From the main page, search 'flexible working' for info about your right to, and options for, flexible working and how to apply.

payandworkrightscampaign.direct.gov.uk
Helpline: 0800 917 2368
Many women return to casual or part-time work and some are exploited. This government website details your rights and the helpline can advise on specific questions.

workingfamilies.org.uk
Helpline: 0800 013 0313
The website of the charity Working Families has lots of fact sheets and other info on employment rights, benefits, childcare and other relevant issues for returning to paid work, including help for parents of disabled children. Its helpline can offer more personalised advice.

acknowledgements

There are many people who gave so generously of their time, compassion and medical expertise to help me make this fully updated new edition as accurate and informative as possible. Special thanks to Dr Virginia Beckett, consultant obstetrician and gynaecologist, Bradford Teaching Hospitals NHS Foundation Trust, midwife Sharon Broad, and most of all, the delightfully scrupulous, clever and rather conveniently pregnant Rough Guides editor, Ruth Tidball (there's attention to detail for you). My grateful thanks also to midwife and maternal and child nurse Cath Curtin, ultrasound specialists Dr Jacqueline Oldham, Dr Andrew Ngu and ultrasound and fetal diagnostics expert Professor Lachlan de Crespigny. Dr Len Kliman was the original obstetrics consultant, Dr John Mills the paediatric advisor on premature babies. IVF specialists Dr Lyndon Hale, Dr Kate Stern and Dr Robert Lyneham helped with the info on assisted fertility. Many staff at the Murdoch Children's Institute provided invaluable info and fact-checking on genetics and screening, including Deborah Dalton and genetics specialists Associate Professor Jane Halliday and Dr George McGillivray. I would also like to thank Julie Gibbs, Lesley Dunt, and Rough Guides commissioning publisher Andrew Lockett, who were all instrumental in taking extra time and allocating resources to do this book properly, with meticulous research and care. That is increasingly rare in book publishing. The UK's Chief Medical Officer, Dr Liam Donaldson, requested of this author and others that their pregnancy books include specific information warning parents about the dangers of jaundice after birth. I have complied. Other details of acknowledgments, including some from way back in the original edition, can be found in *Up the Duff: The Real Guide to Pregnancy*, published by Penguin Australia. And of course none of this would be possible at all without Geoff and Oofty Goofty.

index

A

abdominal exercises 154

abnormalities in baby 54, 113, 115–19
  screening for 130
  see also Down's syndrome; rubella

abortifacients 44–5, 113

abortion *see* miscarriage; termination

abuse and violence 6
  help 449

activity during pregnancy *see* exercise

acupuncture 306, 349, 429

addictions 55–8

advice
  bad 177–8
  confusing 179
  hints from mothers 5, 178, 232–3
  unsolicited 85, 162, 175–9, 182–3, 196, 198–9

'afterpains' 366

age
  and Down's syndrome risk 116–17
  and infertility 14, 432
  older mums 14–15, 116–17
  young mums 457–8

AIDS *see* HIV

air pollution 59

alcohol 8, 18, 31, 33, 48, 56, 142, 166–7, 190

allergies 34

amniocentesis (amnio) 20, 128–30
  miscarriage risk 130
  procedure 129

amniotic fluid 31, 129, 130, 158, 262, 271, 290, 340

amniotic sac 40, 138, 272, 326, 330

amniotomy 348

amphetamines 56

anaemia 37, 154, 263

analgesics 261, 366

antacid medications 260

antenatal, definition of xx

antenatal care 104–7

antenatal classes 222–5, 268–70, 277–9, 289–91, 304–5, 314–15, 324–5
  men's questions 269–70, 291
  women's questions 269

antenatal clinics 104

antenatal tests 68–9, 125
  see also tests

anti-abortion campaigners 455

antidepressant medication 405

Apgar test 281, 358

areolae 80, 166, 168, 372

aromatherapy 44–5, 306

'arsenic hour' 325

artificial rupture of the membranes 348

aspirin 57, 433

assisted conception 436, 438–47
  emotional aspects 444
  medical and legal aspects 444
  websites and books 437, 447
  see also IVF

attachment in breastfeeding 372, 411

attachment-parenting philosophy 285, 420

B

baby
  big babies 313
  bonding with 141, 292, 371, 400
  late 338, 347–8, 349
  measuring growth 75
  with special needs 130, 457
  see also newborn baby; premature baby; sex of baby

baby bathtime 243–4, 253

baby beds 241–2, 288

'baby blues' 136, 212, 324, 402

baby care 385, 393–5, 421–2
  websites and books 122–3, 394, 395, 421–2
  see also bottlefeeding; breastfeeding

baby carriers 245, 393

baby-changing bags 245, 412–14

baby clothes 205
  basic newborn wardrobe 230–1
  borrowing 232
  hints from mothers 232–3
  materials 232, 233, 284
  for premmie baby 284
  safety 232
  sizes 197, 232–3
  summer baby 231
  winter baby 232

baby equipment 240–6
  safety 240, 251, 254

baby excursions 412–14

baby massage 393

baby monitors 245

baby names 319, 336–7

baby restraints (car) 12, 177, 240–1, 316

baby sleeping-bags 231, 241, 385

baby walkers 147, 246

baby yearning 436

babygros 230, 231, 232

backache 181, 186, 260–1

Balaskas, Janet 222

bathtime, baby 243–4, 253

beds, baby 241–2, 288

benefits 14
  registering for 384

bibs 231, 253

birth *see* childbirth; labour

birth centres 96, 99, 102–3, 107–8, 295, 297

birth certificate 384

birth defects
  and excessive vitamin A 32, 58, 177
  in IVF 115, 440
  following rubella 6
  see also dangers to baby

birth music 98, 307, 317

birth notice 383

birth place 98–104
  websites 108–9

birth plan 291–3, 304–5, 315, 324, 328, 334–5

birth position 278, 293

birth record 293, 351

birth registration 383–4

birth team 98–9, 104–7
  websites 108–9